# AMERICAN DIABETES ASSOCIATION COMPLETE GUIDE TO DIABETES

### 4TH EDITION
#### COMPLETELY REVISED

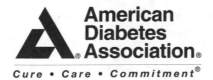

American Diabetes Association®

*Cure • Care • Commitment*®

*Writer,* Nancy Touchette, PhD; *Director, Book Publishing,* John Fedor; *Book Acquisitions,* Sherrye Landrum; *Managing Editor,* Abe Ogden; *Editor, 4th Edition,* Rebecca Lanning; *Production Manager,* Melissa Sprott; *Composition,* Circle Graphics, Inc.; *Cover Design,* Koncept, Inc.; *Printer,* Port City Press.

Printed in the United States of America
1 3 5 7 9 10 8 6 4 2

The suggestions and information contained in this publication are generally consistent with the *Clinical Practice Recommendations* and other policies of the American Diabetes Association, but they do not represent the policy or position of the Association or any of its boards or committees. Reasonable steps have been taken to ensure the accuracy of the information presented. However, the American Diabetes Association cannot ensure the safety or efficacy of any product or service described in this publication. Individuals are advised to consult a physician or other appropriate health care professional before undertaking any diet or exercise program or taking any medication referred to in this publication. Professionals must use and apply their own professional judgment, experience, and training and should not rely solely on the information contained in this publication before p rescribing any diet, exercise, or medication. The American Diabetes Association—its officers, directors, employees, volunteers, and members—assumes no responsibility or liability for personal or other injury, loss, or damage that may result from the suggestions or information in this publication.

♾ The paper in this publication meets the requirements of the ANSI Standard Z39.48-1992 (permanence of paper).

ADA titles may be purchased for business or promotional use or for special sales. To purchase this book in large quantities, or for custom editions of this book with your logo, contact Lee Romano Sequeira, Special Sales & Promotions, at the address below or at LRomano@diabetes.org or 703-299-2046.

American Diabetes Association
1701 North Beauregard Street
Alexandria, Virginia 22311

**Library of Congress Cataloging-in-Publication Data**

American Diabetes Association complete guide to diabetes.—4th ed.
    p. cm.
  Includes index.
  ISBN 1-58040-237-2 (alk. paper)
  1. Diabetes—Popular works.  I. Title: Complete guide to diabetes.
  II. American Diabetes Association.

      RC660.4.A485 2005
      616.4'62—dc22
                                        2005002996

# Contents

# Foreword

For the past 65 years, the American Diabetes Association has led the way in helping to improve the lives of people with diabetes. Over the past decade, the Association's *Complete Guide to Diabetes* has been the premier tool for people learning the basics of diabetes management. This new edition is packed with helpful ideas for people with diabetes, their families, and other caregivers. Each chapter has been revised to bring you the latest diabetes treatment and research available. Written in plain language, the *Complete Guide* gives you all the facts you need to manage your type 1, type 2, or gestational diabetes.

You can use the revised *Complete Guide* to find updated information on the new insulins and oral medications now available to treat diabetes. Expanded sections explain the role of blood glucose monitoring, intensive management, insulin plans, and the meters, pumps, pens, and other tools currently used in diabetes care. You'll also find practical advice on food, nutrition, and physical activity to help you integrate healthy choices into your diabetes care plan. Individual chapters on diabetes complications, diabetes and sex, coping, and family matters contain a wealth of additional information.

The new edition also offers detailed discussions of the current health care system, school and workplace issues, and the laws and policies that affect people with diabetes. An expanded resources section and a new and improved diabetes medical management plan complete the volume.

Whether you are just now learning about diabetes or have years of experience with it, the *Complete Guide* provides the information you need. I encourage you to read and use this book to improve your diabetes care. For additional information, you can call the American Diabetes Association at 1-800-DIABETES (1-800-342-2383) or contact your health care team.

**Karmeen Kulkarni, MS, RD, BC-ADM, CDE**
President, Health Care & Education
American Diabetes Association

# Acknowledgments

The American Diabetes Association is grateful to the following health care and legal experts, whose thorough reviews greatly enhanced this book.

**Martha M. Funnell, MS, RN, CDE**
Michigan Diabetes Research and Training Center
University of Michigan Medical School
Ann Arbor, Michigan

**Robert M. Anderson, EdD**
Michigan Diabetes Research and Training Center
University of Michigan Medical School
Ann Arbor, Michigan

**Shereen Arent, JD**
National Director of Legal Advocacy
American Diabetes Association

**Tom Boyer**
San Francisco, California

**Nathaniel Clark, MD**
National Vice President, Clinical Affairs
American Diabetes Association

**Katie Hathaway, JD**
Legal Advocate
American Diabetes Association

**Morey W. Haymond, MD**
Baylor College of Medicine
Houston, Texas

**Lee Ann Holzmeister, RD, CDE**
Tempe, Arizona

**Crystal Jackson**
Legal Advocacy Paralegal
American Diabetes Association

**John M. Miles, MD**
Mayo Clinic
Rochester, Minnesota

**David S. Schade, MD**
University of New Mexico School
  of Medicine
Albuquerque, New Mexico

**Clara Schneider, MS, RD, RN**
Arlington, Virginia

**Geralyn R. Spollett, MSN, C-ANP,
  CDE**
Yale University School of
  Medicine
New Haven, Connecticut

**Holly Whelan, MPA**
Manager, Health Insurance
  Advocacy
American Diabetes Association

# Introduction

The mission of the American Diabetes Association is to prevent and cure diabetes and to improve the lives of all people affected by diabetes. To further this mission, the Association has written this book for all people who want to better manage their diabetes. The *American Diabetes Association Complete Guide to Diabetes,* 4th Edition, will help you to be an educated health care consumer by reading labels, asking questions, and actively participating in your own health care. You'll learn what steps to take to keep your blood glucose (sugar) levels close to normal. By managing your diabetes, you can prevent or delay many of the complications of diabetes.

No one cares as much about your health or knows as much about your life as you do. But you can't do it alone. Successful diabetes management is a team effort. Your health care providers form a support team dedicated to your good health. Learn as much as you possibly can about diabetes and how it affects you. Ask all the questions you need to have answered and become your own advocate. Your provider, diabetes educator, or dietitian can listen to your needs, help you meet your goals, and provide you with information, but it is up to you to make the day-to-day choices and decisions.

Whether you have recently been diagnosed or have been living with diabetes for years, whether you have type 1 diabetes, type 2 diabetes, or gestational diabetes, your concerns are probably the same: to learn to live with diabetes, to maintain a high quality of life, and to mesh the day-to-day management of diabetes into your routine. At first, the idea of trying to "master" the disease may seem overwhelming. Diabetes management can often be frustrating, even if you're an old hand at it. The trick to living with diabetes is to take it one step at a time. Don't try to do everything at once. Decide what goals are most important, and work on these first. For example, you may want to start by routinely monitoring your blood glucose before you begin to fine-tune your levels. Or you may want to get your walking program up to five times a week before you make any changes in your meal plan. Once your first goal becomes a habit, then you can work on some of your other goals.

The *American Diabetes Association Complete Guide to Diabetes*, 4th Edition, presents information that can help you live well with diabetes. Every time you learn something more about diabetes, you increase your opportunity to live a long and healthy life. But learning about diabetes is only part of the recipe for living well with diabetes. The rest centers on self-knowledge. The best diabetes care plans are personal. Therefore, the more you know about who you are and what you want, the better you can tailor your diabetes care to fit your life.

## How to Have a Healthy Life with Diabetes

- Understand that high blood glucose levels can cause serious complications.
- Create a health care team, consisting of a knowledgeable diabetes care provider, a dietitian, a diabetes educator, doctors, and other specialists.
- Be assured that, with the help of your health care team, you can learn to manage your diabetes.
- Learn all you can about diabetes: read, ask lots of questions, and attend diabetes education programs.
- Keep up-to-date on diabetes research and equipment. Obtain the supplies you need to care for your diabetes.
- Know yourself. Investigate whether fatigue, mood swings, or other problems are related to your blood glucose levels.

# What Is Diabetes? 1

*When you or someone you love has diabetes, you discover that you must think about a part of life that others take for granted. You are constantly striving to reach a subtle balance between glucose and insulin. The more you learn about diabetes, the better you can be at your balancing act and the better your life can be.*

## Types of Diabetes

There are three main types of diabetes. The most common are type 1 diabetes and type 2 diabetes. A third type of diabetes, gestational diabetes, occurs during some pregnancies.

All types of diabetes result in too much sugar, or glucose, in the blood. To understand why this happens, it helps to understand how the body usually works. When you eat, your body breaks down your food into simpler forms such as glucose. The glucose goes into your bloodstream, where it travels to all the cells in your body. Your cells use glucose for energy. Insulin, a hormone made by the pancreas, helps move the glucose from the bloodstream to the cells.

People with type 1 diabetes make very little insulin or no insulin at all. People with type 1 diabetes must take insulin shots in order to live. In contrast, people with type 2 diabetes and women with gestational diabetes do make insulin. But for some reason the cells in their bodies are resistant to the action of insulin or their bodies don't make enough insulin. In all types of diabetes, the glucose does not get into the cells that need it and builds up in the bloodstream instead.

About half of the time, type 1 diabetes starts during childhood or the early teenage years. For this reason, it used to be called *juvenile-onset diabetes*. If your symptoms first appeared during your early teenage years, your health care provider probably suspected diabetes right away. If you were a young child when the disease developed, it might have occurred so fast that you went into a coma, before anyone suspected diabetes. Type 2 diabetes most often develops in adulthood and used to be called *adult-onset diabetes*. Usually, it does not appear suddenly. Instead, you may have no noticeable symptoms or only mild symptoms for years before diabetes is detected, perhaps during a routine exam or blood test. *Gestational diabetes* only appears during pregnancy in women with no previous history of type 1 or type 2 diabetes and usually goes away after pregnancy. Pregnant women are tested for gestational diabetes, usually during the 24th week of gestation. After pregnancy, 5 to 10 percent of women with gestational diabetes are diagnosed with type 2 diabetes. Women who develop gestational diabetes have a 20 to 50 percent risk of developing type 2 diabetes in the next 5 to 10 years.

All people with diabetes have one thing in common. They have too much sugar, or glucose, in their blood. People with very high blood glucose levels share many similar symptoms:

- extreme thirst
- a frequent desire to urinate
- blurred vision

## Body Mass Index Table

| | Normal | | | | | | Overweight | | | | | Obese | | | | | | | | | | Extreme Obesity | | | | | | | | | | | | | | |
|---|---|---|---|---|---|---|---|---|---|---|---|---|---|---|---|---|---|---|---|---|---|---|---|---|---|---|---|---|---|---|---|---|---|---|---|---|
| BMI | 19 | 20 | 21 | 22 | 23 | 24 | 25 | 26 | 27 | 28 | 29 | 30 | 31 | 32 | 33 | 34 | 35 | 36 | 37 | 38 | 39 | 40 | 41 | 42 | 43 | 44 | 45 | 46 | 47 | 48 | 49 | 50 | 51 | 52 | 53 | 54 |
| **Height (inches)** | | | | | | | | | | | | **Body Weight (pounds)** | | | | | | | | | | | | | | | | | | | | | | | | |
| 58 | 91 | 96 | 100 | 105 | 110 | 115 | 119 | 124 | 129 | 134 | 138 | 143 | 148 | 153 | 158 | 162 | 167 | 172 | 177 | 181 | 186 | 191 | 196 | 201 | 205 | 210 | 215 | 220 | 224 | 229 | 234 | 239 | 244 | 248 | 253 | 258 |
| 59 | 94 | 99 | 104 | 109 | 114 | 119 | 124 | 128 | 133 | 138 | 143 | 148 | 153 | 158 | 163 | 168 | 173 | 178 | 183 | 188 | 193 | 198 | 203 | 208 | 212 | 217 | 222 | 227 | 232 | 237 | 242 | 247 | 252 | 257 | 262 | 267 |
| 60 | 97 | 102 | 107 | 112 | 118 | 123 | 128 | 133 | 138 | 143 | 148 | 153 | 158 | 163 | 168 | 174 | 179 | 184 | 189 | 194 | 199 | 204 | 209 | 215 | 220 | 225 | 230 | 235 | 240 | 245 | 250 | 255 | 261 | 266 | 271 | 276 |
| 61 | 100 | 106 | 111 | 116 | 122 | 127 | 132 | 137 | 143 | 148 | 153 | 158 | 164 | 169 | 174 | 180 | 185 | 190 | 195 | 201 | 206 | 211 | 217 | 222 | 227 | 232 | 238 | 243 | 248 | 254 | 259 | 264 | 269 | 275 | 280 | 285 |
| 62 | 104 | 109 | 115 | 120 | 126 | 131 | 136 | 142 | 147 | 153 | 158 | 164 | 169 | 175 | 180 | 186 | 191 | 196 | 202 | 207 | 213 | 218 | 224 | 229 | 235 | 240 | 246 | 251 | 256 | 262 | 267 | 273 | 278 | 284 | 289 | 295 |
| 63 | 107 | 113 | 118 | 124 | 130 | 135 | 141 | 146 | 152 | 158 | 163 | 169 | 175 | 180 | 186 | 191 | 197 | 203 | 208 | 214 | 220 | 225 | 231 | 237 | 242 | 248 | 254 | 259 | 265 | 270 | 278 | 282 | 287 | 293 | 299 | 304 |
| 64 | 110 | 116 | 122 | 128 | 134 | 140 | 145 | 151 | 157 | 163 | 169 | 174 | 180 | 186 | 192 | 197 | 204 | 210 | 216 | 222 | 228 | 232 | 238 | 244 | 250 | 256 | 262 | 267 | 273 | 279 | 285 | 291 | 296 | 302 | 308 | 314 |
| 65 | 114 | 120 | 126 | 132 | 138 | 144 | 150 | 156 | 162 | 168 | 174 | 180 | 186 | 192 | 198 | 204 | 210 | 216 | 222 | 228 | 234 | 240 | 246 | 252 | 258 | 264 | 270 | 276 | 282 | 288 | 294 | 300 | 306 | 312 | 318 | 324 |
| 66 | 118 | 124 | 130 | 136 | 142 | 148 | 155 | 161 | 167 | 173 | 179 | 186 | 192 | 198 | 204 | 210 | 216 | 223 | 229 | 235 | 241 | 247 | 253 | 260 | 266 | 272 | 278 | 284 | 291 | 297 | 303 | 309 | 315 | 322 | 328 | 334 |
| 67 | 121 | 127 | 134 | 140 | 146 | 153 | 159 | 166 | 172 | 178 | 185 | 191 | 198 | 204 | 211 | 217 | 223 | 230 | 236 | 242 | 249 | 255 | 261 | 268 | 274 | 280 | 287 | 293 | 299 | 306 | 312 | 319 | 325 | 331 | 338 | 344 |
| 68 | 125 | 131 | 138 | 144 | 151 | 158 | 164 | 171 | 177 | 184 | 190 | 197 | 203 | 210 | 216 | 223 | 230 | 236 | 243 | 249 | 256 | 262 | 269 | 276 | 282 | 289 | 295 | 302 | 308 | 315 | 322 | 328 | 335 | 341 | 348 | 354 |
| 69 | 128 | 135 | 142 | 149 | 155 | 162 | 169 | 176 | 182 | 189 | 196 | 203 | 209 | 216 | 223 | 230 | 236 | 243 | 250 | 257 | 263 | 270 | 277 | 284 | 291 | 297 | 304 | 311 | 318 | 324 | 331 | 338 | 345 | 351 | 358 | 365 |
| 70 | 132 | 139 | 146 | 153 | 160 | 167 | 174 | 181 | 188 | 195 | 202 | 209 | 216 | 222 | 229 | 236 | 243 | 250 | 257 | 264 | 271 | 278 | 285 | 292 | 299 | 306 | 313 | 320 | 327 | 334 | 341 | 348 | 355 | 362 | 369 | 376 |
| 71 | 136 | 143 | 150 | 157 | 165 | 172 | 179 | 186 | 193 | 200 | 208 | 215 | 222 | 229 | 236 | 243 | 250 | 257 | 265 | 272 | 279 | 286 | 293 | 301 | 308 | 315 | 322 | 329 | 338 | 343 | 351 | 358 | 365 | 372 | 379 | 386 |
| 72 | 140 | 147 | 154 | 162 | 169 | 177 | 184 | 191 | 199 | 206 | 213 | 221 | 228 | 235 | 242 | 250 | 258 | 265 | 272 | 279 | 287 | 294 | 302 | 309 | 316 | 324 | 331 | 338 | 346 | 353 | 361 | 368 | 375 | 383 | 390 | 397 |
| 73 | 144 | 151 | 159 | 166 | 174 | 182 | 189 | 197 | 204 | 212 | 219 | 227 | 235 | 242 | 250 | 257 | 265 | 272 | 280 | 288 | 295 | 302 | 310 | 318 | 325 | 333 | 340 | 348 | 355 | 363 | 371 | 378 | 386 | 393 | 401 | 408 |
| 74 | 148 | 155 | 163 | 171 | 179 | 186 | 194 | 202 | 210 | 218 | 225 | 233 | 241 | 249 | 256 | 264 | 272 | 280 | 287 | 295 | 303 | 311 | 319 | 326 | 334 | 342 | 350 | 358 | 365 | 373 | 381 | 389 | 396 | 404 | 412 | 420 |
| 75 | 152 | 160 | 168 | 176 | 184 | 192 | 200 | 208 | 216 | 224 | 232 | 240 | 248 | 256 | 264 | 272 | 279 | 287 | 295 | 303 | 311 | 319 | 327 | 335 | 343 | 351 | 359 | 367 | 375 | 383 | 391 | 399 | 407 | 415 | 423 | 431 |
| 76 | 156 | 164 | 172 | 180 | 189 | 197 | 205 | 213 | 221 | 230 | 238 | 246 | 254 | 263 | 271 | 279 | 287 | 295 | 304 | 312 | 320 | 328 | 336 | 344 | 353 | 361 | 369 | 377 | 385 | 394 | 402 | 410 | 418 | 426 | 435 | 443 |

Source: Adapted from *Clinical Guidelines on the Identification, Evaluation, and Treatment of Overweight and Obesity in Adults: The Evidence Report.*

■ a feeling of being tired most of the time for no apparent reason

People with type 2 diabetes may also experience leg pain that may indicate nerve damage or poor circulation. Many people with type 1 diabetes and some people with type 2 diabetes also find that they lose weight even though they are hungrier than usual and are eating more.

Type 2 diabetes tends to develop in people who have extra body fat. Where you carry your excess fat may determine whether you get type 2 diabetes: extra fat above the hips (central body obesity) is riskier than fat in the hips and thighs for developing type 2 diabetes. And leading an inactive "couch potato" lifestyle can also lead to diabetes. This lifestyle also contributes to obesity.

Three-fourths of all people with type 2 diabetes are or have been obese—that is, they have a body mass index of 30 or above (see the BMI chart for adults on page 5). A BMI of 25 to 29.9 is considered overweight.

If you have recently been diagnosed with diabetes, you are not alone. Approximately 18.2 million Americans—about 6.3% of the population—have this disease. About 1.3 million people are diagnosed with diabetes each year. Of all cases of diabetes, 90 to 95 percent are type 2 diabetes. And more than one-third of all people with type 2 diabetes are unaware they even have the disease. Because of the nature of type 2 diabetes, it is possible to have mild symptoms (what you feel) or signs (what the doctor can detect) of type 2 diabetes for years before diabetes is detected. In contrast, few cases of type 1 diabetes go undetected for long. The symptoms of type 1 diabetes are severe enough that the person goes to the doctor for help.

## Who Has Diabetes?

About 18.2 million Americans have diabetes. This is more than 6 percent of the people in the country. An estimated 900,000 to 1.8 million people have type 1 diabetes. It is hard to get an exact count of the number of people with diabetes because we have no nationwide diabetes registry. Type 1 diabetes is more common in Caucasians than in African Americans, Hispanic Americans, Asian Americans, and American Indians.

About 16 to 17 million people have type 2 diabetes. Nearly 6 million people are undiagnosed. (And 16 million more people have **pre-diabetes**—a condition in which blood glucose is higher than normal but not at diagnostic levels.) Type 2 diabetes is common in older people. More than 18 percent of Americans over the age of 60 have it. It is more common in some ethnic groups than others. In those age 45 to 74, approximately 25 percent of Mexican Americans and Puerto Rican Americans have type 2 diabetes, more than 13 percent of African Americans have type 2 diabetes, and about 16 percent of Cuban Americans have type 2 diabetes. It is even more common in American Indians. In some tribes, almost half of adults age 30 to 64 have type 2 diabetes.

About 135,000 women develop gestational diabetes each year. Of these, about 40 percent get type 2 diabetes within 15 years.

## Tests for Diabetes

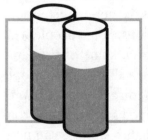

Although your health care provider may suspect that you have diabetes because of your symptoms, the only sure way to tell is with blood tests. Blood tests are used to diagnose both type 1 and type 2 diabetes, as well as gestational diabetes. These blood tests may be repeated to confirm the diagnosis.

The blood tests are based on the fact that diabetes causes your blood glucose levels to be above normal some or all of the time. Your blood glucose levels may be high even though you haven't eaten recently.

**Random plasma glucose tests** are the simplest way to detect diabetes. This test measures the amount of glucose in the blood at any given time and is done without fasting. If you have obvious symptoms of diabetes and the amount of glucose in your blood is 200 mg/dl or higher, you have diabetes. Symptoms of diabetes include frequent urination, intense thirst, blurred vision, unexplained weight loss, and extreme tiredness.

The preferred method for diagnosing diabetes is the **fasting plasma glucose test**. In diabetes, extra glucose remains in the blood, even after fasting. For this test, you will be asked not to eat or drink anything but water for at least 8 to 10 hours. Then, a sample of your blood is taken from a vein and the amount of glucose present in the blood is measured. Normally after fasting, the amount of glucose is less than 100 mg/dl. But when the amount of blood glucose is greater than 126 mg/dl, diabetes is suspected. A firm diagnosis of diabetes is made when two fasting plasma glucose tests, done on different days, are over 126 mg/dl.

If your test results are greater than 100 mg/dl but less than 126 mg/dl, you may have **impaired fasting glucose (IFG)**. Some people also have **impaired glucose tolerance (IGT)**, a condition in which blood glucose levels are higher than normal (140 mg/dl to 199 mg/dl) 2 hours after the start of an oral glucose tolerance test (GTT). If you have IFG and/or IGT, you may be diagnosed with pre-diabetes. This is not diabetes, but sometimes occurs before diabetes develops. Some people with pre-diabetes never get diabetes. However, some of the same problems that result from having diabetes also occur in people with pre-diabetes. If you have been diagnosed with pre-diabetes, you will want to have your blood glucose tested routinely and to watch for symptoms of diabetes. Also, you need to talk with your provider about reducing your risk of heart disease. Keeping your weight in the healthy range and exercising regularly will lower your chances of developing diabetes.

Certain pregnant women are at high risk for developing gestational diabetes. These are women who are 25 years of age or older, are overweight, have a parent or sibling with diabetes, or are Hispanic, American Indian, Asian, or African American. Women who had gestational diabetes in a previous pregnancy have a greater risk of developing it again.

If you have any of these characteristics, you will be screened for gestational diabetes with a **glucose challenge**. This is done between the 24th and 28th weeks of pregnancy. At this time, the hormones of pregnancy naturally begin to cause temporary

**FACT OR MYTH?**

### "I used to have type 2 diabetes, but now I have type 1 diabetes. I started taking insulin last year."

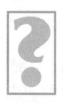

Lots of people, more than 40 percent of adults with diabetes, use insulin. Because there are about 90 adults with type 2 diabetes to every 5 adults with type 1 diabetes, this means there are a lot of people with type 2 diabetes taking insulin. People with type 1 diabetes must use insulin to make up for their pancreas no longer making it. You don't necessarily have type 1 diabetes just because you need insulin. Many people with type 2 diabetes take extra insulin to overcome their body's resistance to the insulin already being made by the pancreas.

Type 1 and type 2 diabetes, while having a lot in common, have different causes. The type of diabetes you have does not change as you age or if you lose or gain weight or change treatments.

insulin resistance that lasts until the baby is born. The glucose challenge helps you find out whether your body is able to overcome the insulin resistance on its own. You are given a glucose drink to finish at a certain time, without regard to eating. If the glucose in your blood 1 hour later is 140 mg/dl or above, you may have gestational diabetes. You will need a full glucose tolerance test for a firm diagnosis.

## Type 1 or Type 2?

If tests reveal that you have diabetes (and you're not pregnant), the next question is whether you have type 1 or type 2 diabetes. Although the symptoms and blood test results can be similar for both type 1 and type 2 diabetes, the causes are very different.

FACT OR MYTH?

**"Having a sweet tooth runs in my family. My dad got diabetes from eating too much sugar."**

 Eating too much of anything causes weight gain, which leads to obesity. Having a certain genetic background predisposes you to diabetes. Being overweight can be the trigger that causes type 2 diabetes to show itself. Whether the excess pounds are from eating candy or bagels or meat loaf makes little difference.

Eating too much sugar doesn't cause diabetes. But eating too much sugar isn't healthy for anyone. It can cause tooth decay and, with the increase in calories, lead to excess pounds. Sweets contain lots of carbohydrates and sometimes fat, which may fill you up without giving you much nutritional benefit. Having a candy bar before lunch makes it easier to pass up the vegetable soup.

It will help your provider to know whether there has been type 1 or type 2 diabetes in your family. Your age is not the only clue about what type of diabetes you have. It's true that most people younger than age 20 who show signs of diabetes have type 1 diabetes and that most people diagnosed with diabetes when they're over age 30 have type 2 diabetes. But there are exceptions. In recent years, an increasing number of children and teens have also developed type 2 diabetes. In a few cases, families carry a genetic trait for developing type 2 diabetes as young people. And in some American Indian families, obesity is so prevalent that children as young as 10 years old have type 2 diabetes.

- If you are overweight or obese, it is more likely that you have type 2 diabetes.
- If you suddenly developed signs of diabetes, such as frequent urination, unusual thirst and hunger, and weight loss, perhaps after an illness, and are a young adult or child, it is more likely that you have type 1 diabetes.
- If you are not overweight and there are ketones in your urine, it is more likely that you have type 1 diabetes (see Chapter 5 for more on ketone testing).
- If you are African American, Native American, Asian American, or Hispanic American, are older than 50, are overweight, and haven't been feeling quite "right" for a long time, it is more likely that you have type 2 diabetes.
- If you take insulin injections, you could have either type 1 or type 2 diabetes.

## Who Gets Diabetes?

The risk factors associated with type 1 or type 2 diabetes are different. For both type 1 and type 2 diabetes, having a family history of diabetes puts you at a higher risk for developing the disease than a person with no family history of diabetes. How-

## Do You Have MODY?

Other types of diabetes also exist that do not fit the type 1 or type 2 profile. For example, maturity-onset diabetes of the young (MODY) usually affects young adults, but can also affect teens and children. It can be misdiagnosed as type 1 in younger patients. Adults with MODY develop diabetes at a younger age than most type 2 patients and do not tend to be overweight or sedentary. In the past, people with MODY were often told they had a form of type 2 diabetes. We now know that MODY is caused by a genetic mutation that leads to impaired insulin secretion. Insulin resistance, which is often found in type 2 diabetes, does not usually occur in MODY.

If you have MODY, you may be able to manage your blood glucose levels through diet and exercise alone, at least for a while. However, therapies that work for people with type 2 diabetes do not always work for people with MODY. You may have more success with insulin therapy or oral agents that stimulate insulin secretion.

ever, many people with type 1 diabetes have no known family history of the disease. Type 1 diabetes is more common among whites than among members of other racial groups. In contrast, members of American Indian, African American, and Hispanic ethnic groups are at higher risk for developing type 2 diabetes.

A major difference in the characteristics of individuals with type 1 and type 2 diabetes is the age of onset. Typically, type 1 diabetes develops in individuals under the age of 40. Half of all people diagnosed with type 1 diabetes are under the age of 20. In contrast, most of the people diagnosed with type 2 diabetes are over the age of 30, although type 2 diabetes is on the rise among children and teenagers. The risk for type 2 increases with age. Half of all new cases of type 2 diabetes are in people age 55 and older.

Type 2 diabetes is more common in overweight and obese individuals, whereas body weight does not seem to be a risk factor for type 1 diabetes. Type 2 diabetes is often found in women with a history of giving birth to babies weighing more than 9 pounds and in women who were previously diagnosed with gestational diabetes. In both men and women, high blood pressure and very high concentrations of fats (cholesterol) in the blood are more common in people with type 2 diabetes.

You can't get diabetes—either type 1 or type 2—from exposure to someone who already has diabetes, or from something you ate. And although diabetes may reveal itself after an illness or a stressful experience, these situations may have only sped up the appearance of the disease.

## Causes of Type 1 Diabetes

Insulin is produced by the beta cells in the pancreas. In people with type 1 diabetes, the immune system mistakenly destroys these cells. The body responds to the beta cells as if they were foreign invaders. This is called an *autoimmune response.* Autoimmune responses also occur in other diseases such as multiple sclerosis, lupus, and thyroid diseases such as hypothyroidism (Hashimoto's disease) and hyperthyroidism (Graves' disease). Researchers do not know exactly why this happens. But for diabetes, researchers have found many factors that appear to be linked to type 1 diabetes. These include genetics, autoantibodies, viruses, cow's milk, and oxygen free radicals.

### Genetics

Scientists have long suspected that genetics play a role in type 1 diabetes. If your mother or father had diabetes, for example, you are more likely to develop the disease than someone without a family history. Also, type 1 diabetes seems to be more common in certain racial groups. Caucasians, for example, are more likely to develop the disease than are people from other racial backgrounds. Type 1 diabetes occurs in less than 1 of 100,000 people in Shanghai, China, but occurs in more than 35 of 100,000 people in Finland.

Everyone is born with a set of instructions that tells the cells in your body how to grow, live, and function. These instructions lie in the particular chemical sequence of units known as bases, which make up the DNA in every cell in your body. Each cell in your body contains 46 chromosomes, which are made up of DNA and protein. Each DNA strand is like a long string that contains millions of bases. Along the strand lie the genes, unique segments of DNA that tell your cells what kind of protein to make.

But just as books sometimes contain typographical errors, so too does the sequence of DNA. If there is a mistake, or mutation, in the DNA within a gene, then a faulty protein may be made that can't do its job. Scientists are trying to determine how mistakes in specific genes cause diabetes. If mutated genes occur in germ cells—the eggs and sperm—then the DNA mutations can be passed on from generation to generation.

Researchers have identified several different genes that might make a person more likely to develop type 1 diabetes. However, they have not found one single gene that makes all people who inherit it develop the disease. Instead, it seems that there are several genes known as "diabetes susceptibility" genes.

One particular set of genes that may predispose a person to diabetes is responsible for a set of proteins known as the human leukocyte antigens, or HLAs. These genes code for certain proteins called *antigens,* which identify a person's own cells as "self." They tell the immune cells not to destroy the cells that are part of a person's body. Scientists believe that some HLAs incorrectly tag a person's own beta cells as "non-self." Then the immune cells, which normally destroy foreign invading cells, destroy these cells. This is called *autoimmunity*—an immune attack on a person's own cells. In type 1 diabetes, the beta cells of the pancreas are destroyed in an autoimmune attack, and the body can no longer make insulin. This destructive process occurs over many months or years.

Each person has many kinds of HLA genes, and thus there are many types of HLAs. Each person inherits one of each kind of HLA gene from each parent. One type of HLA gene, known as HLA-DR, is most strongly linked to type 1 diabetes. There are many variations of HLA-DR, but 95 percent of people with type 1 diabetes have the DR3 form, the DR4 form, or both. This makes researchers suspect that having the DR3 and DR4 variants may make a person more likely to get type 1 diabetes. However, this is not the whole answer, because 45 percent of people without type 1 diabetes have the DR3 or DR4 variants. Also, variants of another HLA gene, known as HLA-DQ, may also play a role in type 1 diabetes.

Just because a person inherits a susceptible HLA variant doesn't mean that person will develop diabetes. Most people with DR3 or DR4 variants remain healthy. But if there is a family history of type 1 diabetes, then screening may help predict the risk of developing the disease. For example, brothers and sisters of a person with diabetes who have two of the same HLA-DR variants have a 15 percent chance of getting type 1 diabetes. But if they share only one variant, the risk is only 5 percent. If no variants are the same, the risk of developing type 1 diabetes is 1 percent or less.

The more we study how people get type 1 diabetes, the more we understand that the answers are not simple. No one event or characteristic seems to bring on diabetes. Researchers have identified several other gene clusters on different chromo-

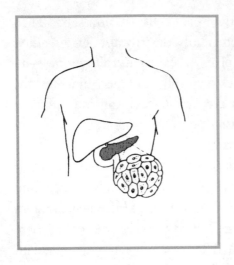

somes in addition to these HLA variants that may also play a role in type 1 diabetes.

## Autoantibodies

The immune system protects you from disease by killing germs and other foreign invaders. It does this largely through the action of white blood cells, or lymphocytes. T lymphocytes, or T cells, can attack foreign cells directly. B lymphocytes, or B cells, produce special proteins called *antibodies* that recognize the shapes of molecules on the surface of specific invaders.

B cells sometimes manufacture antibodies that recognize a person's own cells. These self-recognizing antibodies are called *autoantibodies*. Autoantibodies are found in many people with autoimmune disorders, but three autoantibodies are especially common in people with type 1 diabetes. These antibodies recognize the following:

- islet cells (beta cells are just one type of islet cell in the pancreas)
- insulin
- glutamic acid decarboxylase (GAD, or the 64K protein), a protein made by the beta cells in the pancreas

These three types of autoantibodies all seem to act as markers. Researchers believe that these antibodies contribute to the demise of the beta cells of the pancreas by identifying which cells are to be attacked. It is really the T cells that ultimately destroy the insulin-producing cells of the pancreas. Of people newly diagnosed with type 1 diabetes, 70 to 80 percent have antibodies to islet cells, 30 to 50 percent have antibodies to insulin, and 80 to 95 percent have antibodies to GAD.

The antibodies may be present several years before diabetes is diagnosed. The islet cell antibodies disappear later on. Because these antibodies are so common in people with type 1 diabetes and because they so often appear before the symptoms of diabetes appear, researchers are finding that they are useful in screening people for type 1 diabetes who are at high risk for the disease. Although the risk for developing diabetes may only be 1 to 10 percent for people with a parent or sibling with the disease, a much higher percentage of people who also have antibodies to islet cells develop type 1 diabetes within 5 years. And for many, having combinations of these antibodies and certain HLA genes results in an even higher risk.

## Viruses

Perhaps surprisingly, many scientists also suspect that viruses may cause type 1 diabetes. This is because people who develop type 1 diabetes have often recently had a viral infection, and "epidemics" of type 1 diabetes often occur after viral epidemics. Viruses, such as those that cause mumps and German measles and the Coxsackie family of viruses, which is related to the virus that causes polio, may play some role in causing type 1 diabetes.

A small region of the GAD molecule is almost identical to a region of a protein found in the virus known as Coxsackie B4. The two similar protein regions probably have similar shapes and may be recognized by the same T cells. Thus, to a T cell hunting for foreign invaders, the GAD protein, which is part of the body, might look the same as the Coxsackie virus protein, which is part of an invading cell. After a viral infection by the Coxsackie virus, the T cell, bent on destroying the invading virus, might actually destroy the body's own beta cells that bear the GAD protein. This would destroy the cells that produce insulin and result in type 1 diabetes.

Other theories may also explain how a viral infection might lead to diabetes. Some researchers believe that when a virus infects a body, it might somehow change the structure of the antigens on the surface of the islet cells. If this occurs, then the altered antigen might appear to be foreign to the immune system, and a person's own insulin-producing islet cells might be destroyed.

Another well-known diabetes researcher has a different theory. He believes that diabetes is a relatively new disease caused by a slow-acting virus. Although such a virus has not been found, he holds that the virus causes the immune system to attack proteins in the pancreas. A drastic increase in the number of cases of type 1 diabetes occurred on the island of Sardinia, Italy, in the 1960s and in Finland in the 1970s, and he believes that such a slow-acting virus could be the culprit.

## Cow's Milk

Although it seems unlikely, different kinds of food may play a role in the development of type 1 diabetes. For example, one group of researchers found a connection between being fed cow's milk early in life (before 3 or 4 months old) and type 1 diabetes. They showed that children newly diagnosed with type 1 diabetes have higher amounts of antibodies that recognize a specific protein in cow's milk. These autoantibodies appear to bind to a protein that sometimes appears on the surface of the insulin-producing beta cells in the pancreas after an illness. The researchers speculate that, after an illness, the transient protein may appear on the surface of beta cells. The immune response to the milk protein might be to then recognize the beta cell surface proteins and attack the beta cells, leading to a destruction of the insulin-producing cells of the pancreas and, thus, to type 1 diabetes.

However, other researchers have looked for but not found an increased risk of type 1 diabetes if cow's milk is given early in life and if breastfeeding is done for a short period. Cow's milk is only one kind of food that may play a role in the development of type 1 diabetes. Studies in diabetes-prone rats show that withholding wheat and soy helps delay or prevent diabetes.

## Oxygen Free Radicals

Oxygen free radicals, formed as a by-product of many chemical reactions in the body, wreak havoc wherever they go. Normally, the body has ways of quenching free radicals. But smoke, air pollution, diet, and even genetics can contribute to the formation of excessive amounts of free radicals, which the body cannot always handle. Uncontrolled, the reactive molecules can destroy the body's own cells as well as bacteria. Oxygen free radicals contribute significantly to the aging process and to the development of several other diseases. Researchers have implicated free radicals in the development of amyotrophic lateral sclerosis (ALS), or Lou Gehrig's disease, a degenerative neuromuscular disease.

Some researchers believe that oxygen free radicals may also contribute to type 1 diabetes. Islet cells have very low levels of the enzymes that break down free radicals. Thus, agents that increase free radical production could result in destruction of pancreatic cells. If this is true, then researchers may be able to develop drugs that block the formation of free radicals in the islet cells.

## Chemicals and Drugs

Several chemicals have been shown to trigger diabetes. Pyriminil (Vacor), a poison used to kill rats, can trigger type 1 diabetes. Two prescription drugs, pentamidine, used to treat pneumonia, and L-asparaginase, an anticancer drug, can also cause type 1 diabetes. Other chemicals have been shown to cause diabetes in animals, but scientists don't know for sure whether they have the same effect in humans.

In summary, it is unlikely that either genetics or environmental factors alone cause diabetes. But it does appear that a person could start with a genetic susceptibility—the inheritance of a particular set of genes. If this person is then exposed to some environmental "triggering" factor, such as a virus or a chemical, then diabetes may develop. Although no one is destined to develop diabetes with certainty, a person's heredity may increase the odds.

## Prevention of Type 1 Diabetes

By testing relatives of people with type 1 diabetes for autoantibodies, researchers can often predict who is likely to develop the disease. This could be especially useful as new therapies emerge, because they can be started before damage to the pancreas is too extensive. For example, it was thought that by identifying people who are likely to develop type 1 diabetes at an early stage, researchers might be able to treat them with insulin or drugs that suppress the immune system (anti-rejection medications) and thus prevent the T cells from destroying the beta cells in the pancreas. Recent studies do not support that this is possible at this time.

Some people with a high risk of getting type 1 diabetes have participated in studies to see whether immunosuppressants such as azathioprine or cyclosporine delay or prevent the onset of the disease. These studies suggest that azathioprine or cyclosporine can reduce the dose of insulin needed in people who have already developed type 1 diabetes, if the drug is started at the time the disease is diagnosed. Researchers have also been studying whether insulin can prevent type 1 diabetes. In the Diabetes Prevention Trial (DPT), researchers found that giving insulin by injection or orally does not prevent type 1 diabetes in people at high risk.

Other therapies may also be tested as researchers learn more about the causes of type 1 diabetes. For example, if autoimmunity to GAD turns out to be a primary trigger of type 1 diabetes, it might be possible to develop a vaccine that would protect people from developing the disease.

## Causes of Type 2 Diabetes

The reasons that type 2 diabetes occurs are different from those that trigger type 1 diabetes. Unlike people with type 1 diabetes, who become unable to produce insulin, people with type 2 diabetes produce insulin. But, either the body does not respond to insulin's action (it's resistant) or there is just not enough insulin to go around—or both. Either problem leads to the same outcome: insulin can't deliver glucose to the cells that need it, and there's too much glucose in the blood.

Virtually all cells in the body contain special proteins called *receptors* that bind to insulin. They work like a lock and key. In order for glucose to enter the cell, insulin (the key) must first fit into the insulin receptor (the lock). But for some reason, in some people with type 2 diabetes, there is a faulty lock, or insulin receptor. The key doesn't open the lock, and glucose is shut out of the cell. And in some people with type 2 diabetes, there are not enough locks, or insulin receptors, on the cells to allow enough glucose to enter. But for most people with diabetes, it's not so much that the key doesn't fit the lock, but that insulin doesn't work properly. In rare cases, the insulin is mutated, or built incorrectly, and does not fit the insulin receptor.

Initially, the pancreas is able to produce enough insulin to overcome the resistance. But over the course of several years, the beta cells in the pancreas are no longer able to produce enough insulin or it is released too slowly. Without enough insulin to meet the body's needs, glucose levels rise and diabetes results. Scientists do not know why the pancreas does not function well in these people. Some believe that the system that controls glucose levels in the blood and tells the pancreas to make more insulin does not function properly. Others think that the pancreas, after many years of working overtime to overcome insulin resistance, simply begins to "burn out."

Although researchers do not fully understand why type 2 diabetes develops, they have uncovered many factors that may contribute to the disease.

## Genetics

Genetics also appears to play a role in how type 2 diabetes develops. Like type 1 diabetes, type 2 diabetes also appears to run in families, and it is most likely due to the inheritance of certain genes. The link to genetics seems even stronger in type 2 diabetes than in type 1 diabetes. If a person with type 1 diabetes has an identical twin, there is a 25 to 50 percent chance that the twin will develop diabetes. But if a person with type 2 diabetes has an identical twin, there is a 60 to 75 percent chance that the person will develop diabetes.

More evidence for the role of genes in type 2 diabetes comes from studying certain ethnic groups. Compared with Caucasians, African Americans, Asian Americans, Hispanic Americans (except Cuban Americans), and Native Americans all get type 2 diabetes more often. Native Americans have the highest rate of type 2 diabetes in the world. Hispanic groups, such as Mexican Americans, that share genes with Native American groups (where there has been cultural mixing) have a higher rate of type 2 diabetes than Hispanic groups, such as Cuban Americans, where less intercultural contact has occurred.

Researchers have not yet isolated a single "type 2 diabetes" gene, but they are finding several that may contribute to type 2 diabetes. For example, researchers have identified a protein called *PC-1* that shuts down the insulin receptor, creating insulin resistance. This protein is prevalent in most people with type 2 diabetes, compared with people without diabetes. For some reason, too much of the inhibitor protein is made in some people, and the insulin receptor cannot do its job properly, which can lead to insulin resistance.

Researchers believe that the genes that lead to obesity may also play a role in diabetes. In mice, scientists have identified a gene they called the *obese gene*. The obese gene appears to regulate body weight by making proteins that affect the center in the brain that tells you whether you're full or hungry. When the obese gene is mutated, the mice become obese and develop type 2 diabetes.

## Age, Obesity, and Lifestyle

The most important environmental trigger of type 2 diabetes appears to be obesity. Obesity is defined as having a body mass index of 30 or greater (see p. 5). Genetics may play a role in obesity and, thus, in triggering type 2 diabetes.

In some way, having too much body fat promotes resistance to insulin. This is why, for so many years, type 2 diabetes has been treated with diet and exercise. Losing weight and increasing the amount of muscle while decreasing the amount of fat helps the body use insulin better. There is also a link between type 2 diabetes and where fat is stored. People with central body obesity, which means carrying excess fat above the hips, have a higher risk of developing type 2 diabetes than those with excess fat on the hips and thighs.

Central body obesity, as well as overall obesity, is more common in African Americans than in Caucasians. This may be one reason why type 2 diabetes is also more common in African Americans than in Caucasians.

Age also appears to play a role. Half of all new cases of type 2 diabetes occur in people over age 55. Because people tend to gain weight as they age, many researchers think that the reason more older people develop diabetes is because more older people are overweight.

Leading an inactive, sedentary lifestyle and consuming a high-calorie diet can also lead to type 2 diabetes in susceptible people, presumably by contributing to obesity.

## Prevention of Type 2 Diabetes

The best way to prevent type 2 diabetes is to maintain an active lifestyle and to keep your weight at a healthy level. In the Diabetes Prevention Program (DPP) study, researchers tested whether changing lifestyle habits or taking the oral diabetes medication metformin (Glucophage) could delay or prevent the onset of diabetes in people at high risk for developing type 2 diabetes.

The study evaluated 3,234 volunteers who were overweight and had impaired glucose tolerance (IGT). IGT or pre-diabetes is a condition in which blood glucose levels are higher than normal but not as high as levels in a person with diabetes. The subjects were placed in one of three groups. People in the first group, the lifestyle intervention group, used a low-fat diet and exercised for 30 minutes a day five times a week. People in the second group were treated with 850 mg metformin twice a day, and the people in the third group took placebo pills instead of metformin. The last two groups also received information on diet and exercise. The study ended a year early when researchers found that people in the lifestyle group who lost 5 to 7 percent of their body weight (10–20 lbs) and exercised 30 minutes a day, 5 days a week (usually by walking), had a 58 percent lower incidence of diabetes. Metformin also lowered the incidence of diabetes by 31 percent.

The results clearly indicate that moderate exercise and modest weight loss can go a long way in preventing type 2 diabetes.

## Causes of Gestational Diabetes

Like the other types of diabetes, the exact cause of gestational diabetes is unknown. However, experts do have some clues.

### Hormones

During pregnancy, the placenta, which is the organ that nourishes the growing baby, produces large amounts of various hormones. Hormones are important for the baby's growth. However, these hormones may also block insulin's action in the mother's body, causing insulin resistance. All pregnant women have some degree of insulin resistance.

Gestational diabetes usually appears around the 24th week of pregnancy. This is when the placenta begins producing large quantities of the hormones that cause insulin resistance. The period between the 24th and 28th weeks of pregnancy is the usual time to screen for gestational diabetes.

### Genetics

Because insulin resistance seems to cause gestational diabetes, it is more like type 2 diabetes than type 1 diabetes. And having

## Historical Perspective

For thousands of years, doctors have recognized diabetes as a disease, but did not understand its cause. An early Egyptian medical text written around 1550 B.C., called the *Ebers Papyrus,* describes a condition of "passing too much urine." The Greek physician Aretaeus, who lived in the second century A.D., gave diabetes its name, from a Greek word meaning "siphon" or "pass through." Aretaeus observed that his patients' bodies appeared to "melt down" into urine.

People observed early on that the urine from people with diabetes was very sweet. In fact, one way to diagnose diabetes was to pour urine near an anthill. If the ants were attracted to the urine, it meant that the urine contained sugar. By the 18th century, physicians added the Latin term *mellitus* to diabetes, which describes its sugary taste.

In 1776, scientists discovered that the glucose was in the blood of both people with diabetes and people without diabetes. That led them to suspect that people with diabetes pass glucose from the blood to the urine. But they didn't know how.

Then in 1889—more than 100 years after glucose was found in blood—two German physiologists, Oskar Minkowski and Joseph von Mering, found quite by accident that the pancreas was involved in diabetes. While studying how fat is metabolized in the body, they decided to remove the pancreas from a laboratory dog. Much to their astonishment, the dog urinated again and again. Proving that science rewards a prepared mind, the scientists had the foresight to test the dog's urine for glucose. Sure enough, the dog had developed diabetes when its pancreas was removed.

This led the scientists to suspect that some substance in the pancreas somehow prevented diabetes. As scientists embarked on a 30-year quest to find that magic substance, people with diabetes were subjected to a host of so-called cures, including bloodletting, opium, and special diets. Unfortunately, none of these measures helped the disease. Although some diets did seem to help

## Historical Perspective (*Continued*)

some older people with diabetes, they did nothing for severely affected young patients. These patients typically died within several years of developing the disease.

In 1921, Dr. Frederick Banting, a young surgeon just out of medical school, had a breakthrough. He had the idea to isolate the groups of cells called the *islets of Langerhans* in the pancreas. Banting began his experiments working in the laboratory of a senior faculty member at the University of Toronto, Professor J. J. R. Macleod, an authority on carbohydrate metabolism. Macleod teamed Banting with a young medical student named Charles Best.

Using experimental dogs, Banting's approach was to tie off the pancreatic duct—which connects the pancreas to the intestine. This would destroy most of the tissue of the pancreas, which would no longer be able to secrete its digestive enzymes into the intestine. Banting guessed that the islets of Langerhans secrete something directly into the blood and that these cells would survive. At long last, Banting and Best succeeded in treating a dog with diabetes using extract from the islet cells.

Within 6 months after their success with the diabetic dog, the two scientists injected their extract into Leonard Thompson, a 14-year-old boy who was dying from diabetes, but the boy remained ill. A biochemist working in Macleod's laboratory, J. B. Collip, purified the extract, and the experiment was repeated 12 days later. This time the scientists succeeded, and Thompson, emaciated from diabetes, began to gain weight and lived for 15 years with regular insulin injections, until he died from pneumonia. In 1923, Banting and Macleod were awarded the Nobel Prize in Medicine for their discovery. Feeling that their collaborators had been slighted, Banting shared his prize money with Best, and Macleod shared with Collip. The team had made an important discovery leading to a diabetes treatment that is still in use today.

gestational diabetes increases your chances of someday developing type 2 diabetes (but not of developing type 1 diabetes). Researchers suspect that the genes responsible for type 2 diabetes and for gestational diabetes may be similar.

Gestational diabetes is more common in groups that have more obesity. Obesity can trigger gestational diabetes as well as type 2 diabetes.

Some women show signs of high blood glucose even before the 28th week of pregnancy. It is likely that these women had diabetes that was not recognized before pregnancy. The weight gain and hormonal changes of pregnancy stressed the body and revealed the diabetes. After the pregnancy, these women need to be tested for diabetes, and either type 1 or type 2 diabetes may be diagnosed.

# Diabetes Management | 2

*How you manage your diabetes depends on your personal goals and needs. Here are some options to consider.*

Nan has two small children and is 32. After a flu-like illness, her thirst, weight loss, and almost constant need to urinate brought her to the doctor. She started taking insulin and counting carbohydrates. But she worries about what will happen if she has an insulin reaction when her children need her.

Jesse is a grandfather of four who is 64. Although he tried to keep his weight down and do some walking, his doctor's prediction of diabetes came true. His mother lost both legs below the knee, and eventually her life, because of diabetes.

William is a junior high school student who likes books and dirt bikes. His cousin Sarah, a grown-up, has diabetes. William must take insulin and is worried about all the needles and what his friends will think.

Alvin, 49, knows that he needs to cut back on fried foods to lower his lipid (cholesterol and other fats) levels and help his weight problem. He's thinking of going to a health club.

Anita has gestational diabetes. She is worried for her baby's safe arrival and about her chances of having diabetes permanently.

Marie is an avid shopper and walker at 68 who wants to do more to increase her chances of living longer. She got diabetes at age 40 and has learned how to make insulin adjustments based on her blood glucose readings.

In diabetes, the message that "no two people are exactly alike" comes across loud and clear. Diabetes involves hormone action and metabolism, which vary from one body to the next, plus human behavior, which also varies from one person to the next. Mix the biological processes with the personal preferences, and you end up with an almost endless variety of responses to diabetes. Therefore, everyone with diabetes needs an individualized diabetes care plan.

Despite their differences, Nan, Jesse, William, Alvin, Anita, and Marie all have something in common. They have chosen to meet the basic challenges their diabetes poses. To have as normal a lifestyle as possible, they are working to prevent short-term problems such as blood glucose levels that are too low (hypoglycemia) or too high (hyperglycemia). In addition, they hope to prevent or delay some of the long-term problems diabetes can bring, such as damage to the nerves, kidneys, eyes, or heart and blood vessels.

Here are some ways to meet these goals:

- live a healthy lifestyle, with regular school or job attendance and fun social activities
- avoid extremely high blood glucose levels
- avoid severe low blood glucose or unconsciousness
- keep up normal growth, if you're young
- maintain a healthy body weight and physical fitness
- enjoy normal sexual function

## Designing Your Diabetes Plan

As you and your health care team design your diabetes care plan, you'll need to set some "big picture" goals. Any kind of diabetes treatment should be able to help you meet the basic diabetes management goals listed above. The methods you use to meet these treatment goals almost always include some form of meal and exercise planning and may also include a medication plan (see table on page 32).

Start by thinking about what goals are important to you. You have the best chance of meeting or exceeding your goals if they are meaningful to you and if you tailor your plan to your own style and needs. This can be as simple as finding healthy recipes for your favorite foods at holidays or as complicated as finding out ways to meet the demands of your unpredictable work schedule. Even though most diabetes care plans include diet, physical activity, and insulin or oral medications if needed, you need your own plan. What might work for a sedentary person with type 2 diabetes is not suitable for an active person with type 1 diabetes. Speak up if you feel the plan being offered won't work for you. The best plan to care for your diabetes is the one you can use on a day-to-day basis. Two people may

## Common Treatments for Diabetes

| Type of therapy | Goals of therapy |
|---|---|
| • Meal plans | • Manage weight<br>• Manage blood glucose levels<br>• Manage blood lipid levels<br>• Reduce chances that you'll need additional medications |
| • Exercise plans | • Maintain muscle tone and physical fitness<br>• Lower blood glucose levels<br>• Lower blood lipid levels<br>• Increase sensitivity to medications<br>• Aid meal planning in managing weight |
| • Oral diabetes medications | • Reduce blood glucose levels by improving insulin release, reducing available glucose, and/or decreasing insulin resistance |
| • Insulin injections | • Make up for the body's inability to produce insulin<br>• Reduce blood glucose levels by improving insulin action and overcoming insulin resistance |

have the same type of diabetes, but their management plans can be very different.

When you sit down with members of your health care team to plan your treatment, be sure to consider the following:

- your age and your physical abilities
- what type of diabetes you have
- how long you've had diabetes
- whether you have signs of any diabetes complications
- what kind of lifestyle you lead. For instance, are you a stay-at-home type? Do you like to eat out often or travel? How do your religious or cultural practices affect how you will manage your diabetes? Do you often feel stressed?
- your favorite kinds of exercise, if any, and when you like to work out
- your favorite foods and cooking style
- your occupation. For instance, are you physically active or do you sit most of the day?
- what you know about yourself. For instance, what are your goals? What has and has not worked for you in the past?
- how much support you have from family, loved ones, and friends. For instance, how much time do you spend alone? Are you able to get around by yourself? Is your family available to help you?
- how diabetes has affected you emotionally and psychologically
- how often you have low blood glucose levels and what happens when you do

Your potential diabetes management tools are many. Included in your bag of tricks are insulin, oral diabetes medications, healthy eating habits, regular exercise habits, and a take-charge attitude about your diabetes. Another big player in your diabetes management is self-monitoring of blood glucose (SMBG). This is a tool that gives you an immediate reading of your blood glucose level. When you know your blood glucose level at a given moment, you can make informed diabetes management decisions. Maybe you decide to take a brisk walk when you find your blood glucose level is a little high after lunch. Or perhaps you just don't feel right, and after a test, you know that it's because your blood glucose is low, so you decide to eat a small box of raisins to prevent a severe reaction. You can take as many readings each day as you need and as your budget and fingertips can handle. You can find more information about SMBG in Chapter 5.

## Type 1 Diabetes Management

Because your body no longer makes insulin, insulin injections play a big role in your diabetes care plan. How much insulin you need to take depends on your blood glucose level, or what you predict the level will be after a meal. Naturally, food also plays an important role in your diabetes management plan, because it contributes glucose to your blood. Usually, physical activity can lower your blood glucose level, decreasing your dose of insulin. So, you'll need to account for exercise and physical activity in your diabetes management plan.

### Insulin Therapy

Most people with type 1 diabetes take insulin by injecting it with a needle and syringe or an insulin pen. The goal is to mimic normal insulin release as closely as possible. People without diabetes have a low level of insulin available in the blood most of the time. This is a background, or basal, level of insulin. After meals, a bolus of insulin is released, just enough to clear the glucose in the meal from the blood. To imitate this sequence, you can develop a regular schedule of insulin injections using faster-acting forms of insulin or combinations of both slower-acting and fast-acting forms of insulin (see Chapter 4 for a lot more about insulin and insulin plans).

Some people use insulin pumps to dispense fast-acting insulin at a steady background, or basal, rate and to provide extra insulin to cover meals. Although most insulin pumps in use today are worn on a belt, researchers are working to develop a pump that is placed inside the body. Ideally, scientists would like to make a pump that senses the amount of glucose in the blood and delivers the right amount of insulin, as needed. So far, the most difficult part has been creating a glucose sensor. No matter what method is used, the goal is still the same—to deliver insulin to cells so that they can take in glucose.

Your type of insulin therapy should relate directly to your health and your lifestyle choices. Your chosen therapy may be as simple as keeping your blood glucose levels from shooting too high after meals or falling too low between meals. Or your therapy may be more challenging: trying to keep after-meal blood glucose levels as close as possible to those of someone without diabetes.

Insulin therapy usually consists of taking your insulin in two or more shots a day, using a combination of longer- and shorter-acting insulins. Type 1 diabetes usually cannot be successfully managed with only one or two shots a day. There are too many hours at different times of the day that the blood glucose level is high.

An insulin plan that includes three to four, or even more, injections of insulin per day leads to fewer times when blood glucose levels are high. People who take shots this many times each day usually use a long-acting insulin as the background basal insulin and rapid- or fast-acting insulin to cover meals.

They inject rapid- or fast-acting insulin as a bolus before meals to lower the blood glucose rise that occurs as food is digested.

The food you eat and the exercise you get go hand-in-hand with your insulin therapy. To know how much insulin you'll need to have, it helps to know what your blood glucose level is now (you know this by blood glucose testing), what you're planning to eat (so you'll be able to estimate how much your blood glucose will increase), and what physical activities you'll be doing. Of course, healthy eating and regular exercise are a part of everyone's healthy living plan. But for you, knowing how these two daily features move your blood glucose level up and down is essential.

There is more information about insulin therapy and different insulin plans in Chapter 4, and more about healthy eating is in Chapter 8. Read about exercise for people with type 1 diabetes in Chapter 9.

## Pancreas Transplantation

So far, the only way to treat type 1 diabetes is to give the body another source of insulin. Usually, this is done through injections of insulin. However, new experimental approaches also show some promise.

Patients with type 1 diabetes have experienced positive results from pancreas transplants. Typically, part or all of a new pancreas is surgically implanted in the lower abdominal cavity of a patient. The old pancreas is left alone; it still makes digestive enzymes even though it doesn't make insulin. Most organs are obtained from someone who has died but made provisions to donate organs. People with successful pancreas transplants may no longer need to take insulin and may have normal blood glucose levels. In addition, many of the side effects that often accompany diabetes are also prevented, or at least slowed. Most people with nerve damage who receive a pancreas transplant do not get worse and sometimes show improvement.

The downside to pancreas transplantation is that the body treats the new pancreas as foreign. The immune system attacks the transplanted pancreas. People with pancreas transplants must take powerful immunosuppressant drugs to prevent rejection of the new pancreas. Drugs that suppress the immune system can lower resistance to other diseases such as cancer and bacterial and viral infections. Pancreas transplantation is most often done when a patient is also receiving a new kidney. The pancreas transplant adds little further risk and offers big benefits. However, transplant surgery is risky. Each person needs to carefully weigh the potential benefits and the risks.

## Islet Transplantation

Researchers are testing transplanting only the islet cells of the pancreas. These are the cells in the pancreas that secrete insulin. The islets also sense glucose levels in the blood and dispense the right amount of insulin to the blood.

Scientists believe that transplanting islet cells is less dangerous than transplanting the whole pancreas. They have developed ways to prepare islet cells from the pancreas. Researchers in Canada developed a method of transplanting islets that uses a larger number of islet cells and a new type of drug therapy to suppress the immune system. Islet cell transplantation is now being done in a few specialty centers in the United States. But, immune rejection of islet cells is an even bigger problem than in pancreas transplants. Some scientists surround the cells in a protective membrane before transplanting them. Other scientists are trying to change the cells before transplanting them to trick the immune system into thinking they are part of the body. Sometimes the islet cells are exposed to cold temperatures or ultraviolet light, so that the cells of the immune system cannot recognize the foreign antigens on the surface of the transplanted cells. Another method is to transplant the islet cells directly into the thymus, a gland in the neck, where some immune system cells grow and learn to tell the difference between self and nonself. If exposed to transplanted cells as they mature, immune system cells might think the transplants are part of the body.

The biggest problem with both pancreas and islet cell transplantation is the shortage of organ donors. Only 7,000 bodies are donated for organ transplants each year in the United States—too few to supply islet cells for everyone with type 1 diabetes.

## Type 2 Diabetes Management

You can manage type 2 diabetes by many methods. Not everyone with type 2 diabetes needs pills or insulin at first. Most people who are newly diagnosed begin with new eating and exercise plans. For many, eating healthy portion sizes of low-fat foods and getting a regular workout is all they need to keep blood glucose levels near normal. Others need to add the extra power of oral medications or insulin.

There are many different reasons that people develop type 2 diabetes.

Your muscle and fat cells often are resistant to the action of insulin. In this case, a regular exercise program and weight loss, often in addition to medication, can help. Your beta cells in the pancreas may not release enough insulin to meet your needs. In this case, sulfonylureas or insulin are helpful. Your liver may release too much glucose. In this case, metformin can be helpful.

Sometimes it's possible to figure out which of these problems is causing your high glucose levels. This helps match the treatment to the cause. Most often, type 2 diabetes seems to be caused by a combination of these problems.

Whether you should take oral medication, insulin, or any medication at all and what sort of insulin or medication plan you need depends on how your body is dealing with the glucose it makes. Your treatment plan is based on your usual blood glucose levels. Ideally, you will want to keep your glucose levels as close to normal as possible. This means keeping your blood glucose levels in the 90–130 mg/dl range before meals and less than 180 mg/dl 2 hours after meals.

## Food and Physical Activity

The accepted, tried-and-true treatment for type 2 diabetes is a balance of diet and exercise. Even if you need medications, healthy eating and exercise habits continue to be key in caring for your type 2 diabetes. Most people with type 2 diabetes are advised to lose weight and improve their physical fitness. This can help to lower the body's resistance to insulin. The severity of type 2 diabetes can be greatly reduced by maintaining a healthy body weight. Even a modest weight loss—10 pounds—can have benefits.

By building a healthy lifestyle around a low-fat, well-rounded diet and regular exercise, it is possible to decrease body weight and insulin resistance. Exercise helps by taking some glucose from the blood and using it for energy during a workout, an effect that lasts even beyond the workout. Healthy eating, especially watching the amount of food eaten, helps glucose levels stay lower. As your level of physical fitness improves with regular exercise, so does your body's sensitivity to insulin.

## Oral Diabetes Medications

Your treatment will probably begin with a meal plan and a program of regular exercise, depending on your fasting blood glucose levels. However, you may need more help lowering your blood glucose. Many people with type 2 diabetes use oral medications, along with diet and exercise, to keep their blood glucose on target. The pills work best if you stick with your eating and exercise plans after you start taking them.

One class of diabetes oral medications are sulfonylurea drugs. The effects of sulfonylurea drugs on blood glucose levels were discovered by accident in the 1940s (they were used as antibacterial drugs during World War II). Sulfonylureas lower blood glucose levels by encouraging the pancreas to produce and release more insulin. Scientists have many leads on how these drugs accomplish this.

Seven different sulfonylureas are prescribed in this country: acetohexamide (generic or Dymelor), glyburide (DiaBeta, Glynase PresTab, or Micronase), glipizide (Glucotrol or Glucotrol XL), glimepiride (Amaryl), chlorpropamide (Diabinese), tolbutamide (brand name Orinase), and tolazamide (Tolinase).

Until 1994, sulfonylureas were the only oral medication for type 2 diabetes available to Americans. In December 1994, metformin (Glucophage) was approved for use by the Food and Drug Administration. It belongs to a different class of drugs called the biguanides. Biguanides work differently than sulfonylureas. During times you are fasting, such as overnight, your liver releases glucose so that your cells have the energy they need. Biguanides lower blood glucose mainly by putting a brake on the liver's release of stored glucose. They also hinder the absorption of glucose from food being digested in the small intestine. Biguanides may also lower insulin resistance in the muscles. Because metformin acts to decrease glucose release rather than increase insulin activity, there is little risk of very low blood glucose levels (hypoglycemia). Metformin has the added advantages of helping lower high blood lipid levels and promoting weight loss.

Metformin can be used along with a sulfonylurea or insulin. Because they work in different ways, metformin and sulfonylureas are often prescribed together. Combining different pills works better than either one alone. Metformin is also useful for people who are allergic to sulfa drugs.

Another class of drugs used to treat type 2 diabetes is the thiazolidinediones. Two drugs in this class, pioglitazone (Actos) and rosiglitazone (Avandia), were approved by the FDA in 1999. Glitazones lower insulin resistance, but how they do this is still being studied. If you also take insulin, you may be able to reduce your insulin dose. Extra benefits are lower triglyceride levels and increased high-density lipoprotein (HDL) cholesterol levels.

In 1996, acarbose (Precose) became available for people with type 2 diabetes. Acarbose and miglitol (Glyset) are members of the alpha-glucosidase inhibitor class of drugs. These drugs help keep after-meal blood glucose levels from going as high as they could by temporarily blocking the action of a group of enzymes that helps digest starches. A lot of people who take these drugs complain of intestinal gas and diarrhea, but these side effects often diminish with continued use or dose adjustments.

A final class of drugs is the meglitinides. Repaglinide (Prandin) and nateglinide (Starlix) stimulate insulin release by the pancreas in response to a meal. If you have problems with your blood glucose rising immediately after a meal, these may be good choices for you.

Oral diabetes medications come in pill or tablet form. Make sure you know when, how often, and how much to take before you leave your provider's office or pharmacy. Also, ask about possible side effects and any signs of side effects that you should be on the lookout for.

***Choosing an Oral Diabetes Medication.*** All oral diabetes medications must be prescribed by a health care professional. Your

## Oral Agents for Type 2 Diabetes

| Class | Name | Available as a generic? | Brand names | How often do I take it? When do I take it? |
|---|---|---|---|---|
| **alpha-Glucosidase Inhibitors** *Slow the digestion of starches. After-meal glucose peaks aren't as high* | acarbose | no | Precose | Take acarbose or miglitol with the first bite of each meal. |
| | miglitol | no | Glyset | |
| **Biguanides** *Keep the liver from releasing too much glucose* | metformin | yes | Glucophage | 2 or 3 times a day |
| | metformin | no | Glucophage XR | 1 or 2 times a day |
| | metformin + a sulfonylurea | no | Glucovance | 1 or 2 times a day |
| | | | Metaglip | 1 or 2 times a day |
| **Meglitinides** *Stimulate the pancreas to release more insulin* | repaglinide | no | Prandin | Take right before main meals. |
| | nateglinide | no | Starlix | Take right before main meals. |

| | | | | |
|---|---|---|---|---|
| **Sulfonylureas** *Stimulate the pancreas to release more insulin* | acetohexamide | yes | generic only | 1 or 2 times a day |
| | glimepiride | no | Amaryl | Once a day |
| | glipizide | yes | Glucotrol Glucotrol XL | 1 or 2 times a day |
| | glyburide | yes | Diabeta, Micronase, Glynase PresTab | 1 or 2 times a day |
| | tolazamide | yes | Tolinase | 1 or 2 times a day |
| | tolbutamide | yes | Orinase | 2 or 3 times a day |
| **Thiazolidinediones** *Make muscle cells more sensitive to insulin* | rosiglitazone | no | Avandia | 1 or 2 times a day |
| | pioglitazone | no | Actos | Once a day |
| | rosiglitazone + metformin | no | Avandamet | 1 or 2 times a day |

diabetes care provider will ask about your lifestyle, physical condition, insurance coverage, and personal preferences before prescribing any particular drug or combination of drugs.

- Generally, oral agents are not used by people with type 1 diabetes. They are usually only prescribed for people with type 2 diabetes.
- Not everyone with type 2 diabetes will be helped by oral diabetes medications. Oral medications are more likely to lower blood glucose levels in people who have had high blood glucose levels for less than 10 years, who are using a healthy meal plan, and who have some insulin secretion by their pancreas. The drugs work poorly in people who are very thin.
- You should not take a sulfonylurea if you are pregnant or planning a pregnancy or you have significant heart, liver, or kidney disease.
- During severe infections, surgery, or hospitalizations, you may need to replace your oral diabetes medications with insulin injections, at least temporarily.
- You should probably avoid sulfonylurea drugs if you are allergic to sulfa drugs. Ask your doctor if there is another drug that might work for you. You should not take metformin if you have kidney, heart, or liver disease.
- If you are taking pioglitazone (Actos) or rosiglitazone (Avandia), your liver function should be monitored through blood tests because of the possibility of liver damage in rare instances. These drugs can take some time to work, so be patient.
- Oral diabetes medications vary in price. This may affect your choice of drugs.

***Cautions for Use.*** All sulfonylurea drugs and, to a lesser extent, meglitinides, increase the risk of hypoglycemia, especially if you skip meals or drink too much alcohol. Be sure to talk to your provider about the symptoms to watch for and any precautions you need to take while on your oral medication. Teach your family and friends the warning signs of hypoglycemia. Together, make a plan of action for dealing with unexpected lows.

Oral agents can have other side effects. For example, skin rashes can occur with sulfonylurea use. If you notice any changes in your behavior or your body after starting a course of oral diabetes medications, be sure to tell your provider. If you have side effects, be sure to call your provider and do not just stop taking your medication.

*Drug Interactions.* Talk to all of your providers and your pharmacist about all other medicines, either prescription or over the counter, that you are currently taking or might be thinking of taking. Remember to include vitamins and herbal products. Are there any medicines you take when you are coming down with a cold? in bed with the flu? getting a sudden headache? If you take aspirin or thyroid or high blood pressure medicine, medicine to lower blood cholesterol, or cold or allergy remedies, tell your provider. Sometimes, drugs that are safe by themselves can interact with each other to cause sickness or conditions that can be difficult to diagnose. Some drugs can lower or raise blood glucose levels. This must be accounted for so that your blood glucose levels don't go too low or stay too high. What looks likes hypoglycemia may really be caused by a drug interaction and can be mistreated. Many drugs interfere with the way the body uses and eliminates oral diabetes medications. These drugs can indirectly cause high or low glucose levels.

*Looking Ahead.* After taking an oral diabetes medication for a while, you may find that your fasting blood glucose levels are consistently in the normal range. If you have normal readings for several weeks, it's possible that you can manage your blood glucose levels by meal planning and regular exercise alone. Ask your health care team whether they suggest that you start a trial of not taking your pills. During this trial period, make sure to keep monitoring your blood glucose and stay in close contact with your health care team.

There is a possibility that oral medications won't help you at all. Or they may help, but only for a while. Sulfonylureas stop working for 5 to 10 percent of people within a year. Eventually, they stop working for another 50 percent. If oral medications no longer help you reach your target blood glucose levels, adding insulin to your diabetes care plan is usually the next step.

## Insulin Therapy

Insulin used to be thought of as the last resort for people with type 2 diabetes, but we now know that starting insulin earlier can help keep you healthier longer. It is a big step, but taking insulin does not mean that you have failed to take care of yourself or that your diabetes is worse. It simply means that your body needs more help to keep your blood glucose levels on track. Make sure to pay special attention to instructions, injection techniques, and schedules. If it has been a while since you saw an educator or dietitian, ask for a referral. Learn the symptoms of hypoglycemia, and make sure you know how to treat it in advance.

In people with type 2 diabetes, the body becomes more resistant to insulin as glucose levels remain high. You may have taken insulin when your diabetes was first diagnosed to quickly lower your blood glucose levels. For many people, as the changes in blood glucose levels become less erratic, there is less insulin resistance. You may find that oral diabetes agents, or even a meal plan and exercise program alone, may be enough to keep your blood glucose levels in balance—without added insulin.

Around 30 to 40 percent of people with type 2 diabetes use insulin. You are more likely to use insulin the longer you've had diabetes. A typical plan is two insulin shots per day. In this plan, each dose contains some fast-acting insulin and some longer-acting insulin, either mixed together as one shot or injected with two syringes. The faster-acting insulin lowers the blood glucose level after the next meal, and the longer-acting insulin lowers the glucose levels between meals.

When your morning fasting blood glucose is closer to normal, it can make it easier to keep your blood glucose levels on target all day. If your fasting blood glucose level remains high, you may need insulin. If so, it will probably be given at night. Because your pancreas releases enough insulin to cover your meals, you only need help between meals. One or two injections of intermediate- or longer-acting insulin might work well for you. Another approach is to inject long-acting insulin at supper or bedtime to lower your fasting blood glucose levels in the morning. During the day, you can manage your blood glucose levels with meal planning and exercise and perhaps diabetes pills.

If your premeal blood glucose levels are high during the day, you may need insulin during the daytime as well, to lower glucose levels after you eat. You may take one or two doses of intermediate-acting insulin to cover your basal insulin needs and add injections of rapid-acting insulin before eating to help lower glucose levels after meals. You and your health care team need to arrive at a schedule of insulin types and injection times and doses by trial and error.

Look for more information on insulin and insulin plans in Chapter 4.

**Dad has a touch of diabetes. It's nothing to get worried about.**

Despite what you might read in the newspaper or be told by friends or relatives, there really is no such thing as a "touch" of diabetes. What people may be talking about is type 2 diabetes, which often responds well to healthy eating and regular exercise and may not have yet shown any signs of damaging body parts. Or they may be describing gestational diabetes, impaired glucose tolerance, or pre-diabetes.

The reality is that diabetes is a serious, life-long disease. Describing someone as having a touch of diabetes is like saying a woman is "a little bit pregnant"—it just isn't true because both are "yes or no" conditions.

Once diagnosed, diabetes doesn't go away, although there may be times in your life when it's easier to manage. If this happens, you may be tempted to think your diabetes is cured, but don't forget that there will also be frustrating periods when nothing you do seems to help keep blood glucose levels where you want them. Aging, weight gain, an injury that makes it harder to get regular exercise, or a gradual slowdown of insulin production all make diabetes harder to manage. When these things happen, you'll need to adjust your diabetes therapy to match your body's new needs.

## Gestational Diabetes Management

When you are pregnant, your body needs more insulin than before because of the increased production of hormones that lead to insulin resistance. In gestational diabetes, the pancreas

## Sample Blood Glucose Goals in Gestational Diabetes

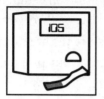 Note that these goals are considered normal for a person without diabetes and are general goals for women with diabetes during pregnancy. Your goals need to be individualized.

- Fasting blood glucose _____95 mg/dl or less
- One hour after a meal _____140 mg/dl or less
- Two hours after a meal _____120 mg/dl or less

is unable to produce enough insulin to overcome this resistance. Gestational diabetes is treated much like type 2 diabetes. Most women start with meal planning and regular exercise. But, if diet and exercise do not keep blood glucose levels very close to normal, insulin is the next course of action. Diabetes pills are not prescribed during pregnancy because of the risk to the baby.

Blood glucose goals are tighter for pregnant women than for most people with type 2 diabetes. This is because of the harmful effects that too much glucose in the mother's blood can have on the growing baby, as well as on the mother. The last half of the pregnancy is when the baby grows larger. Too much glucose in the mother's blood during the last half of pregnancy can lead to a baby that is too large to be delivered safely. This condition is called *macrosomia*. Because of macrosomia, women with gestational diabetes have a higher risk of delivery by cesarean section. Also, the baby may need to be delivered early if he or she grows too large too fast. An early delivery puts the baby at a higher risk for respiratory distress because the lungs are about the last organ to mature. For women who have type 1 or type 2 diabetes before becoming pregnant, keeping blood glucose levels low even before pregnancy decreases the risk of birth defects. Birth defects occur early in pregnancy as the baby's organs are being formed. But gestational diabetes does not usually occur until more than halfway through the pregnancy. By the halfway mark, the baby's organs are already formed. (Chapter 11 has more information about pregnancy and women with preexisting type 1 or type 2 diabetes.)

Women with gestational diabetes are also at higher risk for *toxemia*, a condition in pregnancy in which blood pressure is too high. Swelling of legs and arms commonly goes along with toxemia. Toxemia can be dangerous for the mother and baby and can mean bed rest for the mother until delivery.

Treatment for gestational diabetes is based on the results of your 3-hour glucose tolerance test. If your fasting blood glucose level (taken at the start of the test) was normal (under 105 mg/dl) but your glucose tolerance test results were in the range for gestational diabetes, you may start with nutrition therapy and perhaps with exercise, if you are able. If your fasting blood glucose was over 105 mg/dl, you will probably start insulin therapy, too. Because of the emphasis on keeping blood glucose levels close to normal, you will need to monitor frequently, perhaps four or more times a day.

## Nutrition Therapy

The meal plan during pregnancy is not designed for weight loss. The purpose is to help you eat the right food at the right time and in the right amount to manage your blood glucose. For many women, this is enough to keep blood glucose levels within the target range. Using moderate exercise to lower blood glucose levels can also help. Most women can swim or walk to keep active. You may also focus on limiting the amount of weight you gain, especially if you were obese before pregnancy.

Food choices play a key role in managing gestational diabetes. It's important that you meet with a registered dietitian. You may set a daily calorie goal based on the amount of weight you should gain during the pregnancy. The dietitian may also help you adjust your carbohydrate intake to help manage your blood glucose levels.

## Insulin Therapy

Because normal blood glucose levels are so important during pregnancy, you may need insulin if you are having problems reaching your target ranges. Your insulin resistance is at its highest during the third trimester of pregnancy. Therefore, you may need a fairly large total dose of insulin each day, for example 20 to 30 units. This might be a mixture of faster- and intermediate-acting insulins. This can be given once, usually before breakfast, if fasting blood glucose levels are low. Or the dose can be divided into several injections a day if you need help reducing fasting glucose levels.

Because insulin resistance is so high late in pregnancy, very low blood glucose levels, leading to hypoglycemia, are rare. However, if you seem prone to hypoglycemia, remember that the safest times to exercise are after meals, when you are less likely to develop hypoglycemia.

Don't be alarmed if your total insulin dosage increases as your pregnancy continues. This does not mean your diabetes is getting worse, only that your insulin resistance is increasing, which is to be expected. You may need to make changes in your insulin dosage as often as every 10 to 14 days.

Look for more information on insulin and insulin plans in Chapter 4.

**"Because I have gestational diabetes, my child or I will get diabetes."**

The risk of your child someday developing diabetes is low. This risk seems to go up with the birth weight of the baby. Studies have shown that the larger your baby is at birth, the greater the chance that he or she will develop obesity. Signs of obesity can be seen as early as 7 or 8 years of age. If your child develops obesity during childhood or adolescence, there's also a chance that he or she will develop glucose intolerance, and possibly diabetes, as an adult. Your best bet to keep your child's risk of diabetes as low as possible is to keep your blood glucose levels close to normal while you have gestational diabetes.

However, your risk of getting diabetes permanently is high. Although your blood glucose levels may return to normal after delivery, you need to be checked for diabetes every year. The risk of developing type 2 diabetes 5 to 15 years after gestational diabetes is between 40 and 60 percent, compared with about a 15 percent risk in the general population. Being obese increases the risk to a 3 out of 4 chance.

# Good Health Care and Your Health Care Team 3

*Diabetes care is a team effort that involves you, your family and friends, your providers, and other health professionals. Putting together a diabetes care team takes extra effort, but the payoff is usually worth it.*

Living with type 1 or type 2 diabetes can seem overwhelming. Whether you have just been diagnosed or have had diabetes for a while, many questions often arise. Do I need to take insulin? How often should I test my blood sugar? Should I exercise? What should I eat? How should I take care of my eyes? My feet?

Your health care team is key in helping you answer these questions and learn to manage diabetes. But remember that you are the team captain—you call the shots. So choose team members you trust and who think as you do about diabetes care.

## Getting Started

You may not be used to "shopping" for health care. But if you have a chance to choose your health care team members, take advantage of it and look for health professionals who follow these three R's:

- **Recognize** you as an individual and are willing to help you create a plan that fits your life. Don't agree to a meal plan containing foods you don't like or an exercise program you know you won't do. Tell your health care team what you can and are willing to do. Remember, it's your plan.
- **Respond** to your questions and concerns. You and your family members should be able to ask questions openly and trust that the health professional will take the time to listen and answer you patiently, completely, and honestly.
- **Recommend** the best possible strategies for the care and management of diabetes. All professionals should be aware of and follow standards of care recommended by the American Diabetes Association.

Whatever your preferences, keep in mind that assembling the perfect team and developing a plan may take some time. Your plan will need fine-tuning along the way. Try to choose team members who are easy to reach and willing to adapt to changes along the way.

## The Team Captain: You

In finding your health care team, you will choose professionals with expertise in different aspects of diabetes care. A dietitian can offer you advice to help you reach your weight goals. An exercise physiologist may help you develop an exercise plan that fits your interests, abilities, and schedule. A diabetes nurse educator can teach you how to manage and how to cope with your diabetes.

In the end, though, you are the one who decides whether to use the meal plan, exercise, and take medications. Your health care team can offer you advice, but it's up to you to make the

## Reasons to Contact Your Diabetes Care Team

- You're having frequent or severe low blood glucose levels
- Your blood glucose levels are consistently higher than your targets
- You've noticed a change in your vision
- You're having side effects or have questions about your medicine
- You're having unexplained high or low blood glucose readings
- You're having trouble with your meal or exercise plan
- You develop feelings of numbness or tingling in your hands or feet
- Your skin is dry or you have a sore
- You feel depressed or anxious about having diabetes

day-to-day decisions. After all, you are the team captain, and no one knows you better. You will be the first one to detect any problems. Trust your instincts and listen to your body.

At times, no matter what you do, something may not feel quite right. Maybe your meal plan or diabetes medication needs an adjustment. Your health care team members can't help if they don't know there is a problem. So stay in contact. Your team members are counting on you to let them know what is happening.

As team captain, your job is to choose the other members of your team. Your health care team members are your coaches. You may receive diabetes care from a primary care provider, an internist, a nurse practitioner, a physician assistant, or an endocrinologist or a diabetologist. If you see a diabetes specialist, you also need a primary care provider for your other

| Professional | Degree | Look for | Consult for |
|---|---|---|---|
| Physician (primary care, internist, endocrinologist) | MD or DO | Specialization in diabetes, such as board certification in endocrinology | Medical management of diabetes, including oral agents or insulin, and the detection and treatment of complications |
| Nurse practitioner or physician assistant | APRN, BC-ADM, PA | Specialization in diabetes, such as board certification in advanced diabetes management (BC-ADM) | Management of diabetes, including oral agents or insulin, and the detection and treatment of complications |
| Nurse | RN, BSN, MSN, APRN | Certified diabetes educator (CDE) | Counseling on diabetes self-care, including medicines, blood glucose monitoring, managing sick days, stress, coping, and behavior change |
| Dietitian | RD | CDE is desirable | Helping you to develop or alter your diabetes meal plan, lose weight, or manage health problems (such as cutting dietary sodium or fat) |
| Eye doctor | MD specializing in ophthalmology, or an optometrist | Familiarity with diabetic eye disease | Detecting and treating diabetic eye disease such as retinopathy; ophthalmologists treat eye disease with laser therapy or eye surgery |

| | | | |
|---|---|---|---|
| Podiatrist | DPM | Experience treating diabetic foot problems and routine foot care | Treating foot problems, including calluses, sores, or ulcers; helping you prevent future foot injury |
| Mental health professional | MD (psychiatrist); MS, MEd, or PhD (psychologist); MSW (social worker); LPC (counselor) | Experience in emotional, behavioral, and psychological aspects of diabetes care | Helping you cope with depression, anxiety, or other mental health problems |
| Exercise specialist | Various: BS, MS, or PhD | CDE | Helping you develop and stick with an exercise plan and working with your provider to help you exercise safely |
| Pharmacist | RPH or PharmD | Experience counseling people with diabetes; CDE, BC-ADM, or CDM (certified disease manager) desirable | Providing information and counseling on medications, diabetes products, blood glucose testing, sick days, and referrals to other diabetes specialists in the area |

health care needs. You may also want to find a diabetes educator, a dietitian, and other health care specialists that you may call upon as needed. These specialists could include a pharmacist, an eye doctor, a podiatrist, a counselor (psychologist, social worker, or psychiatrist), and an exercise physiologist.

Sometimes, diabetes professionals will already practice together in a center that specializes in diabetes care. Or your diabetes care provider may routinely work with some of these professionals. If not, you may have to assemble your own group. If your provider doesn't have a diabetes nurse educator or dietitian on staff, ask him or her to recommend one, as well as other professionals you should have on your team.

It's a plus if the members of your team are comfortable communicating with each other. That is often the case if they are recommended by your provider. But you should also pick team members that you feel comfortable with. Don't be afraid to shop around a little and find the team members that best suit your needs.

In assembling your team, don't forget your fans—family and friends that will lend support, help, and understanding on a daily basis. They need to be prepared to deal with your day-to-day routines—what time you test your blood glucose, for example. And you may also need their help should any emergency arise.

Also, don't forget community resources. Many hospitals and community health groups offer classes and support groups for people with diabetes. Here you can receive valuable information and answers to your questions about dealing with the disease. Class instructors and support group members may also be able to provide referrals to other health care professionals that specialize in diabetes care.

## Choosing a Diabetes Care Provider

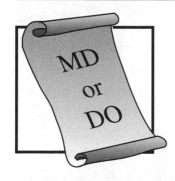

As you start to choose your health professionals, it may help to listen to the experience of other people with diabetes. Consider the stories of James and Helen, decades apart in age, but sharing an initial sense of confusion and a little fear about finding quality care for diabetes.

James had just started college 500 miles away from home when he was diagnosed with type 1 diabetes. Mastering glucose management by blood glucose monitoring, insulin shots, and carbohydrate counting was confusing and a little scary, especially because he was also trying to get used to college life. Being so far from home, he knew he would have to find a new health care provider near campus. He would have to see the provider at least every 3 months, and perhaps more often while he was trying to get his diabetes care plan established. He wasn't sure he could get home that often and wanted someone nearby in case of an emergency. Besides, his familiar family doctor was not an expert in diabetes and suggested that he find a local provider with expertise in managing the disease.

Helen was just starting to plan for her early retirement. Over the past 10 years, she had put on a little extra weight. Between taking care of the kids and working long days at her high-level government job, she had little time for exercise and was always eating on the run. Her health care maintenance had fallen by the wayside also. Although she visited her gynecologist every year or so, she hadn't seen a primary care provider or had a complete physical in nearly a decade. She was looking forward to doing some traveling, taking up some new hobbies, and starting an exercise program when she learned that she had type 2 diabetes.

Both James and Helen needed to find new providers who had experience in coordinating the care for people with diabetes. Although James and Helen had different types of diabetes, they both had similar concerns and needs in finding the ideal doctor. Helen wrote down a list of the important qualities she was seeking and was able to express what she was looking for in a provider:

*"I wanted someone who would really listen to me and answer my questions in English, not medical-ese. So many times, doctors have treated me as though I were a child whose only duty was to obey. Well, I'm the one who has diabetes, and I'm the one who's got to take care of it. I guess I just want a provider who won't talk down to me, who would treat me as another professional."*

James is also concerned about communication:

*"It's hard to talk to doctors sometimes. I mean, a lot of times I nod my head as if I understand something when I really don't. But there's a lot of stuff I'm worried about. Like, someone told me that a lot of men with diabetes become impotent. I want to know if that's true and whether there is anything you can do to prevent it."*

Like James and Helen, you may have personal concerns about diabetes. Before you choose a diabetes care provider, you may want to schedule an appointment to talk with several candidates. Some health care professionals may charge an "interview fee," so be sure to ask about this ahead of time.

Come to your interview with questions you would like answered. If necessary, write them down in advance and don't be afraid to look at them during your interview. Write down answers to your questions during the interview, if need be. Here are some common questions and concerns you might discuss:

- Where did you go to school? Are you board certified in endocrinology or internal medicine? Do you hold professional memberships in associations such as the American Diabetes Association (ADA), the Endocrine Society, or the American College of Physicians?
- What percentage of your patients have diabetes? Are they mostly patients with type 1 or type 2? How many patients like me do you see each month?
- What insurance do you accept? Are you a provider in my PPO plan? If I require a referral to a specialist, do you have colleagues who also participate?
- How often will regular visits be scheduled? What tests are conducted routinely?
- Who covers for you on your days off?
- What procedures should be followed in the event of an emergency? What conditions indicate an emergency? How do I know whether I should call you?
- How hard is it to get an appointment?
- Are you associated with a nurse educator, dietitian, or other health care professionals so that I can benefit from a team approach?
- Are you likely/willing to try new approaches/therapies to diabetes management, or do you prefer to wait until new methods have stood the test of time?

After the interview, take time to reflect on it. How did it feel? Were you comfortable with the practitioner? Did he or she seem concerned about you as an individual? Was the provider willing to work with you to achieve your health goals? Did you feel free to express your feelings? Did you feel that he or she was listening to you? Were you given sufficient time to get all your questions answered or did you feel rushed? Did the provider seem directive or nondirective—is he or she likely to tell you what to do or work with you to reach your goals?

In addition to your interview, you may want to get a sense of the practice from his or her staff and other patients.

Is the office convenient enough for you to get to regular appointments? Maybe the closest endocrinologist is 50 miles away and you would like someone closer. In that case, you might want to find an internist or primary care practitioner with expertise in treating patients with diabetes.

Are the provider's current patients satisfied? Is it easy enough to get an appointment? Does the provider meet his or her appointments? Ask other people who see this provider. You can also contact the ADA for a list of recognized providers (1-800-342-2383; www.diabetes.org) or receive referrals from a physician you know and trust. Your local hospital or community health organization may also provide referrals. Professional medical societies may provide recommendations as well.

Is the office neat and clean? Is the staff polite? Are you accommodated at your scheduled appointment time or are you kept waiting? Are educational materials on display? Is there someone you can call with questions or concerns?

## The Rest of the Team

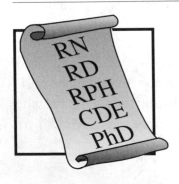

It's unlikely that you will learn all you need to know about managing diabetes in an appointment with your provider. Because diabetes is such a complicated disease that affects many different organ systems in your body, you will benefit from the addition of other health care professionals to your management team. Your best resource for recruiting other team members is your diabetes care provider or certified diabetes educator. It is important not only that your provider communicates with other members of your team, but also that team members are able to communicate with each other about any changes that may arise in your diabetes management plan. To ensure this, make sure that they each have the phone numbers, fax numbers, and e-mail addresses of other members of the team.

### Your Diabetes Educator

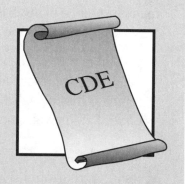

Ron took his insulin faithfully every day—a shot before breakfast and another in the evening. He had apparently mastered near-perfect glucose levels. However, he began to notice hard lumps surrounding the injection site on his abdomen. His primary care physician recommended that he meet with a diabetes nurse educator to work on giving his shots.

Paul had been trying to quit smoking for several years. He sometimes went for weeks or even months without having a cigarette, but he always started up again. Recently, he had been diagnosed with type 2 diabetes. He wondered how his smoking might affect his diabetes and wanted advice on how to quit. His physician put him touch with a diabetes educator.

If you have questions like Ron's and Paul's about managing your diabetes, a diabetes educator can help. She or he can address any of the concerns or questions you may have about

## Finding a Recognized Diabetes Education Program

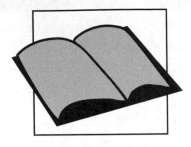

In addition to meeting one-on-one with a diabetes educator, you may also want to participate in a diabetes education program. Your local American Diabetes Association office can refer you to a program that has been recognized as meeting National Standards. This means that it can provide you with quality diabetes education. These programs are covered by Medicare and many insurance plans. Education programs that meet the National Standards cover all of the following topics:

- general information about diabetes and its treatments
- adjusting psychologically to caring for diabetes
- setting goals and solving problems
- understanding your meal plan and incorporating it into your life
- incorporating physical activity into your life
- testing and recording your blood glucose and urine ketones accurately and using the results to manage your diabetes
- managing sick days
- preventing, detecting, and treating long-term complications
- caring for diabetes before and during pregnancy

diabetes. Diabetes educators, for example, may give you background information about the biology of diabetes, teach you how to take insulin or check blood glucose levels, explain how to handle sick days and pregnancy, discuss the effects of various habits on blood glucose levels, and help you learn to cope with stress and how to choose, set, and reach goals.

A diabetes educator is usually a registered nurse (RN), registered dietitian (RD), or pharmacist (RPH) with a special interest and training in caring for people with diabetes. However, physicians, physician assistants, and other health care specialists may also be diabetes educators. The initials CDE (for certified diabetes educator) indicate that the professional has passed a national exam in diabetes education and is up-to-date about diabetes care. CDEs often work in locations where people with diabetes are treated, such as doctors' offices, hospitals, and pharmacies. The American Association of Diabetes Educators can also provide local referrals (see Resources).

## Your Dietitian

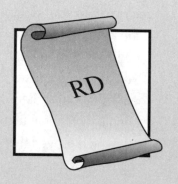

Although Marie had lived with diabetes for 3 years and had managed her diabetes well in the past, she recently noticed that her blood glucose levels had been getting higher. She wondered whether changing her diet might bring her glucose levels closer to normal.

At his last physical exam, Charles gritted his teeth as the nurse pumped the blood pressure cuff tight. He was surprised when he heard the two numbers that indicated his blood pressure was too high. He and his provider decided that the first steps would be to exercise, lose weight, and eat a low-sodium diet to help reduce his blood pressure. His physician suggested a visit with his dietitian for advice on how to cut down on fat and sodium without sacrificing the foods he loved or upsetting his glucose balance.

## How to Afford a Dietitian

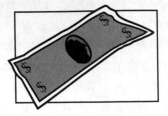

The best way to afford your visit to the dietitian is obvious: get your health insurer to pay. More and more plans are covering services by a dietitian. Medicare now covers medical nutrition therapy provided by a Medicare-certified dietitian. Here are some tips that can increase your chances of getting your claim paid:

- Call your insurer first. You may have an insurer who provides this benefit. If so, ask what paperwork you will need to submit.
- Submit a claim after each visit to the dietitian. Include a written referral from your doctor; it should not prescribe "nutrition counseling" or "nutrition education" but language such as "medical nutritional therapy for diabetes management."
- If you are turned down, resubmit your claim. This time, document how your visit to the RD can save the insurer money. For example, you can cite the Diabetes Control and Complications Trial, which proved that complications can be prevented or delayed with near-normal glucose levels.
- If you are turned down, ask for your claim to be reviewed. Many insurers will tell you "no" at first, only to eventually cover some or all of the claim. In writing, ask for your disputed claim to be reviewed. Follow up with phone calls. Write down the names and titles of the people you call and the dates when you spoke. It pays to be persistent, so continue to write letters and make phone calls until either you or your insurer decides to pay for treatment.

It is recommended that you see a dietitian whenever you are having problems reaching your blood glucose targets. It is a good idea to see a dietitian once a year even if you aren't having problems with diabetes care. A registered dietitian is a member of your health care team who has training and expertise in food and nutrition. For both type 1 and type 2 diabetes, whether or not you take insulin or other medication, a balanced meal plan is critical to living well with diabetes. You and your dietitian can develop a meal plan that has food you enjoy and that will help you balance your food and exercise. You may want help in adapting your diet to special goals, such as losing weight, reducing dietary fat or sodium, or complementing a regular exercise program. Your dietitian can help ensure that your diet achieves these goals and that it accommodates your likes and dislikes, culture, schedule, and lifestyle.

Does your meal plan need a change or adjustment? If you can answer "yes" to any of the following questions, then your meal plan may need a tune-up:

- Has it been more than a year since your dietitian reviewed your meal plan?
- Is your blood glucose level or body weight more difficult to manage than usual?
- Are you bored with your meals?
- Are you planning to start or have you already started an exercise program or changed your insulin regimen since your last nutrition checkup?
- Have you decided to aim for blood glucose levels that are closer to normal?
- Have you been diagnosed with high blood pressure, high cholesterol levels, or kidney disease?
- Are you planning to or have you recently become pregnant?
- Are you entering menopause?

To find a dietitian, ask your diabetes care provider for a referral or contact your local hospital, the ADA, or the American Dietetic Association. In choosing a dietitian, look for the initials RD (registered dietitian). This indicates that the dietitian has passed a national credentialing exam. Many states also require a license, and you may see the initials LD (licensed dietitian) after a dietitian's name. Some dietitians are also CDEs.

During your first visit, your dietitian will assess your dietary needs, a process that generally takes an hour or more. Follow-up visits usually take 30 minutes. Follow-up visits allow for sharing further helpful information, progress checks, and adjustments to your meal plan. Even though your diabetes management may seem to be on target, don't neglect periodic follow-up visits with your dietitian.

Dietitians can advise you on many useful strategies:

- how to use meal planning and carbohydrate counting guides, such as those published by the American Diabetes Association and the American Dietetic Association
- how to count dietary carbohydrate and fat and make adjustments in your insulin dose
- how to read food labels
- how to handle eating out in restaurants
- how to make choices when grocery shopping
- how to handle holidays and other special events
- how to prepare and include foods that are important and meaningful for you and your family

Dietitians may also provide you with a wealth of nutritional resources, such as cookbooks and reading materials, so that you can learn how to prepare easy, nutritious, and satisfying meals for your whole family.

## Your Exercise Physiologist

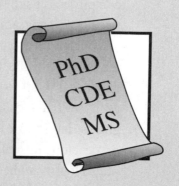

Whenever she exercised, Terry's heart pounded, she broke into a cold sweat, her body grew shaky, and she became exasperated—the classic signs of a hypoglycemic reaction. She was exercising to make herself feel better, not worse. Terry's diabetes care provider referred her to an exercise physiologist, who helped her coordinate exercise with balanced glucose levels and a snack schedule.

Howard, while not completely sedentary, had been traveling a lot lately and over the past year had let his fitness program fall by the wayside. When he learned he had type 2 diabetes, he was determined to manage it through diet and exercise. A former rock climber, he wondered if he dared take up the sport again.

Even when you want to exercise, it's hard to know how to begin. If you haven't been very active in the past, you might want advice on how to get started. If you have a favorite sport or activity, you might want to learn how best to integrate it into your diabetes plan. A professional trained in exercise science and safe conditioning techniques is in the best position to help you design a fitness program you can live with. To find a qualified exercise physiologist, ask your diabetes care provider or other members of your diabetes care team. In choosing an exercise physiologist, look for someone who holds a master's or doctoral-level degree in exercise physiology or a licensed health care professional who has received graduate training in exercise physiology. You may want someone certified by the American College of Sports Medicine to ensure that your exercise physiologist has the skills necessary to design a safe, effective fitness program to suit your needs.

Exercise physiologists can help you design a tailor-made fitness program, set realistic goals, and offer tips for staying motivated to stick with your exercise routine. Whatever your exercise goals—to improve cardiovascular fitness, lower blood glucose levels, lose weight, lower blood pressure or cholesterol, or develop muscular strength and flexibility—your exercise physiologist can help you achieve those goals. Even if you have arthritis, are overweight, experience any complications of diabetes, or have been sedentary and want to become more active, an exercise physiologist can develop an exercise program to accommodate your specific needs. But before embarking on any new exercise program, make sure to clear it with your diabetes care provider. Also make sure that your provider and exercise physiologist are in contact.

## Your Mental Health Counselor

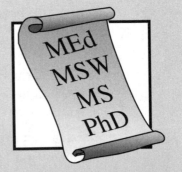

Shelly, a middle-aged woman with type 2 diabetes, prides herself on her success in caring for her diabetes. But whenever she finds that her blood glucose level is higher than she likes, she feels like a failure. She mopes around and thinks, "I can't do anything right."

Everything seemed to be going well for Michael. He had made the final cut on the high school soccer team and had a good shot at starting forward. He had just started dating a girl in his biology class, and he was keeping his grades up. But then he started feeling ill and was diagnosed with type 1 diabetes. What would his team members think? Would he have to give up soccer? Would his new girlfriend think he was some kind of freak?

In addition to creating physical and metabolic problems, diabetes affects a person's thoughts and feelings, often making people with the disease feel as if they have somehow failed. Both Shelly and Michael could probably benefit from seeing a therapist, such as a social worker, family therapist, psychologist, or psychiatrist. Such mental health professionals can help people deal with some of the personal and emotional aspects that are inevitably associated with diabetes.

A **social worker** should hold a master's degree in social work (MSW), as well as have training in individual, group, and family therapy. Social workers can help you cope with many concerns related to diabetes, including problems within the family, coping with workplace situations, and locating resources to help with medical or financial needs.

A **marriage and family therapist** should hold a master's or doctoral degree in a mental health field and have additional training in individual, family, and marriage therapy. These therapists can help you with personal problems in family and marital relationships and problems on the job.

> ## TIP
>
> Having a child or teen with diabetes can be a challenge. Make sure your child's health care team includes a mental health professional. This team member will work with your child and you to identify the behavioral, emotional, and social issues confronting your child and offer support and help for the whole family.

A **clinical psychologist** usually has a master's or doctoral degree in psychology and is trained in individual, group, and family psychology. You may visit a clinical psychologist to help you through a particularly stressful period over the course of several weeks or months, or on a longer-term basis to work through depression, anxiety, or other problems.

A **psychiatrist** is a medical doctor with training in the relationship between physical well-being and mental health. Psychiatrists with expertise in treating people with diabetes can help you understand how the physical problem of diabetes can also affect your mental health. Psychiatrists prescribe medications or hospitalization for emotional problems, if needed.

If you feel that you need some help coping with the emotional burden of diabetes, don't be afraid to talk to your diabetes care provider, who can recommend an appropriate health care professional.

## Your Eye Doctor

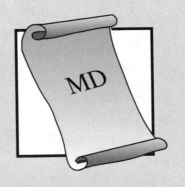

Rose first detected problems with her eyes one afternoon while playing a round of golf. As she was about to tee off, she had difficulty finding the flag on the green, even though it was only a par 3 hole. Instead, she saw strange blotches moving around her field of vision. A quick call to her diabetes care provider assured her that she needed to see an eye specialist.

For anyone with either type 1 or type 2 diabetes, eye care is an important priority. By keeping your blood glucose level close to normal, you can lower your risk for some of the long-term effects of diabetes and preserve your eyesight. An eye specialist monitors changes in your eyes, especially those changes associated with diabetes. He or she then determines what those changes mean and how they should be treated. For example, changes in the tiny blood vessels that supply your retina—the part of the eye that detects light and thus visual images—could be an early sign of diabetic retinopathy. Left untreated, diabetic retinopathy can lead to blindness.

Although your diabetes care provider will look at your eyes during the course of your yearly physical examination, you also need to have them more thoroughly examined by a trained eye specialist. Your eyes need to be dilated for this exam. If you are 10 or older and have type 1 diabetes, you should have a comprehensive examination 3 to 5 years after you are diagnosed with diabetes and yearly thereafter. If you are an adult with type 2 diabetes, you should have a comprehensive eye and visual exam conducted by an eye doctor when you are diagnosed and every year thereafter—even if your vision is fine. Also, if you notice any changes in your vision or you are planning a pregnancy, you should be examined.

Ophthalmologists are physicians qualified to treat eye problems both medically and surgically. Retina specialists are ophthalmologists with further training in the diagnosis and treatment of diseases of the retina. Optometrists are trained to examine the eye for certain problems, such as how well your eyes can focus. While they can prescribe corrective lenses, they do not perform laser surgery to correct retinopathy. If you require surgery, ask your diabetes care provider or regular optometrist for referrals in selecting an ophthalmologist to serve on your health care team.

## Taking Care of Your Eyes

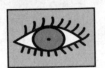 If you are an adult, have a thorough eye exam at the time of diabetes diagnosis and yearly thereafter. If you are over 10 and have had diabetes for at least 3 years, you also need a comprehensive exam once a year.

- After the initial exam, see an eye doctor familiar with retinopathy and other diabetes complications of the eyes once a year for a dilated exam.

- Call your diabetes care provider if you notice changes in your vision, but don't panic. Highs and lows in your blood glucose level may cause temporary blurring in your vision.

- Keep your blood glucose levels close to normal. You will help prevent damage to the small blood vessels that run through your retina.

- Have regular blood pressure checks, and work to keep your blood pressure on target.

- Discuss your exercise program with your eye doctor. Some activities can raise the pressure inside your eyes and lead to bleeding in the retina.

- If you have retinopathy, avoid taking birth control pills because they may affect the clotting of your blood or increase your blood pressure.

- Get early treatment for eye problems! Early intervention, such as laser treatment for retinopathy, cuts the risk of blindness by 90 percent.

Schedule an appointment with an ophthalmologist if you, your diabetes care provider, or your optometrist notice any of the following signs:

- unexplained visual problems, such as spots, "floaters," or cobwebs in your field of vision, blurring or distortion, blind spots, eye pain, or persistent redness
- trouble reading books or traffic signs or difficulty distinguishing familiar objects
- increased pressure within the eye, which could be a warning sign of glaucoma. Some physicians and most optometrists routinely test for this.
- any retinal abnormalities. Most endocrinologists, internists, primary care practitioners, and optometrists will test for this but should refer problems with the retina to an ophthalmologist.
- leaking of blood vessels that supply the retina, which leads to retinopathy, the main cause of blindness in people with diabetes

In choosing an eye doctor, try to find one that has experience treating patients with diabetic retinopathy and is familiar with laser therapy and vitrectomy. Also ask your eye care specialist the following:

- What percentage of your patients have diabetes?
- Do you perform eye surgery? (This is usually limited to ophthalmologists.)
- Are you a retina specialist? (This is important because eye disease in people with diabetes affects the retina, the part of the eye that detects visual images.)
- Will you send regular reports and keep in touch with my diabetes care provider?

### Your Podiatrist

After an early morning jog, Janet noticed a sore on the ball of her foot as she was removing her sock. Her physician's assistant recommended that she see a podiatrist, who confirmed that Janet had a foot ulcer. Fortunately, Janet caught it early enough to be treated.

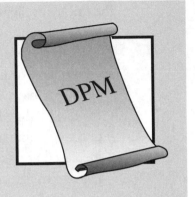

Foot care is especially important for people with diabetes, because they are prone to poor blood circulation and nerve disease in the extremities. In addition, people with diabetes are likely to develop infections that often appear in the feet. Even small sores can turn into serious problems quickly. Any foot sore or callus should be checked by your diabetes care provider or podiatrist. Don't try to treat any foot problems yourself.

Podiatrists graduate from a college of podiatry with a Doctor of Podiatric Medicine (DPM) degree. They also complete residencies in podiatry and can perform surgery and prescribe medication for your feet. Podiatrists treat corns, calluses, and foot sores to prevent more serious problems from developing. They can also show you how to correctly trim your toenails and how to buy shoes that fit properly. To find a podiatrist, ask your diabetes care provider for a referral, or check with local hospitals or your local ADA office. During your initial visit, ask what percentage of his or her patients have diabetes.

## Taking Care of Your Feet

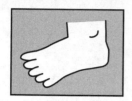 Keep your feet clean and dry. Wash them every day with a mild soap. Dry them off carefully, especially between the toes. If the skin on your feet is too dry, apply a lotion thinly everywhere but between the toes.

- Inspect your feet and between your toes daily. Look for swollen areas, red areas, and cuts or breaks in the skin and feel for very cold areas (this could mean poor blood circulation) and very warm areas (this could mean infection).
- Never go barefoot. Although this is a good rule for everyone, it is really important for people who have lost sensation in their feet. Wear swimmers' shoes whenever you go swimming.
- Make a habit of cutting your toenails to follow the curve of your toe. This helps you avoid ingrown toenails.
- Wear only comfortable, well-fitting shoes. Don't expect to break in new shoes—they should feel comfortable right away. Shoes made of leather help your feet get the air circulation they need to stay healthy.
- If you have a loss of sensation in your feet or have neuropathy, you may not be able to trust how a shoe feels to decide whether the fit is good for you. Find a shoewear specialist who is trained to fit people with diabetes (see Resources).
- Never try amateur surgery on your feet. Have your provider or podiatrist treat calluses, corns, plantar warts, and the like.
- Get early treatment for foot problems! Call your doctor or podiatrist if you have any of these problems:
  - an open sore (ulcer) on your foot
  - a cut or blister that is slow to heal
  - any infection in a cut or blister
  - a red, tender toe—possibly an ingrown toenail
  - any change in feeling, such as pain, tingling, numbness, or burning
  - any puncture wound, such as if you step on a nail or thorn

### Your Pharmacist

Evelyn ached all over. Last night, she barely slept because of her stuffy nose and headache. She decided she needed a liquid night-time cold medicine so she wouldn't have to spend another night like that. At the drugstore, there were so many choices, Evelyn decided to ask the pharmacist to help her choose which medicine would work best for her. Her blood glucose was already running high because of her cold, and she didn't want to raise it any higher.

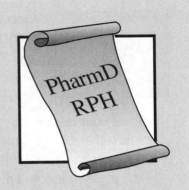

A pharmacist has a wealth of information on medicines: what's in them and how they interact with each other. Pharmacists are highly trained professionals who must know about the chemistry of products they dispense and what effects, both good and bad, medications have on the body. Therefore, they can also give advice on whether and how any medication you take for your diabetes or other conditions could or will affect your blood glucose levels.

It is important to find a pharmacy you like dealing with and stick with it. This way, the pharmacist can keep an accurate and up-to-date profile of your medical history, allergies, and medications. Pharmacists do more for you than fill your prescriptions. They alert you to the potential common or severe side effects of any drug you are going to take. And, with each new prescription, they can review your medication profile to see if any of your current medications might interact with your new prescription. For example, if your pharmacist knows you take a certain kind of sulfonylurea, he or she may recommend a cold medicine with little or no alcohol to avoid any possible inter-action between the two medications. So, in addition to asking your diabetes care provider, you can ask your pharmacist to recommend over-the-counter medicines for colds or other minor illnesses.

## Your Dentist

Ryan didn't worry too much about dental care. He brushed his teeth two or three times a day and rinsed with one of those antiplaque rinses. He knew dental hygiene was important for someone with diabetes, and he tried to floss whenever he could. But it was one of those things that kept slipping his mind. Then one day he noticed that his gums were starting to bleed when he brushed his teeth. Maybe a trip to the dentist was in order.

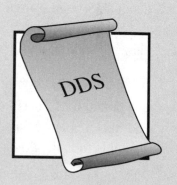

Bacteria, especially those that thrive in the mouth, love sweets. And when you have high glucose levels, your saliva makes your mouth an inviting home for the bacteria that cause gum infections and disease. Having diabetes further complicates matters because it's harder for your body to fight off infections once they start. To prevent gum disease, see your dentist or den-tal hygienist every 6 months for a thorough teeth cleaning. Make sure your dentist knows that you have diabetes and ask him or

## Taking Care of Your Mouth

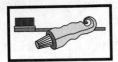 High blood glucose levels can cause severe gum disease and abscesses in young and old.

- Have your teeth cleaned and checked by the dentist at least every 6 months.

- Brush at least twice a day to fight plaque. Use a soft nylon brush with rounded ends on the bristles. Tilt the bristles at about a 45-degree angle against the gum line and brush gently in a scrubbing motion. Brush front and back and also brush the chewing surfaces.

- Brush the rough upper surface of your tongue.

- Use dental floss once a day to remove bacteria from between your teeth. Special floss holders and various types of floss are available to make flossing easier.

- Call your dentist if you find:

  - your gums bleed when you brush or eat

  - your gums are red, swollen, or tender

  - your gums have pulled away from your teeth

  - pus appears between your teeth and gums when the gums are touched

  - any change in the way dentures or partial plates fit

  - any change in the way your teeth fit together when you bite

  - persistent bad breath or a bad taste in your mouth.

her to observe your brushing and flossing techniques to make sure you're doing all you can. In addition to scheduling regular visits, call your dentist if you notice any signs of gum disease.

## Your Dermatologist

When he was a teenager, Robert never thought that dry skin would be a problem. But ever since he had been diagnosed with type 1 diabetes last year, his skin was always dry and itchy. Even his feet cracked and peeled, and nothing seemed to help. His provider referred him to a derma- tologist to find a solution to this common problem.

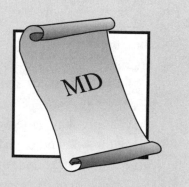

When blood glucose levels are high, the body produces extra urine to rid itself of excess blood glucose. This results in dehy- dration, which causes dry skin. Having diabetes also increases your risk of developing skin infections, especially if your glucose levels are often above normal. For instance, staphylococcal skin infections can cause itchy spots on buttocks, knees, and elbows. Your best weapon against dry skin is to keep your glucose within your target ranges through diet, exercise, and medication.

Should a skin infection or other skin problem develop, see a dermatologist right away, when treatment is most effective. Dermatologists are medical doctors with special training in skin disorders. Your diabetes care provider or local ADA office can provide a referral for a dermatologist, if needed.

## Taking Care of Your Skin

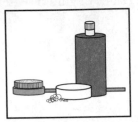

- Keep your skin clean. If you have dry skin, use a superfatted soap such as Dove, Basis, Keri, or Oilatum.
- Dry off well after washing. Be sure to prevent moisture in the folds of the skin, such as the groin area, between the toes, under the breasts, and in armpits where fungal infections are more likely. Try using talcum powder in these moist areas.
- Avoid very hot baths and showers if you have loss of sensation, because you can easily burn yourself without knowing it.
- Prevent dry skin. When you scratch dry, itchy skin, you can break the skin and open the door to bacteria. After you dry off from a shower, you may need an oil-in-water skin cream such as Lubriderm or Alpha-Keri. On cold and windy days, you may need to moisturize often to prevent chapping.
- Drink lots of water, unless your provider advises otherwise.
- Treat cuts quickly. For minor cuts, clean the area with soap, water, and hydrogen peroxide. Do not use antiseptics such as Mercurochrome, alcohol, or iodine because they irritate the skin. Only use antibiotic creams and ointments for a few days without consulting your provider.
- Call your provider if you find any of the following:
  - redness, swelling, pus, or pain that might indicate a bacterial infection
  - jock itch, athlete's foot, ringworm, vaginal itching, or other signs of a fungal infection
  - blisters or bumps anywhere, especially on the backs of your fingers, hands, toes, arms, legs, or buttocks—these are signs of high glucose levels
  - rashes, bumps, or pits near insulin injection sites

## Getting the Most out of Your Health Care Team

You've chosen your health care team. Now what? Your diabetes care provider may already use a team approach and may already be in contact with other team members. If they are not already in touch, make sure all team members know about everyone else on your team. Ask your health care team to consult with each other whenever appropriate. Be sure that they have each other's phone numbers and addresses. If you are making any lifestyle adjustments—quitting smoking, starting a weight loss diet, or taking up jogging, for example—make sure you notify all team members.

Remember, your health care team is there to help you manage your diabetes. They can provide a wealth of information and the resources you need to make the decisions that affect your health. But you are the one who ultimately makes the decisions and puts your health care plan into action.

## The Importance of Communication

To work together as a team, you must be able to communicate with your fellow health care team members. It's not always easy to communicate, especially when you're feeling nervous, worried, or under pressure. Sometimes people can feel intimidated by health care professionals. However, just remember that they are there to help you. But to best help you, they need to know what is on your mind. Only you can tell them how you are feeling and what special concerns you might have. Here are a few tips for establishing a smooth line of communication between you and your health care professional:

- Plan for your visit. Write down questions or concerns you want addressed. Bring your blood glucose record book, a list of your medications, and anything else your diabetes care provider needs to know.

- Share the conversation. Begin the visit by telling your provider what you hope to accomplish and what you want him or her to know. Your provider cannot read your mind or guess what problems you may have.

- If the vocabulary becomes too technical or the concepts too complex and you don't understand, speak up. Ask for an explanation of anything you don't understand. Write down any information or instructions. And don't worry about feeling "stupid" or worry that this is something you should already know. It is important that you thoroughly understand everything that your health care professional is telling you.

- Don't be afraid to bring up sexual or personal topics. Your team members are professionals and are prepared to help you deal with even the most sensitive topics.

- Your emotional health is critical to your well-being. Let your provider know if you are struggling.

- Don't be afraid to discuss money. Health care professionals realize that financial worries can contribute to patient anxiety, and most will be willing to discuss payment options. Tell your provider if you are having trouble paying for your medications or diabetes care supplies, even if you are not asked.

- Consider bringing a spouse or support person to sit in on the visit.

- If you don't feel comfortable with any member of your health care team or feel that you are not communicating effectively, consider interviewing other professionals until you find someone you feel at ease with.

## What to Expect

The first step will probably be to meet with your diabetes care provider. Whether you have type 1 or type 2 diabetes and have just been diagnosed or have lived with the disease for years, your diabetes care provider should provide you with certain basic care. This includes a complete physical exam once each year. A complete medical history should be conducted during the first visit. Your A1C (also known as HbA1c or glycated hemoglobin) should be tested every 3 months, and you need to discuss contingencies and changes with your health care team on an as-needed basis.

## Visiting Your Diabetes Care Provider

Yearly physical examinations are important for everyone as a preventive health measure, but they are especially important for people with diabetes. If you have diabetes, you have a greater risk for developing diabetes complications, including damage to the eyes, kidneys, nervous system, heart, and circulatory system. You are also more susceptible to developing infections. That's why a thorough examination is in order to make sure your whole body is functioning properly.

If you are seeing your diabetes care provider or other health care professional for the first time, you will most likely be asked to provide a medical history. The forms and questionnaires may vary, but all will want the same basic information. Although many questions may refer to matters that you consider private, it is important to answer honestly and trust that your health care team will maintain confidentiality.

Because information related to your medical history will often be hard to recall—when was your last immunization, or

## Diabetes Care Schedule

✓ **Every visit**
- **Blood pressure**
- **Weight**
- **Foot check**

✓ **Every 3 months**
- **A1C test**
- **Regular visits to your diabetes care provider**
- **Regular visits to your dentist**

✓ **Every year**
- **HDL, LDL, triglycerides, total cholesterol:** for average reading; more often if high levels are being treated
- **Kidneys:** microalbumin measured
- **Eyes:** examined through dilated pupils
- **Feet:** more often in patients with high-risk foot conditions (neuropathy, vascular disease)
- **Flu shot**
- **Review meal plan**
- **Update with diabetes educator**

✓ **Every 2 years**
- **HDL, LDL, triglycerides, total cholesterol:** if last reading indicates very low risk

✓ **Once**
- **Pneumococcal vaccine**

how old were you when you contracted mumps?—ask that a questionnaire be mailed to you in advance. That way, you can answer all the questions more accurately and at a leisurely pace. The more complete and correct the picture you provide, the better your health care will be.

Most histories include questions about the health of your close relatives. Think about the general health and specific diseases that have occurred in your family, especially your mother, father, grandparents, sisters, and brothers. You will also be asked to provide a general inventory of your past and present health problems, such as back pain, appendicitis, headaches, and depression. Do not deny or hide any illnesses, such as psychiatric disorders or AIDS.

Dig out a record of your immunizations. You may even need to call past health care providers for dates and names of procedures. Here are a few health-related questions you might be asked:

- What medications are you currently taking?
- Do you smoke? Have you ever smoked? If so, how much and for how long?
- Do you have any allergies?
- Have you ever been pregnant? What was the outcome?
- When were your last chest X-ray, eye exam, and dental exam?
- Have you ever been treated by a psychiatrist?
- Have you recently lost or gained weight? What was your maximum weight? What did you weigh at the diagnosis of diabetes?
- Have you ever been rejected for health insurance or employment for a medical reason?
- Do you use alcohol or any street drugs?

Some of these questions may be difficult to answer. You may not remember or you may not want to be reminded. Make an attempt to overcome your fears of being judged harshly by what you put on the form. A concerned health care professional will use this information to provide you with the best possible care—not to criticize you. What is important is achieving good health.

## Getting Physical

After taking a medical history, your diabetes care provider will give you a complete physical exam. In fact, you need a complete physical once each year. A physical examination usually begins with a discussion. This will include a review of your blood glucose measurements, insulin therapy and other medications, diet, and exercise programs. Bring your provider up-to-date on any changes you have made in lifestyle or habits. Maybe you just quit smoking or started an exercise program. If you feel a need to consult one of the other professionals on your team, now is the time to ask about it. If you feel that there are any parts of your treatment plan that are not working, tell your provider. Also keep your provider informed of what treatment options are successful.

A good physical will also include a close examination of all the parts of your body, from head to toe. Your provider is trained to detect small problems and prevent them from becoming bigger problems and will examine all of the following, and perhaps more:

- **Weight or body mass index.** Talk to your provider about the body weight that you think is best for you and whether you have any difficulty maintaining that weight.
- **Blood pressure and pulse.** Ask what your current readings are and whether these fall within the recommended range. If not, ask what levels are best for you to achieve and how to go about it.
- **Eyes.** Your eyes will be checked for problems and you will be asked about any changes in your vision. Make sure to

TIP

Children whose blood glucose levels are often high sometimes are slow to grow and mature. Height should be measured at every visit, not just the first one. The progress of sexual maturation should also be checked.

keep your provider abreast of any changes that have occurred, even if you are also seeing an eye care specialist.

- **Heart and lungs.** Your provider will most likely listen to your heart and lungs through a stethoscope. Sometimes an electrocardiogram or stress electrocardiogram may be performed to detect symptom-free heart disease. Such tests measure the electrical activity and pumping of your heart muscle and can detect many subtle abnormalities.

- **Feet.** Removing your shoes and socks each time you visit— not just during your yearly physicals—will remind your diabetes care provider to check your feet. You will be checked for calluses, infections, and sores. Using a monofilament to check for sensation, your provider will also look for any loss of feeling that could indicate neuropathy.

- **Skin.** Your skin, your largest organ, will be examined by sight, with special attention to insulin injection sites.

- **Nervous system.** Your reflexes and your sensitivity to the sharpness of a monofilament or pin or the light touch of cotton or a brush will be checked. If you are experiencing any persistent problems, such as dizziness on standing, pain, burning sensation, numbness in your legs or arms, constipation, diarrhea, difficulty urinating, or difficulty with erection or sexual satisfaction, make sure to mention them.

- **Mouth and neck.** Your provider will examine your gums, teeth, mouth, and throat. She or he will feel for swelling in

**TIP**

If you have type 1 diabetes, you have a five times greater risk of also someday developing thyroid disease, which is another type of autoimmune disease. Make sure you have a blood test to detect thyroid disease.

the glands in your neck and ask you about your brushing and flossing habits. The function of your thyroid gland will also be assessed during your initial physical examination.

- **Blood.** A sample of blood will be drawn to test for glucose levels and A1C. A fasting lipid profile, which measures cholesterol and triglycerides, will be performed to determine the levels of these fats in your blood. Your urea nitrogen and serum creatinine concentrations in the blood will also be measured to assess your kidney function.

- **Urine.** Kidney function is also assessed by testing urine for ketones, glucose, and protein. People with diabetes are more likely to have urinary tract infections because of the high concentrations of glucose in urine and the loss of the sensation of knowing when the bladder is empty or full because of neuropathy. If you have any symptoms of infection, a urinary culture may also be performed.

- **Vaccinations.** People with diabetes are more likely to develop complications from the flu or pneumonia. You need a pneumonia vaccine once in your lifetime and a flu shot each year.

- **Other tests.** Some tests may be performed by other members of your health care team. For women, this includes a Pap smear, mammogram, and gynecological and rectal exam. Contraception and pregnancy planning should also be discussed. Men should receive prostate and rectal exams. Both men and women should have their stool samples tested for blood to detect colon cancer.

- **Specific problems.** You may be asked about any unusual concerns you may have, such as a sore shoulder or abdominal pain. If you are experiencing any sexual or personal problems, don't be afraid to bring them up.

Beyond the yearly physical, your A1C should also be checked every 3 months. Measuring your A1C tells you how well your treatment program is working. You need this test whether you use insulin or not. The reading tells your average blood glucose reading from the last 2 to 3 months and can predict the likelihood of future eye, kidney, and nerve disease. Ask for the results of your A1C test. You are aiming for an A1C level of less than or equal to 7 percent. According to research, this reading will help you prevent future complications.

You can use the results of the A1C test to compare with your own self-monitoring records. Be sure to discuss your blood glucose readings (always bring your logbook) at every visit. If your daily blood glucose tests are in range but your A1C is too high, you and your provider need to discuss ways to better manage and monitor your blood glucose levels. It is important to understand why your tests might show good blood glucose readings when your overall blood glucose measure is too high.

Ask about what to do on sick days. Even a mild cold can throw off blood glucose levels, usually by making them higher than normal. Ask what symptoms to be on the lookout for and when you should call your diabetes care provider. What precautions should you take when you feel under the weather?

Other changes in your health may result in return trips to your provider more often than every 3 months. If you're just starting insulin or are changing your dose and your glucose is out of range, you may need to talk by telephone or see your provider as often as every day for a while, until your blood glucose is in range. Or if you are trying to manage high blood pressure, you may need to monitor your blood pressure often and keep records of the readings.

# A1C Testing

***What is the A1C test?*** This test can be done in a laboratory or office or with a mail-in kit you do at home. Blood is collected from a fingerstick or vein. The test measures the concentration of hemoglobin molecules that have glucose attached to them. This tells you what your average blood glucose level was over the past 2 to 3 months. It also tells you your level of risk for the long-term complications of diabetes.

***How do I interpret the results?*** The measure is given as a percentage. A 9 percent level means that 9 percent of your hemoglobin molecules are glycated (sugar coated). People without diabetes have about a 5 percent reading.

***What is glycated hemoglobin?*** Hemoglobin is found in red blood cells. It links up with the glucose in your blood to become glycated. The more glucose in your blood, the more hemoglobin will become glycated. Once glycated, the hemoglobin stays that way until the red blood cell's life is over. This averages about 120 days.

***Why is this test used?*** This test gives you a "long" view of your blood glucose levels because as old red blood cells are dying, new ones are taking their place. If your blood glucose was high last week, then more of your hemoglobin was glycated than usual. Your blood glucose might be back on target this week, but your red blood cells will still be carrying the memory of last week's high blood glucose level.

***How long is the memory of this test?*** Your A1C reading is not a simple average of all the blood glucose level ups-and-downs over the past 2 to 3 months. It is a weighted average. You never have a complete turnover of red blood cells all at once. Some are dying as others are just coming on board. There are always more young cells than old cells. About half are newer cells, ones formed within the last month. So your glucose levels in the last month count for about half of your A1C measure, and cells from the previous 2 to 3 months make up the other half of the measure.

*If my blood glucose levels improve, how long does it take to see results?* It takes about 2 to 3 months to see all the results of an improvement (or worsening) in blood glucose. This is why there's really no need to have the test more often than every 3 months. However, if you are newly diagnosed and may have been far out of range for a while, you may want to have your A1C measured every 2 weeks at first. Significant changes in blood glucose can be seen within 2 weeks. Or, for someone who is pregnant and seeking very tight glucose levels, A1C may be measured every month or two to make sure that the treatment plan is getting results.

*How do my blood glucose testing results relate to my A1C results?* Measuring A1C gives you the big picture. Self-monitoring of blood glucose gives you a snapshot of the moment. Let's say you have type 2 diabetes, and you check your blood glucose twice a day, before meals. The level is usually around 120 mg/dl. But your last A1C was just over 10%, which corresponds to an average daily blood glucose of around 275 mg/dl. This would mean that your after-meal blood glucose levels must be getting pretty high, so some changes in medication dosage, food choices, or portion sizes are in order.

*What should my A1C measure be?* Research has shown that keeping your A1C under 7 percent helps you lower your risk for diabetes complications of the kidneys, eyes, feet, and nerves.

## A1C Measurements

| A1C (%) | Average blood glucose level (mg/dl) |
|---------|-------------------------------------|
| 6 | 135 |
| 7 | 170 |
| 8 | 205 |
| 9 | 240 |
| 10 | 275 |
| 11 | 310 |
| 12 | 345 |
| 13 | 380 |

# Second Opinions

Hermes experienced seven serious episodes involving blackouts, fainting, dizziness, and even cardiac arrest over the course of 2 years. His doctor blamed it on "some latent viral infection" that crops up from time to time. When he asked his doctor for a second opinion, he was told he didn't need one. Finally, after much persistence, his doctor referred him to a diabetes specialty clinic, where his problem was eventually diagnosed and treated. No matter how much you trust your doctor and other health care professionals, there may be times when you would like a second opinion. This could occur when surgery, long-term medication, or other treatments that will drastically affect your lifestyle are recommended. You may also want a second opinion if your doctor says you have a problem for which there is no known therapy or your doctor calls the problem you have incurable.

**TIP**

What to ask when you get a second opinion:

- What is the diagnosis and how was it determined?
- What treatments are available and which are most effective? most risky? most commonly used?
- What treatment do you suggest and why?
- What is the success rate for this treatment?
- Is the condition reversible?
- What are the potential side effects and complications of the treatment and how likely are they?
- Is the problem or treatment likely to affect my blood glucose levels?
- Will the treatment require hospitalization? For how long? Will I need follow-up care?
- Are there any additional costs associated with this treatment, such as repeated blood tests, physical therapy, or postoperative nursing care?
- Is this an experimental treatment? Will I be participating in research? Will I be part of a placebo/control group, or will I receive treatment? If this is the case, you may need to evaluate the potential risks and make sure they do not outweigh the benefits. If this is a research protocol, are more conventional treatments available should this one fail?

Check with your insurance company to determine whether medical costs for a recommended procedure are covered. Also ask whether they cover the cost of a second opinion and whether they pay only their own recommended consultants. Some insurance companies insist on a second opinion before they will fully cover certain treatments.

When searching for a physician to provide a second opinion, first ask your physician or a health care professional you trust. Look for a doctor who is board certified in the field in which you are seeking information, such as cardiology, surgery, or endocrinology. Be sure to tell the physician about your diabetes. If the problem is diabetes related, or you suspect that it is, call the American Diabetes Association for the names of specialists in your area (see Resources). For problems not related to diabetes, try calling the appropriate department of a major medical center or teaching hospital and asking for the names of specialists in the field.

# The Ins and Outs of Insulin $4$

*Get to know insulin. All people with type 1 diabetes and many people with type 2 or gestational diabetes use insulin to manage their blood glucose levels.*

Since its discovery in the 1920s, scientists have learned a great deal about insulin. They know a lot about how it works in people without diabetes. And they also know that when insulin is absent or doesn't do its job, people develop diabetes.

Insulin is a hormone. Hormones are chemical signals made by the body that tell various parts of the body how to do their jobs. Some hormones control how the cells in the body grow. Some control how the body uses food and energy to live. And other hormones help muscles to contract, blood to clot, or the heart to beat.

One of insulin's most important jobs is to help cells use glucose. Insulin acts like a key to unlock the door that lets glucose into the cell. Cells in the body use glucose as a source of energy that they need to live. Without energy, the cells in the body cannot survive. Insulin also helps the body to store extra fuel as fat.

In people with type 1 diabetes, the body does not make enough insulin. This is because most of the cells of the pancreas that make insulin have been destroyed by the immune system. Eventually, all of the cells that make insulin are destroyed and no insulin is produced. That is why type 1 diabetes is also called an autoimmune disorder. People with type 1 diabetes must take injections of insulin in order to live.

In people with type 2 diabetes, insulin is produced, but the cells do not respond to insulin as they should. Glucose has a hard time getting out of the blood and into cells. For some people with type 2 diabetes, diet, exercise, and oral diabetes medication together can help them keep their blood glucose levels on target without insulin injections. But for many people with type 2 diabetes, diet, exercise, and oral diabetes medication are not enough.

## Insulin Type

Insulin is a small protein called a *polypeptide*. It is made up of a chain of small units, known as amino acids. In the early days, only pork and beef insulins were available. These insulins were made from grinding up the pancreases from pigs and cows and purifying the insulin protein. They acted rapidly to lower blood glucose levels. They also were used up rapidly by the body and had to be injected before each meal and at bedtime. Although long-acting animal insulins later became available, the purity and strength of early insulin preparations were not always reliable.

For many years, purified preparations of animal insulins were widely used. However, human insulin is now used most of the time. There is a ready supply of human insulin. It is not harvested from actual pancreases but is made with the help of genetic engineering. The human insulin gene, which tells cells what sequence of amino acids is needed to make the insulin protein, is put into bacteria that multiply rapidly. The bacteria are "tricked" into making human insulin.

Most people who take insulin today use human insulin. Beef insulin is no longer available in the United States and Canada, although pork insulin is. The big advantages to human insulin are that it is easy to make and it is unlikely to cause an allergic reaction. Some people are allergic to animal insulin, because the body sees it as a foreign substance.

## Action Times

People may respond to preparations of insulin and insulin mixtures differently, so it is important to find the types of insulin that work best for you. Each type of insulin has a different action time, a term that describes the length of time it takes to begin acting and how long its effect lasts. The action times of insulin are due to the following three features:

- **onset:** the length of time it takes for insulin to reach the blood and begin lowering blood glucose levels
- **peak time:** the time during which insulin is at its maximal strength in lowering blood glucose levels
- **duration:** the length of time in which insulin continues to lower blood glucose

Before you got diabetes, your pancreas made the insulin you needed to keep your blood glucose in the normal range. The pancreas made a small amount of insulin throughout the day and night that was released in a steady stream. This is the basal insulin level. When you ate and your blood glucose level began to rise, the pancreas released a burst, or bolus, of insulin.

Insulin doses are planned to work as much like the body as possible. Rapid- and short-acting insulins are bolus insulins. Intermediate- and long-acting insulins are basal insulins. Most people with diabetes take both a basal and a bolus insulin.

| Insulin Action | | | |
|---|---|---|---|
| **Insulin type** | **Onset (hours)** | **Peak (hours)** | **Duration (hours)** |
| **Rapid acting** Human lispro or human aspart | Within 15 minutes | 1 to 2 | 3 to 4 |
| **Short acting** Human regular | 0.5 to 1.0 | 2 to 3 | 3 to 6 |
| **Intermediate acting** Human NPH Human lente | 2 to 4 3 to 4 | 4 to 10 4 to 12 | 10 to 16 12 to 18 |
| **Long acting** Human ultralente Insulin glargine | 6 to 10 2 to 4 | — — | 18 to 24 20 to 24 |

The first type of insulin that was made available is known as regular insulin. Regular insulin is short acting and must be injected several times throughout the day. Regular insulin begins working rapidly and is used up fairly quickly by the body. As shown in the table on insulin action times, regular insulin begins to act within an hour. Rapid-acting insulin, lispro insulin and insulin aspart, go to work within minutes. An intermediate-acting insulin, NPH (neutral protamine Hagedorn), contains a molecule known as a protamine, which slows down how fast the body absorbs insulin. Because the insulin reaches the blood more slowly, the onset, peak, and duration times are longer. By using a slower-acting insulin, you can get by with fewer injections each day. For example, a mixture of NPH and regular

TIP

Signs of a local allergic reaction to insulin:

- dents under the skin at injection sites
- redness at injection sites, either persistent or temporary
- groups of small bumps, similar to hives
- swelling at injection sites

insulin injected at breakfast can last until dinnertime. You may not need an injection at lunchtime.

People who are allergic to the protamine in NPH can consider using lente, another intermediate-acting insulin. An even longer-acting insulin, ultralente, provides a continuous level of insulin with a less pronounced peak. In some people, human ultralente insulin may really act more like an intermediate insulin. Insulin glargine is the newest long-acting insulin. It has no peak and works well with rapid-acting insulin taken before meals. Whenever you change insulins, you need to figure out how quickly the new insulin works in your body.

All insulins used for injections have added ingredients. These prevent bacteria and molds from growing and help keep insulin from spoiling. Intermediate- and long-acting insulins also contain ingredients that prolong their action times. If you think you may be experiencing an allergic reaction to your insulin preparation, talk to your provider.

## Premixed Insulin

You might be advised to take a mixture of regular or rapid-acting and NPH insulin in one injection. You can mix them yourself (see Appendix for instructions). Or you may be able to buy the insulin already mixed. Mixtures of regular and NPH insulins come in various combinations that make them more convenient and easier to handle. For example, you can buy a 50/50 mixture of NPH and regular insulin, or you can buy a mixture that contains 30 percent regular insulin and

## Which Short-Acting Insulin Is Best for Me?

Rapid- or short-acting insulins can both be used for bolus doses of insulins. But many people find rapid-acting insulins more convenient.

Rapid-acting insulins can be used by people with either type 1 or type 2 diabetes. The faster action of these insulins makes it easier to time insulin with food. In other words, you can match the rise in blood glucose from food absorption to the rise in insulin in your blood from the rapid-acting insulin.

Rapid-acting insulins are in a form that the body can absorb right away, without having to break it down. With regular insulin, the body needs to reduce the insulin protein chain to a smaller size before it can be absorbed and go to work. It can take over 30 minutes from the time regular insulin is injected until it starts working on cells. With rapid-acting insulins, this time is cut in half, so there's less room for error. It goes to work almost as fast as naturally produced insulin does.

This rapid-acting insulin may give you a lot more flexibility. You can count the carbohydrates in your meal and take insulin to cover that amount. If you eat an extra helping at a meal, you can take care of the carbohydrates with a booster shot right away. You may even be able to wait until you know how much carbohydrate you've eaten to inject these insulins. Also, because rapid-acting insulins don't remain in the body as long as regular insulin does, you may experience fewer episodes of hypoglycemia. Ask your provider whether you could benefit from using a rapid-acting insulin.

| Insulin type | Onset | Peak | Duration |
|---|---|---|---|
| Made by body | Immediate, when needed | 30 to 60 minutes | 2 to 3 hours |
| Human lispro, human aspart | Within 15 minutes after injection | 1 to 2 hours | 3 to 4 hours |
| Human regular | 30 to 60 minutes | 2 to 3 hours | 3 to 6 hours |

**TIP**

Crossing time zones can confuse your insulin schedule. You may need to make a new plan for timing your insulin injections. You may also need to adjust your total daily insulin dose. When traveling east, you get a shorter day and need less insulin. When traveling west, you get more hours in a day and need more insulin. Keep your watch on your home time until the first morning after you arrive in a new time zone. Check your blood glucose level more often than usual. For more on insulin and traveling, see page 108.

70 percent NPH. Preparations containing intermediate- and rapid-acting insulins are also available. Premixed insulins can also be useful for people with eyesight or dexterity problems that make drawing different amounts of insulin from two different bottles difficult. You may want to discuss assistive devices for people with impaired sight with your doctor or diabetes educator.

Even though you can buy mixtures of insulin or can mix them yourself, make sure to talk to members of your health care team before you make any changes in the insulin you take. Never mix types of insulin without the okay from your provider. Mixing insulin with lente or ultralente insulin can be more complicated than mixing with NPH. These longer-acting insulins can interfere with rapid- and short-acting insulins and lead to unpredictable results. Rapid-acting and regular insulins are not always readily absorbed by the body when mixed with slower insulins. If your injection schedule calls for taking both regular and lente insulin at the same time, try to inject them immediately after mixing. Glargine cannot be mixed in the same syringe with other insulins. If you have any questions or notice that you don't get the response you expect from the bolus insulin, talk to your provider. You may need to increase the amount of regular insulin in the mixture or switch to a rapid-acting insulin.

Before you leave your diabetes care provider's office, be sure you understand the following:

- what type of insulin you will be taking and the name of the insulin
- the symptoms of high and low blood glucose that could indicate a problem with your insulin doses
- where you should inject it
- whether you need to prepare any mixtures
- how often to give yourself injections
- the best times of the day to take your insulin
- how to store your insulin

Don't be afraid to take notes or ask questions about anything that's not clear. Even if you have taken insulin before, you might want to review your insulin schedule on a return visit, especially if you are experiencing any difficulties. You might also want to go over any changes in your schedule that were recommended. Make sure you understand how to time injections with mealtimes. Go step-by-step through a typical day. Also talk about how to adjust for an unusual day. What happens if you oversleep, get sick, travel across time zones, or plan to be unusually active?

## Insulin Strength

When insulin was first manufactured, different batches often had different strengths. This made it difficult to know how much insulin was needed to lower blood glucose to the right level. Later, the strength of insulin became standardized, but it was available in several different strengths. This often made it confusing to figure out how much insulin to take.

FACT OR MYTH?

**"Once I open a bottle of insulin, I need to keep it in the fridge."**

 To get the most life out of your insulin supply, keep open bottles "comfortable," not too hot or too cold. If you'll use up a bottle of insulin within a month, keep it at room temperature. If it takes longer than a month to use up, it's best to keep it refrigerated, but warm up the syringe before you inject. Injecting cold insulin can make the injection uncomfortable. Keep unopened bottles in the refrigerator.

Freezing can cause the insulin ingredients to "unmix." Because insulin is a protein, it will unfold (denature) at temperatures above 86°F, including those reached inside a locked car in the summer.

Today, if you buy insulin in this country, you don't have to worry about the strength. Nearly all insulin preparations sold in the United States and Canada today are of the same strength: U-100. This means that they have 100 units of insulin in every cubic centimeter (cc) of fluid. U-40, a more diluted insulin, has been discontinued. U-500, a highly concentrated preparation, is available only by special order for people who have developed insulin resistance and need to take extremely high doses of insulin. Hospitals sometimes use U-500 insulin for emergencies.

Insulin syringes also come in different sizes that match the strength of insulin. If you travel outside the United States, bring along sufficient insulin and matching U-100 syringes. You could end up taking the wrong dose if you don't match insulin strength with the right syringe. If you are planning a long visit outside the country and can't bring along all the supplies you need, remember that you will need to buy U-40 syringes to use the U-40 insulin found in Latin America and Europe. Ask your provider to help you adjust your dosage.

## Buying and Storing Insulin

Don't assume that most pharmacies will charge the same price for insulin. The same insulin at one pharmacy or outlet may be several dollars cheaper than that found somewhere else, so it pays to shop around. You might receive a discount for buying certain quantities at your pharmacy or by ordering through the mail. Be sure to ask your pharmacists whether they offer discounts for large orders. Your insurance company or managed care provider may have an agreement with "preferred pharmacies" to offer insulin at reduced rates. Check with your insurance company or managed care provider to see whether it offers this service. By using these services you may be able to keep your costs down. But if you decide to buy insulin in bulk, check the expiration date. You don't want to buy a big supply of insulin if most of it will expire before you have a chance to use it.

In choosing a pharmacy, convenience may be just as important as cost. You may want a pharmacy that is close by or one that delivers your insulin to you. This can be convenient, especially if you are very busy, ill, or housebound. Also think about the pharmacist. Is the pharmacist easy to talk to? Does he or she seem willing to answer your questions?

Once you find a pharmacy that you like, try to develop a relationship with the pharmacist. Don't just ask for NPH insulin. Ask questions. Check to make sure you have the desired brand and type. You may want to bring along an empty bottle to make sure you get exactly the same thing each time. Before you pay, double-check to see that you have what you

### Storing Insulin

| | | |
|---|---|---|
| Unopened bottles and unused insulin pens or cartridges | → Stored in the refrigerator | → Discard after expiration date on bottle |
| Opened bottles | → Kept at room temperature | → Discard after 1 month |

want. If something doesn't look quite right, or if you are uncertain, be sure to ask your pharmacist.

You don't have to worry about storing the bottle of insulin you are using in the refrigerator in between injections. Store unopened bottles of insulin in the refrigerator. The expiration date on a bottle of insulin applies to bottles that have not been opened and have been stored in the refrigerator. If an open vial of insulin is kept at room temperature for more than a month, the insulin may lose some of its strength. Throw away bottles that have been opened for a month and kept at room temperature. If you go through bottles slowly, write the date you first open a bottle on the label so you know when to toss it. Storage guidelines vary from 10 to 28 days for different types of insulin cartridges and prefilled pens. Read the label or package insert or ask your pharmacist or nurse educator if special storage is needed.

One good reason to store the insulin you're using at room temperature is that injecting cold insulin can make the injection feel more uncomfortable. If your insulin is cold, draw it up into the syringe, then warm it up by gently rolling it back and forth in your hands.

If you are traveling and keep your insulin stored in a cooler, make sure the insulin doesn't freeze or come in contact with ice.

## On the Go with Insulin

- Wear a medical ID bracelet or necklace that says you have diabetes.
- Don't get separated from your supplies. Carry your insulin, syringes and/or insulin pump and infusion sets, lancets, glucose meter, blood and ketone test strips, glucagon kit, glucose gel or tablets, and snacks with you. Check with the airlines to meet security requirements.
- Some states require a prescription only for lispro, glargine, and aspart. Other insulins are available over the counter, as are syringes. In other states, you need a prescription for all insulins and the syringes. If you are traveling and your insulin is lost or destroyed, ask a pharmacist for help.
- Take twice as much insulin and blood testing equipment as you think you'll need. Getting extra diabetes supplies when you're away from home can be difficult.
- Keep insulin out of direct sunlight and protect it from very hot or very cold temperatures. If flying, keep your insulin supply with you instead of packing it in bags that might get too hot or too cold (such as in an airplane baggage compartment).

Storing insulin at temperatures colder than 36°F can cause it to lose potency and clump. Also avoid getting insulin too hot or leaving it in direct sunlight for too long. Insulin can spoil if it gets hotter than 86°F. The general rule of thumb is, if the temperature is comfortable for you, your insulin will be okay, too.

Never use insulin if it looks abnormal. Regular, lispro, aspart, and glargine insulins are clear. If you use clear insulin, always check for any floating particles, cloudiness, or change in color. This could be a sign that your insulin is contaminated or has lost its strength.

Other types of insulin come as suspensions. This means that the material is not completely dissolved, and you might be able to see solid material floating in liquid. However, it should look uniformly cloudy. If you are using NPH or lente, check that your insulin is free of any large clumps of material. Do not use any insulin if you see chunks of material floating around. These changes could mean that crystals or aggregates are forming and the insulin is spoiled or denatured. This can be caused by too much shaking of the insulin bottle or storing insulin at temperatures that are either too hot or too cold.

If you have been instructed to dilute your insulin, use only the diluent recommended by the manufacturer. Properly diluted insulin is good for 2 to 6 weeks stored in the refrigerator.

If you find anything wrong with your insulin right after you buy it, return it immediately. If the condition develops later, try to figure out whether you have handled or stored the insulin the wrong way. If not, talk to your pharmacist about a refund or exchange.

## Using Insulin

Most people with diabetes use a needle and syringe or an insulin pen to take their insulin. Once you learn how, this will be a quick and relatively painless task. If you have problems with your vision or using your hands, there are injection aids that may help solve the problem.

Using a syringe is just one way to take insulin. Advanced delivery systems such as the insulin pump may work better for some people. Some people use an insulin pen, while others use high pressure jet injectors to pass insulin through the skin. Whatever you choose, the basic purpose is the same: to deliver insulin into the fat that lies just under your skin.

Other ways to deliver insulin may become more widely available in the future. Inhaled insulin and insulin patches are being tested. One exciting prospect is an insulin infusion device that is implanted into the body. With this, you might be able to go 2 months without having to worry about refilling it. And scientists hope that one day they will be able to make a device that measures your blood glucose level and delivers the proper amount of insulin automatically.

## Injecting Insulin

Injecting insulin today is a lot less painful than it used to be. You can choose between disposable syringes with lubricated microfine needles and pen devices. There are many other helpful devices that make injecting with a syringe possible for almost anyone.

*Syringes.* Today's smaller gauge needles are slimmer, have sharper points, and are specially coated to slide into the skin smoothly. If you are already using these needles and your injections are still uncomfortable, talk to your diabetes care provider or educator. It often helps to go over your injection technique with them. Trying to relax before injections can help. Tense muscles can make the injection hurt.

Keeping your injection site clean will reduce the risk of developing an infection. But you don't have to use alcohol to clean your skin before injecting the needle. Soap and water works fine. If you use alcohol before injections, make sure the alcohol dries before you inject, or it could cause stinging. See the Appendix for more tips on injections.

*Buying syringes.* The syringe consists of a needle, barrel, and plunger. Syringes come in different sizes. It is important to match the size of the syringe to the dose you'll take with it. You want a syringe that will hold your entire dose of insulin. For example, if you need to take 45 units of insulin, you would want to use a 50-unit syringe to hold all your dose. A 30-unit syringe (the next smallest size) is handy for giving yourself injections of 30 units or less. Likewise, if you need to inject very small doses of insulin, 1/2 unit for example, use syringes that have 1/2 unit marks to keep doses accurate.

Also, check to see whether you can read the markings on your syringe. A 100-unit syringe holds 100 units of insulin in a volume of 1 cc (or 1 ml). Each line marks 2 units of insulin. A 50-unit syringe holds 50 units of insulin in 0.5 cc of liquid, and each line marks 1 unit. A 30-unit syringe holds 30 units of insulin in 0.3 cc, and each line marks 1 unit. You will need to measure out each dose in units. So, if you can't see the lines marked on the syringe, you will have problems getting an accurate dose. There are devices you can buy to make it easier to read the markings on the syringe. Your pharmacist or diabetes educator can tell you what supplies are available to help you. Another good source of information is the American Diabetes Association *Resource Guide* published yearly by *Diabetes Forecast,* the members' magazine of the American Diabetes Association. The *Resource Guide* is also available online at www.diabetes.org/diabetes-forecast.jsp and in single copies from the American Diabetes Association (see Resources).

If you are planning to travel or will be away from home, take along a prescription for syringes. Also ask your provider to write a letter stating that you have diabetes and indicating what type of insulin you use. Some states require a prescription to purchase supplies. If you have problems getting supplies while traveling, try a hospital emergency room.

***Reusing syringes.*** There is no right or wrong answer to the question of whether you should use your insulin syringes over again. It's really up to you. Reusing syringes can save money.

And it creates less medical waste to litter the environment. There is no evidence that you are more likely to become infected if you reuse a syringe—as long as you follow some safety guidelines. If you choose to reuse syringes, the American Diabetes Association offers guidelines for maintaining them properly (see Appendix).

Most manufacturers of disposable syringes recommend that they be used only once. This is because syringes cannot be guaranteed to be sterile if they are reused. If you have poor personal hygiene, are ill, have open wounds on your hands, or have a low resistance to infection for any reason, you should not reuse syringes. Needles also can become chipped or dull after use. Most needles can be used several times before the tip becomes dull. A dull tip is more painful than a new, sharp needle.

The most important advice about syringe reuse is this: never let anyone use a syringe you've already used, and don't use anyone else's syringe—ever.

*Syringe disposal.* How you get rid of your syringe can affect anyone who might come in contact with your trash. This includes the members of your family, neighbors, your trash collector, and people using beaches and other public areas. So it's important that you do it safely. Never toss a used syringe directly into a trash can. Syringes and lancets and any other material that touches human blood is considered medical waste and must be handled carefully. Before deciding what you will do, you might want to check with your local health department. Some towns and counties have special laws or rules for getting rid of medical waste and may offer safe alternatives. When traveling, if possible, bring your unused syringes home. Pack them in a heavy-duty container, such as a hard plastic pencil box.

**TIP**

Each fall, the American Diabetes Association publishes the *Resource Guide,* a supplement to *Diabetes Forecast.* You can also buy the guide separately or view it online at www.diabetes.org/ diabetes-forecast.jsp. The *Resource Guide* lists the latest offerings of diabetes tools from manufacturers.

*Injection Devices.* Talk to your doctor or your diabetes educator if you are having problems with any aspects of insulin injection. There are alternatives to injecting by syringe, such as an insulin pen or jet injector. And there are products available that make giving an injection easier. Ask your educator if you can try out some of the insulin-injection aids before you buy anything. This way you can see if any new product is right for you before you invest your money. Be sure to let them know as well if the injections are causing you a great deal of stress or anxiety.

*Insulin pens.* An insulin pen looks like an ink pen. Instead of a writing tip, it has a disposable needle, and instead of an ink cartridge, there is an insulin cartridge. These pens are popular because they are convenient and accurate in dose. You don't have to worry about filling syringes or carrying them with you when you are away from home. There are two types of pens. You can buy a pre-filled pen that you throw away once the insulin cartridge is empty. Or you can buy a pen that uses disposable cartridges. A variety of insulins are available in pens and cartridges. You decide the number of units you want, set the injector for that dose, stick the needle in your skin, and inject the insulin. This makes them useful for multiple dose schedules. Pen injectors are conveniently portable because you don't have to carry around a bottle of insulin. Some are designed to make it easier for people with visual or dexterity problems to give injections.

**Insertion aids.** An automatic injector shoots a needle into your skin. Some automatically release the insulin when the needle hits your skin. With others, you have to press the plunger on the syringe. An automatic injector can be useful if you have arthritis or other problems that make it difficult to hold a syringe steadily. If you cringe at the thought of injecting yourself or don't like the sight of needles, an automatic injector may be for you.

**Jet injectors.** Jet injectors push the insulin out so fast that it acts like a liquid needle, passing insulin directly through the skin. If you fear needles or take several injections each day, a jet injector may be a possibility.

The downside is that jet injectors are expensive and may not accurately deliver the insulin dose. Check with your insurer about whether it will cover the cost of this device. Although you will save on the cost of needles and syringes, there may be a hefty initial cost. Ask to test a jet injector before buying. Bruising can be a problem, especially in thin people, children, and the elderly, all of whom have less fat under the skin. Jet injectors also need to be cleaned on a regular basis. Ask your doctor, diabetes educator, and others you know who have used them what they think of jet injectors before deciding.

**Aids for the visually impaired.** Several products are available that make it easier for people who are visually impaired. These include

- dose gauges to help you measure your insulin accurately— even mixed doses. Some click with every 1 or 2 units of insulin you measure, and others have Braille or raised numbers.
- needle guides and vial stabilizers to help you insert the needle into the insulin vial correctly. Some of these will also let you set a desired dosage level.

■ syringe magnifiers that can enlarge the measure marks on a
  syringe barrel. One model combines a magnifier with the
  needle guide and vial stabilizer. Another clips around the
  syringe and magnifies the scale.

Some of these aids only fit certain brands of syringes. Make
sure that any aids you purchase will fit the equipment you
already have. Some of these aids can be used along with some
of the devices discussed above. In addition to injection aids, you
can also buy blood glucose meters for the visually impaired (see
Chapter 6).

## Coming Soon: Insulin without Injections

If you are one of the millions of people with diabetes who has
dreamed of a life without needles, several new products are
being tested that could put an end to insulin injections. Inhaled
insulin, insulin sprayed into the mouth, and insulin in a pill are
all being tested (see below). Although none of these products
have made it to the marketplace yet, preliminary results are
encouraging.

*Artificial Pancreas.* A device that serves as an artificial pancreas
continues to be tested and has been shown to be effective in
treating patients with type 1 diabetes. The device consists of a
glucose sensor implanted in the abdominal cavity connected to
an insulin reservoir. When the sensor detects a rise in blood glucose levels, it triggers a release of insulin from the reservoir, thus
functioning much like a healthy pancreas. Preliminary results
show that the artificial pancreas is more effective in controlling
blood glucose levels than insulin injections alone. The device
requires further testing and government approval before making it to the marketplace.

**Insulin Pills.** Oral insulins are currently being tested in human clinical trials. Because insulin is a protein, it gets degraded in the stomach. But new ways of linking the insulin molecule to polymers allow it to escape digestion and become absorbed into the bloodstream. Preliminary studies are promising. The pills appear to have no adverse side effects and can be taken 15 minutes before a meal.

**Insulin Patch.** Insulin is normally too big to be absorbed directly through the skin. But a special battery-operated skin patch is being developed that creates microscopic openings in the skin to allow insulin to pass through and into the bloodstream. The patch uses a two-step process to deliver insulin. First, an electronic patch vaporizes cells on the skin surface. A second patch containing a reservoir of insulin is then applied, and the insulin molecules can be absorbed into the bloodstream over a 12-hour period. The delivery system will require government approval before making it to the marketplace. Potentially, the insulin pill and skin patch could be combined to deliver both basal and bolus doses of insulin.

**Oral Spray.** A new device called Rapid Mist is currently being tested that could deliver an aerosolized version of insulin through the mucus membranes of the cheeks, tongue, and throat. Early results indicate that Rapid Mist, which resembles an inhaler used by people with asthma, is identical to an insulin injection in its ability to lower blood glucose levels.

**Inhaled Insulin.** Several companies are working on liquid or powdered forms of insulin that are inhaled through the mouth and delivered to the lungs. The insulin then enters the bloodstream as a rapid-acting insulin. The products are being tested for safety and efficacy before making it to the marketplace.

## Injection Site Rotation

It is usually recommended that you inject your insulin into your abdomen, but you can use other sites as well, as long as you inject into an area that contains fat. Some people find the abdomen easier to use than the thigh. Wherever you choose to inject, you will want to inject at different sites within that area so that you don't develop problems in and under the skin. You may find that it works best to rotate injection sites within one general area such as the abdomen rather than rotate randomly to sites in different areas of the body. However, some people achieve consistent results by doing all morning injections at one site, such as the buttocks, and all evening injections at a second site, such as the abdomen. You will probably get the most predictable results if you are consistent. That's because insulin is absorbed at different rates in different body areas. That could cause your body to respond to each insulin injection differently and lead to large fluctuations in blood glucose levels. Injecting in the same general area makes your response to insulin more predictable. Once you have used each injection site within a body area, you can start over in the same body area. There are many opinions on the best way to rotate injection sites. Talk to your diabetes educator about the best method for you.

*Typical Injection Sites.* Insulin works best when injected into a layer of fat under the skin, above the muscle tissue. Several areas of the body have enough fat tissue under the skin for insulin injection. The abdomen, except for a 2-inch circle around the navel, is used most commonly. Another suitable area is the top and outer thighs. This is best used when you are in a sitting position. The backs of the upper arms, the hips, and the buttocks also work well. Some people, especially those with a large body size, have other options. For example, the lower

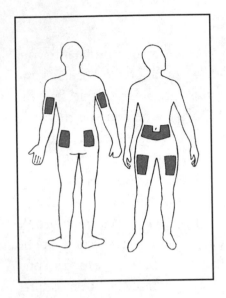

back can also be a good injection site, as long as there is enough fat under the skin. Wherever you choose to inject, keep these basics in mind:

- Divide the body area into injection sites about the size of a quarter. Try to make each new injection at least a finger-width away from your last shot. You may need to devise a way to remember where that last site was. For example, you might inject all of your morning shots on the right side and all of your evening shots on the left.
- When injecting into the arm, use the outer back area of the upper arm, where there is fatty tissue. Avoid the deltoid muscle, the large triangular muscle that covers the shoulder joint. Don't inject into muscle tissue anywhere in the body.
- Inject anywhere there is fat on the abdomen except for the 2-inch space around the navel. This has tough tissue that causes erratic insulin absorption.
- Avoid injecting too close to moles or scar tissue anywhere on the body.
- When injecting in the thighs, shoot for the top and outside areas. If you inject the inner thighs, rubbing between the legs may make the injection site sore. Also avoid the bony area above the knees where there isn't much fat.

**Differences in Insulin Absorption.** Most insulins are absorbed most quickly (and at the most consistent speed) when injected into the abdomen, more slowly when injected into the arms, and slower still when injected into the thighs and buttocks.

After you have been injecting insulin into your abdomen for several weeks, you probably know how long it will take for the insulin to take effect. This predictability can help you better manage your blood glucose.

If you were to suddenly switch to injecting insulin into your thigh, you might experience a different response. You might find that it takes longer for your insulin to take effect. Then it would be more difficult to meet your target blood glucose levels without adjusting what time you inject.

Other factors, such as body temperature, diet, exercise, and level of stress, affect your body's response to insulin. In general, anything that increases the blood flow to an area increases insulin absorption. Your response to insulin could even be the opposite of what you might expect, based on where you inject. For example, playing soccer for 2 hours may cause your insulin to be absorbed more quickly than usual so that your blood glucose level isn't where you expect it to be. So what can you do? Routinely check your blood glucose level. It is the only way to make sure you are having the response you had planned. Then you'll know if your site rotation plan is working for you.

***Exercise and Injection Sites.*** Strenuous exercise of muscles near an injection site can make the insulin act more rapidly than normal. This is because there is an increased flow of blood to exercising muscles. That doesn't necessarily mean that you should stop injecting insulin in the areas of your body you use during exercise. But if you notice that your insulin is peaking faster than you would expect when you exercise, you might want to think about the absorption rate. In general, it's a good idea to avoid strenuous exercise during the peak action times of your insulin. Insulin plus exercise can lead to a low blood sugar (hypoglycemia).

When you exercise, you have to decide whether to eat more or take less insulin. That's because exercise and insulin both decrease the amount of glucose in the blood. And you don't want your blood glucose levels to get too low. Frequent blood glucose monitoring will help you figure out these ups and downs in blood glucose and how to keep things in balance.

***Skin Problems and Injection Sites.*** Two main skin problems can occur at insulin injection sites: lipoatrophy and hypertrophy. With lipoatrophy, fatty tissue under the skin disappears, causing dents in the skin at the injection site. Hypertrophy is the overgrowth of cells, usually fat cells, that makes the skin look lumpy. It can look similar to scar tissue. By rotating the injection site, you can avoid some of these problems. There is also the possibility that some of the problems are caused by the type of insulin you are using.

Lipoatrophy is probably caused by an immune reaction, although its exact cause is not known. Your body is responding to insulin as an injected "foreign" substance. This problem is not common with human insulin. Make sure you are using highly purified insulin, preferably human.

Hypertrophy is not an immune reaction, so you don't have to change your insulin if you are having this problem. But you do need to change injection sites to avoid this. When the same sites are used over and over again, fat deposits can accumulate in the area. This is also called *lipohypertrophy.* You may be reluctant to change because injections seem less painful in these areas. This can be true because the hypertrophy can numb the area. On the other hand, injections can sometimes be more painful in these areas. The abnormal cell growth can limit the absorption of your insulin. Do not inject into the lumps. Insulin action can be restricted by not being able to move through the tissue. Inject away from the lumps and remember to rotate the sites. Ask a member of your health care team to check your injection sites periodically.

## Insulin Pumps

Insulin pumps have come a long way in recent years. These devices are miniature, computerized pumps, about the size of a cell phone, that you can wear on your belt or in your pocket. A pump sends a steady, measured amount of basal insulin through a piece of flexible plastic tubing to a small catheter that is inserted just under the skin and taped in place. This way of delivering insulin is called continuous subcutaneous insulin infusion, or CSII. You can program the pump to send a surge, or bolus, of insulin into your body. You do this just before eating to adjust for the rise in blood glucose that will come as your food digests.

If you use insulin frequently, you have probably thought about getting an insulin pump from time to time. But maybe it seemed too costly or inconvenient. Maybe you didn't like the idea of being hooked to a machine or changing your diabetes care routine so abruptly. Pumps today weigh less than 4 ounces, so they are easy to wear. You can remove the pump for an hour or two for special occasions and still keep your glucose where you want it. The cost of a pump is high. But with a prescription, and persistence on your part, most insurance companies will pay for all or part of it.

***Paying for the Pump.*** Insulin pumps can cost up to $6,000. Monthly maintenance can run $300 or more, including insulin, infusion sets, and blood testing supplies. If your insurance company will cover them, you're all set. But some insurance companies won't pay the start-up or maintenance costs of the pump. What to do?

- Keep asking! Keep in mind that it took many years, much research, and lots of people asking to convince insurance companies to pay for other therapeutic measures, such as prescription footwear, that have long-term health benefits.

- Your provider should be your most convincing advocate. He or she may have to write several letters and make several calls to your insurance company with details of your need for the improved glucose levels that are possible on the pump.
- Ask your diabetes educator to write to your insurance company as well.
- Work on writing effective, informative letters. All letters should stress how lower glucose levels can mean fewer and less severe diabetes complications in the long run—which is also less expensive for the insurance company in the long run.

**How Pumps Work.** The pump is a marvel of technology:

- It beeps if clogged.
- It lets you know when the batteries run low.
- It has dosage limits to stop an accidental overdose.
- You can program it to change the amount of insulin pumped to match your metabolism.

However, insulin pumps are not foolproof. Although they will alert you when a clog stops the flow of insulin, they will not identify a slow flow. Even if you are using an insulin pump, you will still need to monitor your blood glucose frequently.

Pumps use rapid-acting or regular insulin. The insulin is pumped from a filled syringe or cartridge inside the pump through thin plastic tubing to a needle or catheter inserted under the skin. Depending on your insulin needs, the pump can hold a 1- or 2-day supply of insulin. The tubing comes in different lengths, but it is long enough to allow plenty of slack for normal body movement. The insulin pump sends a continuous flow of insulin that trickles through the tube into the injection site at a slow, steady (basal) rate, day and night. The basal rate for pumps can be adjusted from 0.1 to 10 units per hour, depending on your metabolism. Before you eat, you push a button to deliver an extra portion of insulin, called a *bolus*. You can program, or adjust, the size of the bolus, depending on how much carbohydrate you will be eating in your meal. Delivering a bolus of insulin is just like injecting your premeal shot of insulin when you take multiple injections—without the shot! Usually, you won't have to take an extra bolus when you eat between meals, unless the snack is large.

Your diabetes care provider or educator will help you calculate your basal and bolus insulin doses. The total basal dose over a day is some percentage of the total daily insulin dose that you've been injecting, perhaps 40 to 50 percent. The other 50 to 60 percent of your daily insulin dose is divided into the before-meal bolus doses, most of it at breakfast and dinner, and the remainder at lunch and bedtime. You will need to know how these doses were chosen, so you can learn to adjust them for fine-tuning.

A big advantage to using a pump is that you will have flexible insulin coverage for meals and snacks. You will have to spend a lot of time at the beginning to find the best basal rates, to find out when you need to adjust the basal rate, and to figure out how big a bolus you will need for each meal. You'll probably want to learn how to estimate the number of grams of carbohydrate in your meals so you can take the needed number of insulin units. This will help you even out your after-meal blood glucose levels. You'll avoid having big changes in blood glucose levels throughout the day. Eventually, this will lead to a more flexible eating schedule. Pumps still cannot automatically sense your body's need for insulin. It doesn't adjust by

## Unexplained High Blood Glucose Levels on the Insulin Pump

Have you considered these possibilities?

- The insulin: Is it expired? Has it been exposed to extreme heat or cold? Does it look clumped or filled with particles? Is the vial nearly empty? Have you used it for more than 1 month?
- The insertion site: Have you placed the needle in or near a scar or mole? Near your beltline or other area where there's friction from clothing? Does the site hurt? Is it red or swollen?
- The infusion set: Did the needle come out? Is insulin leaking around the infusion site? Is there blood or air in the infusion line? Is there a kink in the line? Did the line come loose from the pump? Has the infusion set been in place for more than 2 days? Think about changing the infusion line.
- The insulin pump: Is the basal rate set correctly? Has the battery run down? Was the cartridge of insulin placed correctly? Is it empty? Was the pump primed with insulin when a fresh cartridge was put in? Is the pump working correctly?

itself. You still need to take blood glucose readings throughout the day.

Where will you attach the needle for the insulin pump? Most people choose the abdomen for insulin delivery. This area is convenient to use and gives a reliable, uniform absorption of insulin. How you insert the insulin needle will be different for different brands of infusion sets. With some infusion sets, you use a needle to insert a catheter and then remove the needle, leaving the soft catheter under your skin. With other sets, you insert a short needle. Pumps are easy to remove temporarily because, after clamping the tubing, you can leave the infusion set (the needle and tubing or the soft Teflon catheter) in place. You reattach only the pump. Some infusion sets even have a quick-release feature.

You don't have to worry that it will hurt when you exercise or if someone bumps into your pump or infusion area. The needle or catheter should be comfortable at all times. If you see any redness or swelling at the infusion site, remove the needle or catheter right away and find a new infusion site. Discuss persistent problems (lasting longer than 24 hours) with your health care team.

Every 1 to 3 days, you'll need to replace the infusion set and move to a new insertion site. This helps you avoid infection at the insertion site or a clog in the infusion set. Place the new insertion site at least 1 inch away from the last insertion site on the abdomen. Just like with syringes, you need to avoid inserting the needle in scar tissue or moles and use a site rotation schedule.

Using the same insertion site too often or for too long can cause the same skin problems that develop when you don't rotate your syringe injection sites. Scarring can occur. Check your injection site every day to make sure no insulin is leaking out.

You'll need to wear the pump almost all the time. If you take the pump off, you'll need to resume a schedule of insulin injections. However, it is possible for you to take off the pump temporarily, but not for more than 1 to 2 hours. Your blood glucose levels will get high again quickly because you don't have any insulin. You may want to unhook during lovemaking or other physical activities that can lower blood glucose level. How long you can keep the pump off without an injection depends on how active you are when the pump is off. A dancer might be able to keep it off during an entire performance because exercise lowers blood glucose levels. Through experience and testing, you will figure out how long you can keep the pump off before you need to put it back on or take an insulin injection.

Like all things worthwhile, using a pump successfully takes practice. You will most likely have problems here and there. Perhaps the most common problem is mysterious high blood glucose levels. This occurs quickly when clogged or kinked tubing stops the flow of insulin and pressure builds up in the infusion line. Your pump will sound an alarm if this happens. This is not the only reason for high blood glucose levels. For instance, an infection or inflammation at the insertion site can develop and delay the absorption of insulin. See the box on page 124 for other things to consider when you have unexplained hyperglycemia on the pump.

**Should You Use a Pump?** Maybe you're already having trouble sticking to your current testing and injection routine. Then a more intense schedule, such as multiple daily injections or an insulin pump, may not be for you. However, the possible benefits may help you find a new level of commitment.

A major advantage of a pump is that you don't have to stop what you're doing to fill a syringe. Your insulin is delivered at the push of a button. You can do this anywhere and at any time. Pumps are also precise. You can set them to pump out as little as one-tenth of a unit (0.1 unit) of insulin per hour.

What are some other reasons for choosing a pump? Maybe you're planning a pregnancy and want the tightest control possible. Maybe you have to work odd hours at your job and it's hard enough to balance work, family, and meals during the week without having to adjust to a new injection schedule every weekend. Maybe you have had unwanted swings in blood glucose when injecting intermediate- or long-acting glucose, and you'd like to keep your blood glucose in check. People who want an insulin plan that adapts to day-to-day changes in their lifestyle might like an insulin pump. Making a list of personal advantages and disadvantages may help you decide. One of the most important factors is your level of commitment to this therapy. It does take work—especially at first. But many people find that the added flexibility and improved control are worth it.

***Choosing a Pump.*** There are several insulin pumps on the market today (see the *Resource Guide*). Your doctor or diabetes educator may prefer one brand over the other. Ask for his or her thoughts on each model. Your best bet may be to talk to other people who use pumps. Find out what they like and what they don't like about each model. Here are a few things you might want to know:

- Is it waterproof? Some models are waterproof and can be submerged for up to 30 minutes. Other models are splash proof or water resistant. Check to see whether you can shower, swim, or dive into a pool with the model you want.
- Can you adjust the basal rate for different times of day? Your pump can alter the rate up to 48 times a day. For example, your basal rate is likely to be greater from 3 a.m. to 7 a.m. than during the rest of the day.
- All pump manufacturers offer a 24-hour toll-free number. You will want to talk to service people about problems when you suspect the pump isn't working correctly.
- What kind of warranty does the manufacturer offer?
- How often do you have to change the batteries? How easy are the batteries to find, and how expensive are they? Batteries usually last 2 to 4 months.
- Do you want a pump that will help you calculate doses based on your blood glucose level and carbohydrate intake?

## Insulin Plans

How often should you inject insulin? There is no answer that is right for all people at all times. Different plans suit different people, depending on how easily managed your blood glucose levels are and how well you understand the way different foods and physical activity, and even stress, affect your blood glucose levels.

With **type 1 diabetes,** the pancreas no longer secretes insulin. The goal of insulin therapy is to mimic a normal pancreas as closely as possible. This often requires multiple daily injections of insulin or the use of an insulin pump and frequent blood glucose monitoring.

**Type 2 diabetes** can cause two different problems. In some people, not enough insulin is produced in relation to how much is needed by the body. Insulin is often needed along with meal planning and exercise. In addition, the cells in the body resist the action of the insulin that is produced. Diet and exercise and oral diabetes medications alone or with insulin may be needed. Therapies for type 2 diabetes may have to take into account both lack of insulin and resistance to insulin. Because their bodies make and release natural insulin, people with type 2 diabetes may be able to manage blood glucose by changing their eating and exercise habits. Others will need oral diabetes medication and still others will need insulin in addition to diet and exercise.

Some women with **gestational diabetes** manage the high blood glucose levels caused by insulin resistance without insulin therapy. Others need the help of insulin.

Insulin plans can use one, two, or three types of insulin. This means using rapid-acting or regular (short-acting) insulin and, for some people, also using a longer-acting insulin. When deciding on an insulin plan, you and your diabetes care pro-

## When Will Insulin Take Effect?

| Type of insulin | When it works | When taken | When it's active | Blood test that shows its effect |
|---|---|---|---|---|
| Rapid or short acting | Rapid: Begins to work within 15 minutes after injection, peaks in about 1 hour, and continues to work for 3–4 hours. Short acting: Begins to work within 30 minutes, peaks 2–3 hours later, and continues to work for 3–6 hours. | With or before a meal | Between that meal and the next meal | After that meal and before the next meal |
| Intermediate acting | Begins to work about 2–4 hours after injection, peaks 4–10 hours later, and is effective for about 12–18 hours. | Before breakfast | Between lunch and dinner | Before dinner |
| | | Before dinner or bedtime | Overnight | Before breakfast |
| Long acting | Begins to work 2–4 hours after injection and usually lasts 20–24 hours. | Before breakfast or before dinner or half dose at each time | Overnight, because short-acting insulin hides its effect during the day | Before breakfast |

vider will consider how to match your personal goals and needs, both medical and practical, to a combination of insulin type, dose, and schedule. You also need to know when the different injections of insulin are likely to have an effect on your blood glucose levels (see the table on page 129).

Most insulin plans try to mimic the effects a normal pancreas could produce (see Graph 1, page 131). A pancreas puts out a steady stream of insulin (a basal or baseline dose) day and night. It also secretes an extra dose of insulin (a bolus) in response to meals. This is the way insulin pumps are usually set up. If insulin injections are preferred, a longer-acting insulin is used to mimic the basal insulin secretion. To substitute for the bolus of insulin, a dose of rapid-acting or regular insulin is usually given before each meal. Which combination of short- and long-acting insulins you use is up to you and your provider. Together, work out a plan that will suit your life and schedule. If your plan is not working out for you, talk to your provider. There are usually many other plans you can try.

## One Shot a Day

A single shot of insulin can sometimes be enough to bring the blood glucose into the target range. Usually, a long-acting insulin such as glargine or intermediate-acting insulin such as NPH is given at bedtime or in the morning. The insulin is used to provide the basal level of insulin. Long-acting insulins provide a steady level of insulin throughout the day and night. Taking intermediate-acting insulin at bedtime helps lower your fasting glucose level. Taking intermediate-acting insulin in the morning provides some coverage for the food you eat as well as basal insulin.

Graph 1 shows what happens during the course of the day for people who do not have diabetes. Graphs 2 and 3 show what happens during the course of the day when these insulins

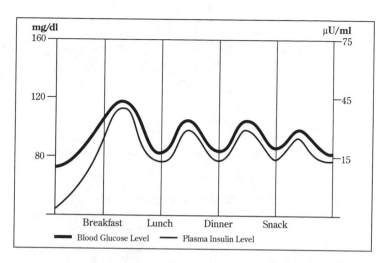

**Graph 1: Typical changes in glucose and insulin levels over 24 hours in someone without diabetes.**

are used once a day. As you can see, there isn't always insulin available from this one injection to provide the bolus of insulin that is needed for meals. Taking one shot a day can also mean that you are more locked into a schedule for your meals. If you take an intermediate-acting insulin, you will need to eat when your insulin is peaking, whether it is convenient or not.

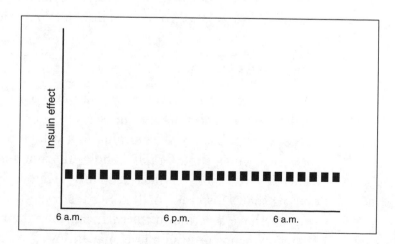

**Graph 2: One shot of long-acting insulin.**

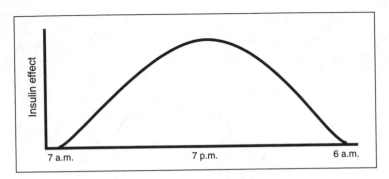

**Graph 3: One shot of intermediate-acting insulin.**

If you take one shot of long- or intermediate-acting insulin, there are several ways to get the bolus of insulin you need for meals. Some people with type 2 diabetes may be able to make enough insulin to cover the post-meal increase in blood glucose. For these people, providing the basal insulin helps their pancreas to do its job better. Another option is to take oral diabetes medications. These medications can provide the coverage needed for meals. Still another possibility is to take a combination of insulins. You can take a rapid- or short-acting insulin along with your morning shot of NPH insulin. This gives you a bolus of insulin to cover your breakfast meal. You can either use pre-mixed insulins or mix two types of insulin in one injection.

## More than One Shot

You may get better coverage by splitting your one shot of insulin into two shots. These can be given in the morning and in the evening. Usually, the morning shot will be a bigger dose than the evening shot. Graph 4 shows the amount of insulin available if you split your intermediate dose into a morning and evening shot. However, you'll notice that even with this plan, you may have a period in the early morning, between 3 and 10 a.m., when your insulin level may be low.

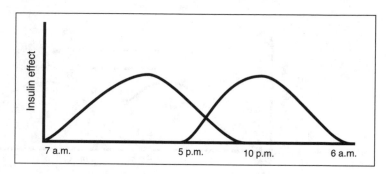

**Graph 4: Intermediate-acting insulin split into two shots.**

One way to improve your coverage is to also mix rapid- or short-acting insulin with each intermediate dose (see Graphs 5 and 6). The rapid-acting or regular insulin provides the mealtime bolus. If you use rapid-acting, the insulin is taken with meals. Doses with regular insulin are taken about 30 minutes before breakfast and dinner, as shown in Graph 6. As you can see in these graphs, as the rapid-acting or regular insulin

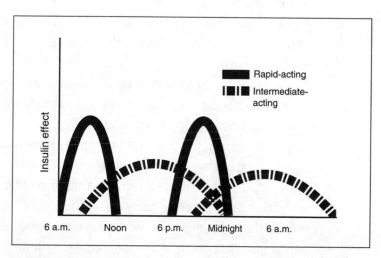

**Graph 5: A combination of intermediate- and rapid-acting insulins.**

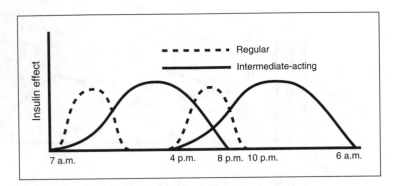

**Graph 6: Split and mixed regular and intermediate-acting insulin in two shots.**

decreases, the intermediate insulin starts to work. Just when the intermediate insulin starts to wear off before dinnertime, another mixed dose is given. Again, the rapid-acting or regular insulin kicks in early, and the intermediate insulin picks up the slack to carry you through the night.

It may take a little experimenting and consulting with your health care team to figure out how to best mix rapid-acting or regular and intermediate-acting insulins. The ratio may change until you are getting the results that best suit you. You may find it convenient to buy a premixed insulin, such as a 70/30 or 75/25 mixture. Or you may prefer to split and mix the doses yourself. This lets you change the amounts of rapid-acting or regular and NPH independently of each other. You may find this helpful when trying to account for activity level and food intake.

If you are using a two-shot plan using split and mixed doses of intermediate-acting and rapid-acting or regular insulin, you will need to keep close tabs on your body's response. This means that you need to monitor your blood glucose levels before and after meals. You may need to monitor at other times as well. A two-shot program gives you better coverage than a single-shot plan but still keeps you closely tied to a regular meal schedule and a regular pattern of activity. This is because you cannot make short-term adjustments in longer-acting insulins. Only rapid-acting or regular insulin can be adjusted immediately to respond to a blood glucose level or change in schedule.

If you find that your blood glucose level is fine at bedtime but high in the morning, you may want to move your evening insulin shot from dinnertime to bedtime. This will make insulin available a little later during the course of the night to keep your glucose levels in range. Make sure that your glucose levels are on target during the evening hours if you try this adjustment.

You may find that you have low blood glucose in the early morning (around 2 or 3 a.m.) with the two-shot plan. If this is the case, think about a three-shot plan. With this, you would give yourself a mixture of rapid- or short-acting and intermediate-acting insulin at breakfast, a rapid- or short-acting insulin at dinner, and an intermediate-acting insulin at bedtime. The insulin levels throughout the day are shown in Graph 7.

The more often you inject insulin, the more opportunities you have to fine-tune your control. You also have more freedom and flexibility with your schedule and food choices. One such plan uses three or four shots a day. A common example is to take rapid-acting insulin before all meals. The dose is based

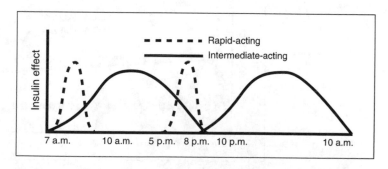

**Graph 7: Three shots: split and mixed morning dose, rapid-acting dinner dose, and intermediate-acting evening dose.**

on the carbohydrates eaten at that meal. A long-acting insulin such as glargine provides the basal dose of insulin (see Graph 8). The injections of rapid-acting insulin provide the bolus for the three meals. To make this plan work for you, you need to monitor your blood frequently. Then you can adjust the amounts of rapid-acting or regular insulin given before each meal to

- cover the carbohydrates in your meal;
- lower a high blood glucose level not sufficiently lowered by the previous rapid-acting injection;
- anticipate the rise in blood glucose caused by the next meal.

The goal is to keep your blood glucose levels within your target range.

## Timing Your Insulin Injections

Knowing when to give your injection, or take your premeal bolus by pump, can be confusing. Rapid- and short-acting

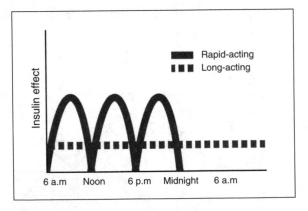

**Graph 8: Three rapid-acting doses and one long-acting dose.**

## Examples of Insulin Plans

| Before breakfast | Before lunch | Before dinner | Before bedtime |
|---|---|---|---|
| | | | Intermediate or long acting |
| Mixture of rapid or short and intermediate acting | | | |
| Mixture of rapid or short and intermediate acting | | Mixture of rapid or short and intermediate acting | |
| Mixture of rapid or short and intermediate acting | | Rapid or short acting | Intermediate acting |
| Rapid or short acting | Rapid or short acting | Rapid or short acting | Intermediate acting* |
| Rapid or short acting | Rapid or short acting | Rapid or short acting | Long acting** |

*The intermediate-acting dose can also be given before dinner.
**The long-acting insulin dose can be taken at bedtime or before dinner or split in half, with half taken before breakfast and half before dinner.

insulins are taken before meals or very big snacks to counter-act the increase in blood glucose that will occur as food is absorbed. Rapid-acting insulins begin to work in about 5–15 minutes. You can take your injection just before you eat. Taking your injection more than 15 minutes before meals can result in a hypoglycemic reaction. Regular insulin takes about 15–30 minutes to start working. If regular insulin is taken too close to the start of a meal, the food will cause blood glucose levels to go too high before the insulin has had a chance to be absorbed for use.

How much in advance of your meal you need to take your regular insulin depends on your blood glucose level before the meal. Try checking about 45 minutes before you plan to start eating. If your blood sugar level is high, you need to inject your regular insulin quickly to help counteract your already high blood glucose level before food sends it even higher. You may also want to postpone your meal for a short time. If your blood sugar level is low, you need to wait to inject regular insulin closer to the time you'll start eating. Inject at the end of the meal if your blood sugar level is 50 mg/dl or lower. If you can't check your blood glucose, a general guideline is to take regular insulin 30 minutes before your meal.

## Intensive Diabetes Management

Intensive insulin therapy is defined as taking three or more injections a day. But it's more than just taking shots. It also means more blood glucose checks and spending more time thinking about and caring for your diabetes. So why would you do it? Well, more shots and more monitoring give you more flexibility and spontaneity. It can also keep your blood glucose levels more even and on target. You'll feel better now and lower your risk for future complications. But is it for you? Ask yourself the following:

- Am I unhappy with my blood glucose levels?
- Do my blood glucose checks frequently show unexpected levels, high or low?
- Are my glucose checks frequently out of range?
- Do I have any signs of the complications of diabetes?
- Do I lack the amount of energy I need to participate in all my activities—both day and night?
- Do I want more flexibility in my lifestyle for timing meals, exercise, and other activities?

If you answer "yes" to any of these questions, you may want to investigate the idea of intensive diabetes management. See Chapter 7 for more information.

# Keeping Your Glucose on Target | 5

*Each day, you try again to solve the diabetes challenge: how to keep blood glucose near normal with so many things pushing it up or down.*

## Why Monitor Your Glucose?

Why should you have to pay special attention to your glucose levels? If you take insulin or oral diabetes medications regularly and watch your diet, shouldn't that take care of everything? Probably not. Blood glucose levels change throughout the day. This is true for both type 1 and type 2 diabetes:

↑ Food pushes the blood glucose level up.
↓ Insulin or an oral diabetes medication brings it down.
↑ Stress drives it up.
↓ Exercise can bring it down.
↑ Illness makes it rise.

Diet, activity, stress, and overall general health all affect blood glucose levels. Everyone with diabetes responds somewhat differently to each of these. It would be wonderful if there was a magic formula to tell you how to arrive at the right blood glucose level. Instead, you'll need to discover how each of these factors affects your blood glucose level. Knowing how much to eat, how much to exercise, and how much insulin or medication to take is not always easy. You are likely to feel frustrated at times. Look to your health care team for support. They can also help you learn to understand the meaning of your self-monitoring results and what to do about them.

## You're in Charge

Monitoring your blood glucose allows you to make decisions about your diabetes management. You wouldn't want to guess which road to take on a car trip—why guess how much insulin to take or how much to eat? Your blood glucose check can act as your road map, telling you which turns to take.

Here's something else to keep in mind: If your blood glucose levels swing too high or too low during the course of the day, you could develop some serious problems. Some of these problems can be risky in the short term and result in a life-threatening crisis. For example, if your blood glucose levels drop too low and you don't treat it, you could become unconscious. High blood sugar may not cause an immediate emergency but may lead to severe complications over time. People with a history of chronic high blood glucose levels can develop debilitating eye disease, kidney disease, circulation problems, or nerve disease.

The best way to lead a healthy life is to take charge of your diabetes. You do this by managing glucose levels with food, exercise, and medication. And the single most important thing you can do for yourself is keep track of the amount of glucose in your blood on a regular basis. Instead of saying "I feel great" or "I feel lousy," take measurements and keep records. These records tell you how well your diabetes plan is working. Monitoring is the only way to know how your body responds to food, insulin, activity, and stress. Without knowing this, you can't make changes in your diabetes care plan. Trial and error—and a little patience—will help you reach your glucose goals.

## What Affects Glucose in the Blood?

### Food

Your body breaks down the carbohydrate in the food you eat to glucose. Glucose travels through your blood to nourish every part of your body. When you eat, the amount of glucose in your blood goes up. How much your blood glucose rises after a meal depends on many things. Different foods have different amounts of carbohydrate and will produce different amounts of glucose. How much of a food you eat at one time changes how much glucose is produced. Carbohydrates come in several forms that take various amounts of time to be digested and that affect the blood glucose differently. Fat or protein can slow down digestion and the rate at which glucose levels rise. High-protein foods can raise blood glucose levels but do so more slowly than foods containing mostly carbohydrate.

One way to take charge is to learn how the food you eat affects your blood glucose levels. You may be surprised at how your glucose levels respond to different foods. Measure your blood glucose 1 to 2 hours after you eat particular foods. Do you find that your blood glucose rises faster with carrots than with sweet potatoes? Or faster with mashed potatoes than with ice cream? What about a serving of meat versus a slice of bread? By figuring out how your body responds, you can make adjustments in your plan, so that your blood glucose will not rise too high, too quickly.

You will want to match what you eat with the amount of insulin or oral diabetes medication in your blood. It may take you a while to learn how your body responds to the insulin you take and to the food you eat. A registered dietitian or nurse educator can help you balance your diet and insulin intake. If you are taking other medications to help lower your blood glucose, your dietitian can also help you balance your food intake and response to medication. Work with your dietitian to make a plan that fits your tastes and culture. If there are particular foods you want, be sure to make a plan that includes them. You need a plan that you can use on a daily basis.

## Insulin

As your body digests the food you eat, glucose builds up in the blood. In people without diabetes, glucose signals the body to release insulin. Insulin then lets glucose into the cells that need it. Without insulin, cells in the body can't get the energy they need to live and grow. In people with type 1 diabetes, the body no longer makes insulin. Glucose can't get to the cells that need it. In people with type 2 diabetes, the body makes and releases insulin, but the insulin has problems in getting enough glucose into the cells that need it.

The body carefully balances the amount of glucose and insulin in the blood. It works almost like a thermostat. When there is too much glucose in the blood, insulin is released. Insulin reduces the amount of glucose in the blood. Then, when glucose levels drop, insulin is no longer secreted. The body balances the amount of insulin and glucose to keep glucose at a fairly even level throughout the day. It keeps a little bit of insulin ready to go to work at a moment's notice. For meals, it releases the right amount of extra insulin in time to clear glucose from the blood before the glucose levels climb too high.

People with diabetes need to try to strike a balance between insulin and glucose, much like the body does naturally. Too much insulin, and glucose levels may fall too fast or too low. Too little insulin, and glucose builds up in the blood. By testing blood glucose levels before and after meals, you can learn how much a given dose of insulin will reduce your blood glucose level.

If you use regular insulin, timing your injections and meals is important. If you eat too soon after an injection of regular insulin, your glucose can climb too high. If you wait too long after an injection, your blood glucose can fall too low. This is also a consideration if you are taking any type of sulfonylurea or glitinide, oral diabetes medications that lower glucose by increasing insulin release. Also, where you inject insulin can affect timing. Many people have found that they get the most reliable timing in insulin action when they use the abdomen as the injection site.

For best results, inject regular insulin 30 to 45 minutes before you eat. Rapid-acting insulin can be injected at or just before mealtime.

You also need to match the amount of insulin you take to the amount of food you eat. If you inject the usual dose of insulin and then eat more than you had planned, you may end up with high glucose. On the other hand, if you don't eat as much as you thought you would, your blood glucose level will drop too low.

Even if you eat the same amount and exercise the same amount every day, you won't always be able to predict how your body takes in and uses the insulin you inject. The amount of insulin your body absorbs can change by 25 percent or more from day to day. This is especially true for NPH insulin. So don't be surprised by differences. The way to adjust for these changes is to test your blood glucose and increase or decrease your next insulin dose.

For more information on food, see Chapter 8.

## Exercise

If you are used to exercising and you have just been diagnosed with diabetes, you might be wondering whether you will be able to continue your workouts. (Of course you will!) If you are not yet in the swing of things, it's time to think about beginning an exercise program. Everyone needs to be physically active—it's good for your overall health. It can help prevent heart disease and other health problems. Regardless of your type of diabetes, exercise can have many positive benefits.

Not only does exercise make you feel and look good, it improves blood flow and muscle tone. It can even help you handle stress. Aerobic exercise gives your heart and lungs an especially good workout. It makes your heart pump harder and gets the blood flowing through even your smallest blood vessels. This helps prevent the circulation and foot problems that people with diabetes can get. Walking is something that almost everyone can do and is very effective as an all-around exercise.

When you exercise, your muscles work harder and use up the glucose they have stored for fuel. When the glucose stored in muscle runs low, glucose from the blood is used. Exercise can help use up some of the glucose that builds up in the blood. And exercise has another bonus for people with diabetes. It seems to make muscles and other tissues more sensitive to insulin, so less insulin is needed to move glucose out of the blood and into muscle cells. If you exercise regularly, you may be able to eat a little more or inject a little less insulin. Some people with type 2 diabetes find that they no longer have to take insulin or other diabetes medication once they start a regular exercise program. However, to be safe, talk it over with your health care team before you start an exercise program or make changes in your diet, insulin, or medication.

If you have type 2 diabetes, you can count on regular exercise to help with your weight and to increase your body's sensitivity to insulin and other medications. Exercise may be just as important as eating healthy meals. For people with type 1 diabetes, exercise can lower your risk of cardiovascular disease, help with weight, and allow you to use less insulin on the days you work out. But instead of using exercise to manage your diabetes, it is something you must account for in terms of food and insulin. For example, on days you have a 1-hour aerobics class after dinner, you may need to eat extra carbohydrates at dinner or inject less insulin.

You need to take special precautions when you exercise. You want to make sure that your blood glucose levels don't drop too far too fast. This can also happen in the hours after exercise, although this is more common in people with type 1 diabetes. This is when your muscles take glucose from the blood to restore their glucose reserves. So even if your glucose level seems on target right after exercising, don't assume it will stay that way during the hours following your workout. It's a good idea to check blood glucose levels several hours after exercise as well.

On the other hand, if you have type 1 diabetes and your blood glucose levels are too high (over 250 mg/dl) when you exercise, activity may cause your blood glucose level to go up rather than down. Hard exercise with too little insulin can make the liver release stored glucose. If you have type 1 diabetes and your blood glucose is greater than 250 mg/dl, test your urine for ketones. Do not exercise if significant ketones are present. Use caution if your blood glucose is greater than 300 mg/dl, even if no ketones are present. Ask your health care team for guidelines about exercise and blood glucose levels.

For more on exercise, see Chapter 9.

## Stress

Everyone seems stressed out these days. And living with diabetes adds even more stress to your life. People with diabetes sometimes try to do more than everyone else, just to prove that diabetes doesn't make them any different. But you, too, need to allow yourself enough time to relax and recover from the stresses of everyday life.

Stress can produce hormones that can shoot your blood glucose levels up and out of your desired range. Stress can also be a hidden contributor to unexpected swings in blood glucose levels. The effect of an angry driver who cuts you off on the interstate can't be as easily measured as grams of carbohydrate, units of insulin, or calories burned during exercise. When you can't figure out why your blood glucose level is so high despite "doing everything right," think about the stresses in your life. Also, think about how you respond to stress. Do you eat when you are under stress? This can bring up blood glucose levels. Do stressful situations make you more active than usual? This response can decrease blood glucose levels.

## Illness

When you're sick, your body is also stressed. To deal with this stress, your body releases hormones that help you fight the illness. But these hormones also counteract the effect of insulin in lowering blood glucose and cause blood glucose levels to go up. Sickness can cause your diabetes to go out of control. Extremely high blood glucose levels caused by illness can also lead to diabetic ketoacidosis in people with type 1 diabetes and to hyperosmolar hyperglycemic syndrome (HHS) in people with type 2 diabetes. (See the section on emergencies on page 161.)

Blood glucose monitoring is especially important during any bout of sickness. Even if you have type 2 diabetes and only

## Sick-Day Action Plan

Before your next illness, decide on an action plan with your health care team. Include the following:

- When to call the doctor.
- How often to monitor your blood glucose.
- Whether you should test your urine for ketones. Ketones are produced when fats instead of glucose are used for energy. Most commonly, this is a sign that not enough insulin is available to help your body break down glucose. (Less commonly, when carbohydrates are very restricted, ketones can appear in the blood. This is called *starvation ketosis*.) When blood glucose levels are high during illness, ketones can appear if extra insulin is not given.
- Medication changes that might be needed. You need to know how much extra insulin to take to bring down unusually high blood glucose levels. If you take oral diabetes medications, you need to know whether you should continue taking them or increase or decrease the dose.
- Whether you need to have anti-nausea suppositories or over-the-counter cold or flu or cough medications on hand, which ones are good choices, and when to take them.
- How to choose foods and fluids during your illness.

monitor once a day, you may want to keep a closer check during times of illness. Be sure to talk to your health care team before you get ill about what you should do in the event of illness. You and your health care team can work together to come up with a plan to help you handle common illnesses such as colds or the flu.

Along with eating chicken soup and drinking lots of liquids, here are a few things you can do when you are feeling under the weather:

- If you have type 1 diabetes, continue to take your insulin—even if you can't eat. You may even need extra insulin to take care of the excess glucose your body releases when you are sick. Ask your provider about what blood glucose levels call for a change in your insulin dose.
- Monitor your blood glucose and ketone levels about every 3 to 4 hours. If the levels are too high or you are pregnant, you may need to monitor more often.
- Make substitutions for your usual food if nausea and vomiting are making it difficult to eat. Try to eat or drink your usual amount of carbohydrates. Talk to your dietitian about ways to cover your basic eating plan. Prepare a sick-day plan before you even become sick. Try to keep some comforting foods like soup or frozen fruit bars on hand, especially during the cold and flu season.
- Drink plenty of caffeine-free liquids. If you are losing fluids by vomiting, from fever, or from diarrhea, you may need nondiet soft drinks or sports drinks with sugar or carbohydrate. This can help prevent the hypoglycemia caused by not eating or taking extra insulin. If vomiting or diarrhea is severe, try sipping 3 to 6 ounces an hour to keep your blood glucose even.
- Keep a thermometer on hand and a small supply of common sick-day medications that are safe to take. Be sure to read the labels.

Some cold medicines sold over-the-counter to treat colds and flu can affect your blood glucose level. Many cough and cold remedies labeled "decongestant" contain ingredients (such as pseudoephedrine) that raise blood glucose levels and blood pressure. Talk to the pharmacist or your provider before you take any over-the-counter medication.

In addition, some cough and cold remedies contain sugar and alcohol. Make sure you read the label and find out exactly what "active ingredients" as well as "inactive ingredients" any medication contains. A small amount of sugar or alcohol is probably fine, as long as you are aware you are taking it. If you will be taking frequent or high doses of a particular medicine, try to find a sugar-free version. Alcohol is a common ingredient in nighttime cold medications, but alcohol-free alternatives are available.

Pain medications are also usually safe in small doses. You don't have to worry about taking an occasional aspirin for a headache or fever. Also, many people with diabetes take a daily coated "baby" aspirin to protect against cardiovascular disease. This is safe for people with diabetes. Ibuprofen is not safe for anyone with kidney disease. People with diabetes should not take ibuprofen unless a provider advises it. This drug could cause acute renal failure in people with kidney problems.

***It's Time to Call Your Provider.*** Call your diabetes care provider if you experience any of the following:

- You have been sick for 1 or 2 days without improvement.
- You have had vomiting or diarrhea for more than 6 hours.
- You have moderate to large amounts of ketones in your urine.
- You are taking insulin and your blood glucose levels continue to be over 250 mg/dl or the level determined by you and your provider.
- You have type 2 diabetes, you are taking oral diabetes medication, and your premeal blood glucose levels are 250 mg/dl or higher for more than 24 hours.

- You have signs of extreme hyperglycemia (very dry mouth or fruity odor to the breath), dehydration, or loss of mental competence (confusion, disorientation).
- You are sleepier than normal.
- You have stomach or chest pain or any difficulty breathing.
- You have any doubts or questions about what you need to do for your illness.

When you call, you need to have some information ready. Keeping records during your illness will make it easier to figure out how sick you are. This will also help you and your provider keep track of your progress in getting well. Tell your provider the following information:

- your blood glucose level and your urine ketone results, starting when you first realized you were ill
- what insulin doses and diabetes pills you have taken and when you took them
- other medications you have taken
- how long you have been sick
- your temperature
- how well you can take foods and fluids
- if you have lost weight while sick
- any other symptoms you may have
- your pharmacist's phone number

## Monitoring Your Blood Glucose

You can keep your long-range diabetes management goals, such as staying healthy, on track by making and aiming for shorter-term goals. Shorter-term goals in diabetes management usually focus on measurements of your blood glucose level that you take yourself, which is called self-monitoring of blood glucose.

## Who Needs It?

If you have type 1 diabetes or you have type 2 diabetes and you take insulin, you need to monitor. If you have type 2 diabetes and take oral diabetes medications, check with your health care

FACT OR MYTH?

### "I can tell my blood glucose level without checking."

 Some people with diabetes claim they have a sixth sense: knowing their blood glucose level. It would be a wonderful sense to have, but it's just not reliable. Checking your blood glucose is the only way to go.

However, you can learn more about sensing the clues your body or behavior gives about your blood glucose level by attending a class or series of classes on hypoglycemia prevention and recognition. This education can be very valuable to anyone with diabetes, but especially for people who have stopped recognizing symptoms of severe low blood glucose (hypoglycemia unawareness). Just as jet pilots can be trained to recognize and react to signs of oxygen deprivation, you can become better aware of your cues of possible hypoglycemia:

- autonomic: heart rate, trembling, sweating
- mental: slow thinking and lack of concentration and coordination
- mood: irritation or aggression

You are more likely to develop hypoglycemia if you have missed a meal, taken your insulin early, eaten later, or worked out harder or longer than normal.

Cues for hyperglycemia are much harder to detect. Look for increased thirst and urination and blurry vision.

team about whether and how often you need to monitor. If you have gestational diabetes and take insulin, you need to monitor. Insulin and oral diabetes medications are powerful drugs that lower blood glucose. You can tell how well they are doing their job by keeping track of your blood glucose. It can help you figure out how much medication you need to take to keep your after-meal blood glucose levels in your target range. Monitoring will also let you see how exercise affects your blood glucose. Also, when you use these medications, you are at risk for low blood glucose levels. Monitoring will tell you if your blood glucose is low, so you don't have to guess. It can also guide you in deciding how much carbohydrate you need as a treatment.

If you have type 2 diabetes or gestational diabetes and manage it with an eating and exercise plan, you don't need to worry about low blood glucose levels. However, monitoring blood glucose may be helpful to you. It gives you feedback on how well your diabetes care is working. Positive feedback may be a wonderful source of encouragement for you. You can see the effects of your exercise program or food choices on your blood glucose levels. For pregnant women, it guides the treatment adjustments that will help keep you and your baby healthy.

## How Much Monitoring?

How often you decide to measure your blood glucose depends on your reasons for checking it. If you use the results to adjust your next insulin injection or your food intake, then you need to check your blood glucose level each time before you inject or eat a meal. This would mean three to four checks a day. You might also monitor after meals to see if you gave the right insulin dose.

On the other hand, you may only be taking one or two insulin shots each day or oral medications. If this is the case, you may decide to monitor just two times each day.

If you aim for blood glucose levels close to normal, it's essential to monitor at least four, and sometimes eight, times a day. You would check before and after each meal and before bedtime every day and in the middle of the night (around 3 a.m.) about once a week. Studies have shown a relationship between the number of blood checks a day and A1C levels. When monitoring drops to less than four tests a day, glucose levels worsen.

Blood glucose levels in people with type 2 diabetes are often more stable over the course of a day. If you take oral diabetes medications, you don't need as many blood checks as someone taking insulin. You can't use the results to fine-tune your next dose. You will monitor frequently while you are trying to find the best dose of medication for you or when there's a change in your care plan (such as a new exercise routine). Finding the best dose of oral medication can be as tricky as finding the right amount and timing for insulin injections. While you are making adjustments, you could be surprised by unexpected hypoglycemia. During this period, check your blood glucose once or twice a day (before breakfast and one other time during the day). Occasionally, you may want to check 2 hours after meals to see how well the medication is working with your meal plan. Your monitoring records will help you and your health care team decide what changes, if any, are needed. But once your blood glucose levels are closer to normal, monitoring one or two times a day may be fine for you.

If you manage your type 2 diabetes without medications, once your blood glucose levels are stable, you might monitor once or twice a day, three or four times a week, or not at all. But you can always check when you're curious about what your blood glucose level might be, such as after a special dinner or an extra-strenuous workout.

How often you monitor depends on how often you're willing to prick your finger, how you use the information, what your schedule permits, and what supplies you can afford. More frequent monitoring means you have to spend more money on supplies.

Sometimes you might not be feeling quite right and you don't know why. Monitoring your blood glucose may tell you what the problem is. Maybe you're feeling sweaty and a little shaky after a 3-mile run. Maybe you're just tired from the workout, or maybe you're having a low blood glucose reaction. Without monitoring, you may tend to eat because you think your blood glucose level is too low, when it is really too high. Only by monitoring your blood glucose can you tell what your body really needs.

Over time, you will gain confidence in your ability to manage your diabetes. You may think it's okay to monitor less often. Beware! It's tempting to think you can tell what your glucose level is by the way you feel. But research shows that most people cannot guess their glucose level reliably. Guessing is dangerous, especially if your blood glucose levels tend to swing with little warning.

## When to Check Your Blood Glucose?

Once again, this depends on your particular reasons for monitoring. You have many choices. Check whenever you like. However, if you are on the lookout for patterns, there are standard times to check your blood glucose:

- before breakfast, lunch, and dinner (or an especially big snack)
- before you go to bed
- 1 to 2 hours after breakfast, lunch, and dinner (or an especially big snack)
- at 2 or 3 a.m.

## When to Do Extra Blood Glucose Checks

- when you're ill
- if you suspect low blood glucose
- before you drive (if you take insulin)
- when you have trouble recognizing the warning signs of hypoglycemia
- when you're physically more active than usual
- if you start taking a nondiabetes medication that affects blood glucose levels or your ability to recognize low blood glucose warning signs
- if you have insulin reactions at night or wake up with high blood glucose levels
- when you are changing your insulin plan, your meal plan, or your exercise routine
- when you have lost or gained weight
- when your levels have been outside your target range more often than in your range

If you have type 2 diabetes or gestational diabetes managed without medications, you can learn a lot by checking your blood glucose levels regularly. It helps you keep track of your diabetes and see how all your efforts are working. One approach is to measure your fasting (prebreakfast) blood glucose levels routinely. It can also help to check your blood glucose at different times during the day—for example, before and after exercise, before and after meals, or at bedtime. This gives you a better idea of what is happening with your blood glucose levels.

## Blood Glucose Goals

| Time of check | Recommended levels |
|---|---|
| Before meals | 90 to 130 mg/dl |
| After meals | less than 180 mg/dl |

## Choosing Your Blood Glucose Goals

Choosing blood glucose goals can be easy. You can simply use the guidelines supported by the American Diabetes Association (see table on this page). However, these goals may not be easy for you to reach. Or they may not be right for you. Why not see what your blood glucose levels are before and after meals and compare them to the goals in the table? Then choose a realistic goal for the short term.

Whether you have type 1 or type 2 diabetes or gestational diabetes, the goal of diabetes care is the same: to keep blood glucose as close as possible to that of a person without diabetes. For many people with diabetes, getting normal blood glucose levels (like a person without diabetes) just isn't realistic or even desirable. For instance, if you are elderly and live alone, you may be more concerned with preventing severe low blood glucose than avoiding long-term complications. Talk with your health care

**TIP**

Blood glucose goals for children are looser. For example, the target range may be 100 to 200 mg/dl. Most children under the age of 6 or 7 are not yet able to be aware of and respond to oncoming low blood glucose, and it's very important to limit episodes of low blood glucose. Tailor goals to the age and abilities of the child and be flexible with goals as the child grows.

team about your goals and how to reach them. Choose goals based on your needs, lifestyle, and health. You will be able to reach realistic goals. You will not be able to reach unrealistic ones, and setting but not reaching them will only hurt your self-confidence.

Perhaps you can make changes, a few at a time, to slowly lower your blood glucose levels. Here are some things you may want to change:

- how much food you eat
- the kinds of food you eat
- how much exercise you get
- how much insulin or medication you take

Write down an acceptable blood glucose range for you at this time. The range could be something like 70 to 200 mg/dl. This means that any reading under 70 mg/dl is too low. Anything over 200 mg/dl is higher than you want. This range includes lower blood glucose levels for before meals and somewhat higher glucose levels 1 or 2 hours after meals. As you work toward reaching your goals, you will see the high end of the range come down.

## Dealing with Your Blood Glucose Numbers

After monitoring your blood glucose levels, don't forget to keep track of your results. Although a reading that is too high or too low can alert you to a dangerous situation, it's the patterns in blood glucose readings throughout the day or from day to day that give you clues about how to manage your diabetes. The only way to see the patterns in blood glucose levels is to record your results.

Ask your diabetes care provider or educator for a record book with an easy-to-use format. You can also make your own.

Some blood glucose meters store 10 or 20 or over 1,000 test results. This saves you from having to write the results down each time, but you will still have to see if there are any patterns in your blood glucose readings by charting out the results. Make sure to show the members of your health care team the results of your monitoring. Let them know if you are pleased or not with the results and what you want to do to change your results.

When you are new to blood glucose monitoring, your concern is doing it correctly. But even if you are getting consistent results, you may want to have your diabetes educator watch you do a check, to make sure you're doing everything properly. There's information on blood checking accuracy in Chapter 6.

Sometimes you will be faced with an unexpectedly high or low reading. Try to figure out what could have caused it. You might already know why the reading could be higher than usual. If you have a series of high or low results that you can't explain, contact your health care team.

As you get the hang of monitoring, you will come to know what to expect your readings to be at certain times of the day. If your readings are consistently higher or lower than your target, or if you get a reading that is unexpectedly high or low, this could indicate a problem. Discuss with your health care team in advance what you should do if your readings are way off scale. If you detect patterns in your glucose levels that indicate a need to adjust your plan, let the team know. For example, you may find that your blood glucose levels tend to be high when you check in the morning. This could be because your body is "rebounding" from a very low blood glucose level while you sleep. Try checking your blood around 3 a.m. If you discover hypoglycemia, treat it as you normally would.

Monitoring can be frustrating. Despite all your best efforts, you may sometimes come up with readings that are too high or low for no apparent reason. But if you find that you're avoiding monitoring, ask yourself why. Are you feeling anxious or discouraged about your diabetes? If so, ask for some help from your health care team. They are convinced of the importance of monitoring to your health. They may be able to help you track down the culprit. Maybe it's time for a change in your plan. But you won't know if you give up on monitoring.

## Emergencies

Dealing with high and low blood glucose levels is a fact of life with diabetes. People with type 1 diabetes are more susceptible to swings in blood glucose levels than are people with type 2 diabetes. But all people with diabetes should be aware of possible emergencies that can occur. It is important that you learn to recognize the warning signs and to have a plan for dealing with them. Discuss with your health care team what you should be on the lookout for and what you should do if you suspect an emergency situation may be developing. Also talk to your family, friends, and coworkers about what to do in an emergency. If you are in danger, you may not always be able to handle the situation yourself. Being prepared is your best bet, and frequent monitoring of blood glucose will alert you in time to prevent most emergencies.

Emergencies can be caused by glucose levels that are either too high or too low. The most common condition is hypoglycemia, or low blood sugar. This is a problem for those taking insulin or oral diabetes medications (sulfonylureas). Dangerously high levels of blood glucose can lead to diabetic ketoacidosis (DKA) in people with type 1 diabetes. People with type 2 diabetes can develop hyperglycemic hyperosmolar syndrome (HHS) if glucose levels climb too high. DKA is rare in people with type 2 diabetes; HHS is rare in people with type 1

## Brittle Diabetes?

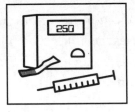 You used to hear the term "brittle dia-betes" often—before blood glucose moni-toring became possible for everyone. It refers to wide, unpredictable swings in blood glucose. Now, it's rarer for people with diabetes to be unaware of these swings and frustrated about why they can't manage their blood glucose levels.

Why do blood glucose levels swing so widely? The changes can be created by several factors, working alone or together. The amount of time it takes for food to be absorbed is different every time you eat. Insulin you inject is absorbed at different rates from under the skin. The stresses and strains of everyday living create the release of different amounts of stress hormones at different times.

Has glucose monitoring made brittle diabetes extinct? For most people, yes. A regular program of monitoring yields plenty of clues about why your blood glucose levels go up and down. But some people's bodies have exaggerated responses to food, med-ication, and stress. They may inject the same dose of the same insulin at the same time of day and eat about the same thing every day, but their blood glucose levels are high one day and low the next. Extreme swings in blood glucose level are primarily a problem for people who inject insulin.

Figuring out why this happens takes some doing. Here are some places to start looking for answers:

- **Timing of insulin injections:** When do you take your insulin? If you take regular insulin, are you giving your shot a full 30 to 45 minutes before you eat? Would a rapid-acting insulin work better for you?

### Brittle Diabetes? (*Continued*)

- **Insulin dose:** Are you sure you are measuring your dose accurately? Would using an insulin pen or pump help?
- **Injection sites:** Are you on a regular rotation schedule? Most insulins are absorbed at the most consistent rate from the abdomen.
- **Injection depth:** Do you inject your insulin at the same depth each time?
- **Blood flow:** Do you inject into areas where muscles are at work? Do you smoke? Working muscles and warm temperatures speed up absorption. Cool temperatures and tobacco slow down absorption.
- **Food intake:** Are you able to accurately count the carbohydrates in your food? Does your carbohydrate-to-insulin ratio need to be adjusted?
- **Hypoglycemia:** Do you have frequent bouts of very low blood glucose? Your body's natural defenses to this (glucose release from the liver) can be spoiling your insulin's work.
- **Neuropathy:** Do you have nerve damage that affects your absorption of food? Nerve damage can slow digestion or can produce unexpected bouts of diarrhea.
- **Dehydration:** Do you have sustained periods of high blood glucose that drain your body of fluids? The less water in your body, the harder it is for your insulin to flow into tissues.

diabetes. Both DKA and HHS can lead to coma, shock, respiratory distress, and death, if not treated promptly.

## Hypoglycemia

Hypoglycemia is not unusual for people with diabetes who take glucose-lowering medications, such as sulfonylurea or insulin

## Causes of Hypoglycemia

- too much insulin
- too little carbohydrate
- too much exercise
- a delayed meal
- alcohol on an empty stomach

(then it's called an "insulin reaction"). It occurs when blood glucose levels get too low. At the beginning of a hypoglycemic reaction, you might feel dizzy, sweaty, shaky, or faint. If untreated, you could lose consciousness or have seizures.

On average, people with type 1 diabetes have one or two episodes of hypoglycemia each week. It is much less common among people with type 2 diabetes. Hypoglycemia is usually caused by insulin doing its job too well. In people without diabetes, the body stops releasing insulin before glucose levels fall too low. But if you inject insulin, there is no way to shut it off.

Another interesting, if frustrating, fact about diabetes is this: The body's use of insulin is inconsistent. Even if you always give yourself the same dose of insulin or oral diabetes medication, you could end up with more than enough insulin to handle the glucose in your blood. This can happen even when you are doing everything, including eating, the same as usual.

How much insulin your body needs can change. This depends on many things:

- how much food you eat
- what kind of food you eat
- how much exercise you get
- when you exercise versus when you take your medication
- where you're injecting insulin

## Looking for Hypoglycemia

The symptoms (what you feel) and signs (what someone else can see) of hypoglycemia are divided into two groups:

- those caused by the effect of low blood glucose on the autonomic nervous system: shakiness, nervousness, sweating, irritability, impatience, chills and clamminess, rapid heartbeat, anxiety, light-headedness, and hunger
- those caused by the effect of low blood glucose on the brain: sleepiness, anger, stubbornness, sadness, lack of coordination, blurred vision, nausea, tingling or numbness in the lips or tongue, nightmares, crying out during sleep, headaches, strange behavior, delirium, confusion, personality change, seizures, and unconsciousness

- the state of your health
- how much stress you're under

It's impossible to control all of these things perfectly each day, no matter how hard you try. And insulin will do its job of clearing glucose from the blood even if it means that blood glucose levels fall too low. Hypoglycemia usually occurs just before meals, during or after strenuous exercise, or when insulin is peaking. Sometimes you may even get hypoglycemia during the night when you are sleeping.

*Low Blood Glucose Symptoms.* It's important that you learn your own signs of hypoglycemia. Different people may have different feelings, so it is important to know what signals your body gives during a low glucose reaction. The only sure way to know whether you have hypoglycemia is to test your blood glu-

**TIP**

How do you know whether you have had a hypoglycemic reaction during the night? Certain symptoms may tell you. Do you find your pajamas and sheets damp with sweat in the morning? Have you had restless sleep and nightmares? When you wake up, do you have a headache or still feel tired? Do you have ketones in your urine in the morning without a high blood glucose? You may want to test your blood around 2 or 3 a.m. a few times and try to match your results with your food, exercise, and medication doses from the previous day and evening. This will help you pinpoint what is really going on.

cose. Your signal to check may include shakiness, nervousness, sweating, chills and clamminess, rapid heartbeat, trouble concentrating, headache, dizziness, light-headedness, moodiness, clumsiness, tingling in your face or lips, extreme hunger, or irritability. These symptoms can happen at any time. You could even wake up in the middle of the night with a nightmare because of hypoglycemia.

Each person's reaction to low blood glucose can cause a different set of symptoms. It's unlikely that you will have them all, and you will probably have the same symptoms each time. Some of the symptoms, such as nervousness, shakiness, hunger, and light-headedness, are considered early warning signs. They are called *autonomic symptoms* because low blood sugar affects the autonomic nervous system of the body to create these symptoms. The autonomic nerves control many of the things the body does automatically, without your having to think about them: opening blood vessels, making your heart beat, and controlling your breathing. Sometimes, you might not notice the autonomic symptoms at all. Or you might be anxious about a test or new job. Or your heart may be beating faster because you just got a speeding ticket.

Some of the symptoms of hypoglycemia appear because of the effect of prolonged low blood glucose on the brain. These include anger, sadness, lack of coordination, and blurred vision. It may be hard to know if you are irritable because of hypoglycemia or because you had a fight with a friend. When in doubt, don't wait for the symptoms to go away. Check your blood glucose, because that's the only way you can tell for sure.

## Hypoglycemia Unawareness

Some people lose the ability to know when their blood glucose level has fallen to a dangerous level. They are missing the early warning signs of hypoglycemia. For them, the first symptom of low blood glucose can be impaired thinking.

Hypoglycemia unawareness seems to occur more often in people who intensively manage their blood glucose. It is common in pregnant women. There is some evidence that frequent bouts of low blood glucose can bring on hypoglycemia unawareness. Avoiding even mild hypoglycemia can help restore awareness of symptoms. Sometimes this means increasing blood glucose goals to higher numbers.

If you or your health care team suspect that you have hypoglycemia unawareness, you need to establish some safety nets:

- Increase the number of times you test your blood glucose every day.
- Always test before driving.
- Discuss your hypoglycemic episodes with your health care team so you can look for patterns to use as warning cues.
- Educate more of the people you're with every day about hypoglycemia and how to help you.
- Wear an ID bracelet for diabetes.
- Ask for a prescription for glucagon, and be sure those around you know how to use it.

Some people have a hard time detecting oncoming hypoglycemia. If you have had episodes of low blood glucose often, especially if you have had diabetes for many years, you could lose the ability to feel the early warning signs of hypoglycemia. People who tend to miss the early symptoms are said to have *hypoglycemia unawareness*. If you have hypoglycemia unawareness, you can have a severe hypoglycemic episode and not recognize it. People who intensively manage their diabetes increase their chances of having low blood glucose reactions. Having many episodes can cause you to stop sensing the early warning signs of hypoglycemia. This can lead to even more episodes of very low blood glucose. For these reasons, blood glucose testing has added importance for people using intensive diabetes management and for people who have hypoglycemia unawareness.

Hypoglycemic symptoms can serve as important clues to whether you are having a low glucose reaction. But they are not always the full story. Sometimes the symptoms could be due to something else. Unless you check your blood glucose level, you could overtreat or overreact, causing glucose levels to soar.

Maybe you have read that hypoglycemia occurs when your blood glucose levels fall below 70 mg/dl. But many people may have blood glucose readings below this level and feel no symptoms. Others may start to have symptoms of hypoglycemia when their blood glucose levels are higher than 70 mg/dl. All this can be very confusing. To start, ask your provider or educator what glucose levels to look out for when you suspect hypoglycemia. Make note of the symptoms you are experiencing. You will soon learn what level is too low for you.

**Treatment.** If you think you are having a hypoglycemic reaction, you need to check your blood glucose level. Talk to your health care team about the blood glucose level at which

TIP

One way to gauge how much glucose to take during a hypoglycemic reaction is to do a glucose check. When your blood glucose is about 100 mg/dl or less, eat or drink your favorite fast-acting sugar. Wait 15 minutes, then recheck. Did your blood glucose rise 25, 30, or 50 mg/dl, or more? This will give you an idea of how to treat your hypoglycemia. You'll be less likely to overtreat low blood glucose if you can predict how much your treatment will increase blood glucose. Ask your health care team what blood glucose levels to aim for following treatment of hypoglycemia.

you should begin treatment. Although it's best to check before treating, this may not always be possible. What if you don't have your monitor with you? Should you wait until you get home? No! Eat or drink something immediately. Never wait until you get home, especially if you have to drive.

When you are having severe hypoglycemia, you need to eat or drink a sugar that can be rapidly absorbed from your digestive tract and into your blood. But that doesn't mean you need to go overboard. You'll feel worse later on if you send your blood glucose levels soaring. There are many choices of fast-acting sugars. Keep in mind that the fat in chocolate or candy bars slows down absorption.

You're best prepared for low blood glucose if you carry around a measured amount of "pocket sugar." This should be about 15 grams of carbohydrate (1 fruit or 1 starch exchange). The easiest and most convenient fast-acting sugar is found in glucose tablets or gel, available at pharmacies. Two to five glucose tablets or one package of glucose gel (check the labels to be sure of the dose) will usually bring quick relief.

After taking your quick-fix treatment for hypoglycemia, recheck your blood after 15 minutes. If you still have low blood glucose, you may need to take another dose of 10 to 15 grams of carbohydrate. If your next meal or snack is more than 30 minutes away, have a follow-up snack after you have treated your hypoglycemia.

You need to wear medical ID jewelry or carry a medical information card. This gives others the information they need to help you during hypoglycemia. Keep a source of fast-acting sugar in your car, purse, or briefcase and close to your bed in case of a nighttime reaction. If you use insulin or sulfonylurea, you need to be prepared to treat low blood glucose at any time.

*Severe Hypoglycemia.* If symptoms of hypoglycemia go unnoticed, or are ignored, you could develop severe hypoglycemia. When your blood glucose level is very low for too long, your brain does not get enough glucose and you can lose consciousness. This is a real emergency. The best way to deal with severe hypoglycemia is to take precautions so that it doesn't happen in the first place. Be alert to your symptoms and treat yourself right away. Don't wait to see if it gets worse or put off treatment until a more convenient time. Also, your family, friends, coworkers, and whoever you spend time with need some training. Either you or a member of your health care team

## Fast-Acting Sugars for Hypoglycemia

Each of these has about 15 grams of carbohydrate for treating hypoglycemia:

- 2 to 5 glucose tablets
- 2 tablespoons of raisins
- 1/2 cup regular soda
- 4 ounces orange juice
- 5 to 7 LifeSavers
- 6 jelly beans
- 10 gumdrops
- 2 large lumps or teaspoons sugar
- 2 teaspoons honey or corn syrup
- 1 tube (0.68 ounces) Cake Mate decorator gel
- 6 to 8 ounces skim or 1% milk

**TIP**

If you live alone, you may be concerned about having a severe hypoglycemic reaction while you are sleeping. Your best bet is to monitor your blood glucose levels before you go to sleep and occasionally during the night. If your blood glucose level is dropping, eat a small snack before going to sleep.

should instruct them on the signs of severe hypoglycemia and what to do should it develop. If you are elderly and taking oral diabetes medications (sulfonylureas) or insulin, you are at especially high risk for developing severe hypoglycemia.

During a hypoglycemic reaction, you can become so confused and irritable that you refuse help. Those around you may have to be persistent to get you the help you need. They can save you from a coma and a trip to the hospital by insisting that you take some form of glucose quickly. Your life will be easier and safer if those with whom you spend the most time can spot a low glucose reaction and know what to do about it.

If you become unconscious, someone else must take over. You will not be able to eat or drink anything. But your blood glucose levels need to go up immediately. The safest remedy is to get a glucagon injection. Your helper should call for emergency help at once if he or she does not know how to inject glucagon. Glucagon is a hormone made by the pancreas that causes the liver to release glucose. It also inhibits insulin release. Glucagon will not work on someone who has no glucose stored in the liver or on people with type 2 diabetes. This can happen in cases of starvation or chronic hypoglycemia or in people who are alcoholics.

If you are prone to hypoglycemia, you'll need to train someone you trust to inject glucagon. Talk to your provider about whether you should buy a glucagon kit, which is available by prescription. If so, ask your family or close friends to learn with you how to use glucagon so they know what to do. The kit has a special glucagon syringe that is filled with a diluting solution. Kits usually last a year before the glucagon and diluting solution expire (check the date on the box). However, if you pre-mix the glucagon in diluting solution, the mixture only lasts about 48 hours if kept refrigerated.

After you have been treated with glucagon, you may vomit, so your head needs to be turned to the side. You should respond to glucagon within 5 to 15 minutes. When you are awake enough to chew and swallow, you should have some clear fluid, such as 7-Up, to settle your stomach and then eat a snack, such as a roll with peanut butter or half of a cheese sandwich. If you do not respond to the first shot within 15 minutes, your helper should get emergency help right away. Glucagon can be repeated after 20 minutes.

If you have such a low blood glucose level that you have to take glucagon, be sure to let your health care team know. Also tell them if you are having frequent bouts of even mild hypoglycemia. By working together, you might find a pattern in your insulin, diet, or activity routine that may be causing the hypoglycemia. With clues, you and your health care team can do some problem solving and decide on some changes to prevent severe hypoglycemia.

*Pregnancy.* Many pregnant women choose to manage their diabetes intensively. In addition, many also become desensitized to low blood glucose levels, and some experience hypoglycemia unawareness. Thus, they are more likely to have mild and moderate bouts of hypoglycemia. That's why it is so important to develop and keep up a blood glucose monitoring routine and to check your blood glucose when hypoglycemia is most likely, in between meals and in the middle of the night. You need to treat any blood glucose level under 70 mg/dl.

If you are pregnant and become unconscious, special precautions are necessary. The baby may be harmed more by high blood glucose and ketone levels and by drastic changes in blood glucose than by the hypoglycemia itself. Therefore, you may need only half of the normal dose of glucagon at the beginning of a severe episode of hypoglycemia. After 15 minutes, if you do not regain consciousness or your blood glucose levels do not rise, you need another shot and someone should call 911 for emergency help. Make sure that those with whom you spend time know that you are pregnant and know what to do if you develop severe hypoglycemia. Ask your health care provider about the dose of glucagon you need.

**Exercise.** Exercise lowers blood glucose levels, so you have to be extra careful to avoid hypoglycemia during exercise. Try not to overdo it by working out really hard, especially when you are alone. Instead, exercise at a pool or gym where others are around. If you can't get to a gym, jog or cycle with a friend. If you'll be burning a lot of calories, you may need a snack beforehand. For more information about matching food needs to exercise, see Chapter 8.

If you do feel as though you are becoming hypoglycemic while you are exercising, stop at once! Don't say, "I'll just do one more lap," or "Just 5 minutes more won't hurt." Test your blood glucose level right away and treat the hypoglycemia if you need to. If you want to continue your workout, eat a snack, take a 15-minute break, and check to make sure your blood glucose has come back up (>100 mg/dl) before starting back. If you don't, your blood glucose level may drop again, quickly. Studies show that hypoglycemia is even more likely to occur 4 to 10 hours after your exercise than during the activity or shortly after. When you first begin an exercise program, you will need to monitor your blood levels after exercise to find out how your body responds.

*Sexual Activity.* If you are prone to hypoglycemia when you exercise or at night, you may also have a low blood glucose reaction following sexual activity. This can be especially true if you are intimate at night. This is when your blood glucose levels typically dip, so you may need to adjust your insulin or have a snack before or after sexual activity. Be especially careful if you are combining sexual activity with alcohol.

*Heart Disease.* Hypoglycemia can cause your heart to beat faster than normal. If you have heart disease, talk to your provider about how hypoglycemia might affect you. You may need to keep your blood glucose levels a little higher to reduce the risk of developing hypoglycemia.

*Alcohol.* Alcohol lowers blood glucose levels. Normally, when your blood glucose levels begin to drop too low, your liver will convert stored starch to glucose. This helps protect you from a severe reaction temporarily and gives you time to recognize and treat hypoglycemia. But alcohol interferes with this process. If you drink alcohol, you may have a severe hypoglycemic reaction with little warning. There's more information about alcohol and your meal plan in Chapter 8.

*Dawn Phenomenon.* Your body has a normal mechanism that wakes you up and gives you energy to start the day. Your body responds to this wake-up call of the growth hormones. These hormones depress the activity of insulin, allowing blood glucose to rise between around 4 and 8 a.m. This is called the dawn phenomenon. The dawn phenomenon can be one reason for blood glucose readings and ketone levels that are high when you wake up.

If high morning blood glucose levels seem to occur mysteriously, discuss the problem with your health care team and talk about the best way to treat it. You may need to eat less food at breakfast or the night before or increase your prebreakfast or evening insulin dose.

## Hyperglycemia

Having high levels of glucose in your blood over time may lead to the complications of diabetes. But blood glucose levels can also become dangerously high in the short term and cause a life-threatening situation that could result in coma or death. It is important to know what the warning signs are and how to treat hyperglycemia.

*Type 1 Diabetes.* Having too little insulin in your body leads to too much glucose. A rare and serious, but often preventable, emergency can arise from high blood glucose levels. Diabetic ketoacidosis (DKA) occurs when you don't get enough insulin, and is mostly a problem for people with type 1 diabetes. Any time your body doesn't have enough insulin, muscles can't take in the glucose that they need. They feel starved, so your body breaks down fat for energy. Ketones are the by-products of this breakdown. If ketones form faster than your body can get rid of them in the urine, they build up in the blood. These acidic products poison the blood. At the same time, glucose spills into your urine, your kidneys produce more urine, and you get dehydrated. When you have dehydration and ketones in the blood, you've got DKA.

It can start innocently enough: you miss a dose of insulin, the insulin you've been using has gone bad, or your insulin pump tubing gets clogged. But an undetected high blood glucose level can progress to a coma, shock, pneumonia, difficulty breathing, and even death. Small children can also develop swelling of the brain (cerebral edema). DKA can occur in people with type 1 diabetes who have not yet been diagnosed and can also develop during periods of stress or illness. When the body has to deal with a bacterial infection, a sickness such as the flu, or a stressful situation, hormones cause the liver to release stored glucose. These hormones also block the effects of insulin.

Sometimes when you are sick and can't eat, you may think, "I shouldn't take insulin today." Even though you aren't eating, your body still needs insulin to cover its 24-hour insulin needs. Plus, you are likely producing extra glucose. So, in addition to your usual dose of insulin, you may actually need extra insulin. Drinking plenty of fluids will also help.

Sick days call for more frequent blood glucose monitoring and urine testing for ketones. Do both at least every 4 hours until you're feeling better. Any time you feel queasy or are vomiting, even if your blood glucose isn't high, you need to check your urine for ketones. A buildup of ketones can cause nausea.

Pregnant women also test for ketones frequently. Daily urine ketone testing can help detect elevated levels and prevent DKA, which can be very dangerous for the developing baby. See chapter 11 for more information about pregnancy and diabetes.

If your urine shows trace or small amounts of ketones, it's a sign that you need more insulin or carbohydrate (depending on your glucose readings). If your urine has moderate or large amounts of ketones, call your health care team immediately or use the plan that you and your team made ahead of time. You probably need to take extra rapid- or short-acting insulin right away. Drink plenty of sugar-free fluids as well to prevent dehydration. If urinary ketones do not promptly go down, or if you are vomiting and can't stop, you need emergency help at once. Make sure that those who spend time with you know what to look for and what to do if you have signs of DKA.

*Signs of DKA.* DKA often gives plenty of warning before it happens, but it can also occur with little warning. If you regularly check your blood glucose several times during the day, you won't miss the most important warning signs: high blood glucose and ketones in your urine. Test your urine for ketones whenever your blood glucose is over 300 mg/dl or you feel ill. Call a member of your health care team if you have moderate to large ketones, even if your blood glucose levels are not significantly increased. Signs of DKA include the following:

- lack of appetite
- pains in your stomach
- vomiting or feeling sick to your stomach
- blurry vision
- fever or warm, dry, or flushed skin
- difficulty breathing
- feelings of weakness
- sleepiness
- a fruity odor on your breath
- classic signs of hyperglycemia: intense thirst, a dry mouth, and the need to urinate frequently

*Type 2 Diabetes.* Compared with people with type 1 diabetes, people with type 2 diabetes have less dramatic swings in blood glucose levels. But they can sustain high blood glucose levels over prolonged periods without even knowing it. This can wear on the body and may cause diabetes complications. By monitoring your blood glucose levels regularly, you can guard against chronic hyperglycemia.

Acute hyperglycemia can occur in people with type 2 diabetes and is life threatening. Hyperglycemia in people with type 2 diabetes does not usually produce ketones. But blood glucose levels can soar to over 600 mg/dl and even as high as

1,000 mg/dl. This sometimes happens before diabetes is diagnosed. Extreme hyperglycemia can cause a coma.

Hyperosmolar hyperglycemic syndrome (HHS) occurs almost exclusively in people with type 2 diabetes. It can happen to people who manage their diabetes with diet and exercise only, those who use oral diabetes medications, and those who use insulin. It most often occurs among people who don't use insulin. One-third of all cases of HHS are caused by undiagnosed diabetes. HHS results from stress, infections, heart attacks, strokes, and even diuretics. Sometimes even something simple, such as not being able to get a glass of water when you want one, can contribute. This occurs more often in people who have restricted mobility, such as the elderly, or in people who cannot take adequate care of themselves. Also, as you age, your sense of thirst diminishes and it's harder to drink enough fluids.

HHS occurs because as blood glucose levels go higher and higher, urine output goes up, and dehydration sets in. This process may go on for days or weeks. Extreme dehydration eventually leads to confusion and lack of ability to even get a drink or make it to the toilet. With that much glucose in the blood, plus the fluid loss, blood gets thicker. Eventually, the severe dehydration leads to seizures, coma, and death.

**Signs of HHS.** If you experience any of the following signs, you need to check your blood glucose level at once and call your provider. Be sure those around you know what to do, because you may not be able to react.

- dry, parched mouth
- extreme thirst, although this may gradually disappear
- sleepiness or confusion
- warm, dry skin with no sweating

■ high blood glucose. If it's over 300 mg/dl on two readings, call your health care team; if it's over 500 mg/dl, have someone take you to the hospital immediately.

If you are checking your blood glucose levels even once a day, you'll be alerted to high blood glucose levels well before the process that leads to HHS gets going. Because illness can make blood glucose levels rise, you'll want to test three or four times a day when you're sick. It's also very important to drink plenty of alcohol-free fluids. You may need to take insulin, even if you don't ordinarily use it.

Besides illness, certain situations can increase your risk for HHS.

■ **Medications.** Ask your provider, pharmacist, or other member of your health care team about glucocorticoids (steroids), diuretics, phenytoin (Dilantin), cimetidine (Tagamet), and beta blockers, especially Inderal. If you take any of these medications, you may need to monitor your blood glucose regularly and adjust your diabetes medications accordingly.
■ **Treatments.** HHS can occur in people having peritoneal dialysis or intravenous feedings because of the large amounts of glucose used. If you're on either of these treatments, you need frequent blood glucose checks.
■ **Nursing homes.** About one-third of the cases of HHS occur in people living in nursing homes. This can happen when residents are confused or have to wait for staff to offer them something to drink, and they may get dehydrated. Family members may have to educate staff to the patient's needs and ask for regular blood glucose monitoring.

# Diabetes Tools | 6

*The average person with diabetes spends more than $2,500 each year at the pharmacy. You'll need medications, test strips, a blood glucose meter . . . so it pays to make informed choices.*

Mastering the lifestyle skills—food, exercise, and stress management—is key to managing your diabetes care plan. But that's only half the battle. Taking charge of your diabetes also means mastering the science and technology that underlie the disease.

This means understanding the medical basis of diabetes and becoming familiar with the tools of the trade. All of the various supplies that can help you manage your diabetes form a sort of high-tech toolbox. This toolbox consists of everything from the simple fingerstick lancet to the latest computerized blood glucose management systems.

As with any tool, each piece of equipment must be carefully chosen to suit your individual needs. Once chosen, you need to learn to use and maintain the equipment in your diabetes toolbox. It may seem a bit overwhelming at first, but your health care team is there to help you with these challenges. Talk to them. Ask them what they would recommend and what their other patients like or dislike about various tools and systems.

The best catalog for a diabetes toolbox is the American Diabetes Association *Resource Guide,* available online and published every year by the magazine *Diabetes Forecast* (see Resources). This guide lists and describes all available diabetes care tools on the market. The next best references are the regular advertisements and the Shopper's Guide section in *Diabetes Forecast.*

You can find information about insulin and insulin pumps in Chapter 4.

## Blood Glucose Meters

In your efforts to take charge of your diabetes, your blood glucose meter is essential. Only by keeping close tabs on your blood glucose levels and recognizing when they are out of range can you take steps to remedy the situation.

There are many different brands of blood glucose meters on the market today that detect how much glucose is in the blood. These meters measure an electric current in the blood that depends on the amount of glucose present. With these meters, blood is placed on or in a small area of a test strip or disk. A special enzyme transfers electrons from glucose to a chemical in the strip, and the meter measures this flow of electrons as current. The amount of current depends on how much glucose is in the blood. This weak current flows through the strip and is measured in the meter. The meter produces an electronic reading of blood glucose levels (mg/dl).

There are glucose meters on the market that allow you to take blood from other parts of your body, not just your fingertips. Check the American Diabetes Association *Resource Guide* for more information. Noninvasive glucose meters are in various stages of development, so watch for them.

There are also several meters that check more than blood glucose. One meter measures blood glucose and ketones. Another measures blood glucose, ketones, and lipids, including cholesterol, triglycerides, and HDL.

All meters perform the same basic job of measuring the amount of glucose in blood. But all meters are not created equal, even among meters of the same type. Some models may fit your needs better, depending on your particular lifestyle. To choose the right meter, you may want to consider several aspects.

### Insurance Coverage

Before you invest in any meter, check with your insurance plan or company health program. They may pay for only specific meters or have a cost allowance. Also find out if you are covered for the test strips and the quantity allowed.

### Your Budget

You may be surprised when you go to buy replacement strips for your meter. The meter that seemed like a bargain at the time of purchase may turn into a major expense when it comes time to pay for strips, especially if you don't get reimbursed for them by your health care insurance. In the long run, the strips will cost you more than the meter itself. Most meters will only use one kind of strip. Make sure you check the cost of the strips your meter uses before you buy it. Check the American Diabetes Association *Resource Guide* and ads for lists of companies that sell less costly strips.

### Ease of Use

Some blood glucose meters are about the size of a credit card. Some even come as small as a flash drive for your computer.

Others are more like a calculator. You may find the smaller models difficult to manipulate. If you have trouble with small hand and finger movements, you may want to consider a larger meter. However, these might be heavier and more difficult to carry around. Also, consider what strips you need to use for your meter. Some come packaged in a vial, while others are individually wrapped in foil. The foil wrappings can be more portable but also more difficult to open, so you may want to avoid brands that require this type of strip.

## Test Site

Alternative test site or forearm blood glucose monitoring is now available with some meters. Studies have shown a good match between fingerstick and forearm methods in people who are fasting. But fingerstick readings do tend to be higher than forearm blood glucose readings after meals. This may be due to less vigorous blood flow in the forearm. Some studies have shown a difference in readings taken from a finger compared to the forearm when blood glucose is low. Read the manufacturer's instructions or ask your diabetes educator. It may be safer to do a finger check if you feel the symptoms of a low blood glucose.

## Your Schedule

If your life is a constant battle with the clock, stay away from devices that require too much time. Some meters can measure blood glucose just 5 seconds after a drop of blood lands on the strip. These devices can be especially useful when you test often or in work and social situations where a few seconds here and there really do make a difference. If you are always on the move, there is a meter and insulin pen combination available.

## Your Vision

Whether you have severe visual impairment or just have a hard time focusing on small print, you may want to bear this aspect in mind when choosing a meter. There are products for visually impaired or disabled users. For example, meters are available with voice guides. Otherwise, look for a meter with a large digital display if you have difficulty reading the numbers.

If you have any degree of color-blindness, test-drive a few different models. Make sure that you have no trouble reading the digital display.

If you have even some vision loss, perhaps a close companion or family member can help. Make sure that he or she is trained in the use of your meter and the other components of your diabetes toolbox.

## Support System

If you are using a meter for the first time, consider one that offers a video that teaches you how to do the reading. A picture or visual image can make a seemingly complicated procedure crystal clear. Also make sure that the company has a 24-hour toll-free number to call, should you have questions about the meter. Sometimes a quick phone call may clear up a simple problem. Also check that your health care team is familiar with the model you purchase and that supplies are easily available in your area or by mail order.

## User-Friendliness

Make sure your meter or monitoring system is easy to handle. Several features can make meters easier to use. Some models require a smaller-sized drop of blood. Ask how much blood is required for each model you might be considering. With some models, too little blood may give a faulty reading and you may need to repeat the test. This can be inconvenient at best but could be more of a problem for those with poor circulation in their hands or who must check blood glucose in cold environments. Ask your diabetes educator to show you how different meters work and to help you pick out one that is best for you.

## Accuracy

Testing strips can vary from batch to batch. There may be differences in the amount of chemical on the strips in each batch. So, when you open a new batch of strips, you must standardize or calibrate your meter to make up for these small differences. If you don't calibrate, all your results with the new strips may read higher or lower than they really are. Instructions for calibration are included in every new package of strips. Some machines calibrate all by themselves—you don't have to do anything when you open a new batch of strips or the disk.

Almost all meters provide a standard solution known as a "control" solution. It contains a known amount of glucose to help check for accuracy. If you measure the amount of glucose in this standard solution in your meter and your meter shows a reading that is either too high or too low, your machine could be giving you a faulty reading. The manufacturer's instructions will tell you how often to check the control solution for best results. If you are having a problem with accuracy, first check to see if your problems are being caused by old or damaged test strips. Then call the manufacturer of your meter. There may be something wrong with your meter. You can usually order a vial of standard glucose solution by calling your machine's manufacturer. Date your control solution when you open it, and remember that it is good for one month.

FACT OR MYTH?

**"I've been monitoring my blood glucose level for years. With all my practice, I get accurate results every time."**

 Researchers have found that practice, at least in the area of blood glucose monitoring, does not make perfect. Fresh from training by a diabetes educator, people start off getting accurate results. But, as time goes by, they begin to get sloppy. Accuracy actually decreases over time.

You can avoid this source of error in your blood monitoring results by having your technique checked by your provider or diabetes educator. Here are some potential problem areas for you and your health care team to watch:

- **Your blood.** Are you getting enough blood on the test strip? To increase blood flow, wash your hands in warm water, hang your hand down, and massage your hand from your palm out to the fingertip before pricking. You may find it less painful to prick the side of your finger rather than the fleshy pad. For some strips, once the drop is on the strip you can't add more blood.
- **Test strips.** Are your strips fresh? Be aware of the expiration date. Avoid exposing the strips to light and moisture. Are you calibrating your meter to each new batch of test strips? There are variations from one batch to another, even when they are made by the same manufacturer.
- **Your meter.** Check your meter regularly with the control solution specified by the meter's manufacturer. Look in the instructions that came with the meter if you've forgotten how to do this. If your meter can be cleaned, do it periodically. You may find a buildup of blood, dust, and lint that can affect the readings. The instructions that came with the meter will tell you about your meter and how to use it accurately.

Getting accurate readings also depends on your blood monitoring technique. There are easy ways to figure out how well you are using your meter. Take your meter with you when you visit your diabetes care provider or diabetes educator and have him or her watch your technique. Or measure your blood glucose level with your own meter when your blood is drawn for laboratory glucose tests. Record your results. The two readings are best compared when you are fasting. If you have just eaten, the comparison may not be accurate, because shortly after a meal, fingertip (capillary) blood glucose can be higher than that drawn from a vein.

When your lab-tested blood results are available, compare the numbers. The box of strips should tell you whether your current meter gives a plasma or a whole blood reading. If you are not sure, call the manufacturer and ask. If you are using a meter that tests whole blood, your results will be different from the lab's results. When blood from your veins is tested, a sample is sent to a laboratory. There, the blood is spun down, and blood cells, platelets, and cell debris are removed, leaving the plasma. The amount of glucose in the plasma is measured, and these numbers can be 15 percent higher than whole blood glucose readings you measure on your meter. For instance, if the lab results are 150 mg/dl, your technique and meter are accurate if your results were within the 127 to 173 mg/dl range. If your result was off by more than 15 percent, go over your technique with your diabetes educator or provider. If he or she can't find any reason why your technique should be causing a problem, it's time to suspect that something may be wrong with your meter. Call the manufacturer and ask about getting a replacement meter.

Almost all meters now calibrate your blood glucose level to give you a plasma blood glucose level. You can compare this result directly with your lab test results.

## Meter Size

If you're on the move and don't relish the idea of lugging around a lot of excess baggage, consider investing in a very small meter. They slip easily into a shirt pocket or small purse. But be careful—smaller meters are easier to lose. If you do opt for the smaller version, make sure it's easy to handle.

## Meter Memory

Some meters can store up to 3,000 glucose readings. If you carry your meter around with you during the day, you may want one that stores results in its memory. If your meter has a date and time feature, make sure it is correct. (Call the manufacturer if you are not sure how to set the date and time.) At night you can jot down the day's readings in your logbook so you can look for patterns and have it to take along on your trip to your provider or diabetes educator. On the other hand, if you take all of your readings at home with your logbook close at hand, meter memory may be less important. Either way, writing down your numbers helps you to better understand and use your results.

## Data Management Systems

Diabetes management is much more than blood glucose readings. And data management systems can do much more than store blood glucose readings. These systems can store many test results and information on time, date, insulin doses, exercise, and food intake. Some will store or calculate grams of carbohydrate in food and insulin doses. Some even have built-in alarm clocks. Some systems can load all of these data into your or your health care team's computer while others are part of the meter. PDA systems are also available. Surprisingly, data management systems don't cost too much more than regular meters. These systems can give you a detailed picture of your overall diabetes management plan. Before you buy a system, check to see if your health care team uses or recommends one system over another. Also call the manufacturer's toll-free number and ask them exactly what you will be getting. They should be willing to answer any questions you may have.

You can also buy computer programs or PDA systems that take data management one step further. You can enter the data through an electronic download from your system. The program can then provide a trend analysis, averages, graphs, printouts, and more. This can make it easier for you and your health care team to pinpoint any problem areas that might arise. Check ads in the American Diabetes Association *Resource Guide* for these products.

Don't buy a high-end blood glucose data management system unless you can afford the extra cost. Many people find that they can get along with a good logbook. This is especially true if you have type 2 diabetes and monitor less often. However, if you have type 1 diabetes and are managing your diabetes through intensive treatment, you might decide it is worth the extra cost.

## Language

Some meter systems can display in English, Spanish, and even up to seven other languages. Others use symbols instead of words to display information.

## Battery and Machine Replacement

Yes, glucose meters need batteries, too. But each model handles batteries differently. For some models, you can buy the battery and insert it into the meter yourself. Some of these batteries can be fairly expensive and difficult to find. Other meters use standard equipment batteries—the same kind you might use in your flashlight or remote control. And some meters have no replaceable batteries. Before you buy any meter, find out what type of replacement battery it uses, whether the batteries are easy to find, and how expensive they are. With daily use, batteries generally have to be replaced every 1,000 readings. Most manufacturers will tell you how long the meter's batteries will last. Some companies will replace batteries for you, and others simply replace the whole meter. You can order the new meter by express delivery. The company supplies an envelope to ship back the old meter. Usually, you miss testing for no more than 2 days.

## Blood Contamination

Contamination can be a serious concern if you have a blood-borne illness such as hepatitis or HIV infection. If this is the case, choose a system that will keep the handling of blood samples to a minimum. Don't share lancet devices or meters in which blood can contaminate the device.

## Convenience

If you commute to work, or split your time between two locations, you might want to buy two meters (make sure they use the same brand of test strip). You can keep one at home and the other at work. Lugging your meter back and forth every day can be a bit of a nuisance. Not only will you avoid the inconvenience, you will also avoid the hazard of forgetting to bring the meter back home or to work with you. If you use two meters, finding ones with memory will be less of an issue. It will be easier to look for patterns if you use one logbook to record the results from tests of both meters.

If the meter of your dreams turns out to be a real lemon, take heart. Many companies will provide you with a rebate for the return of any meter even from other companies. This rebate is good toward the purchase of their meter. Look for ads in *Diabetes Forecast* for companies that offers such trade-in deals. But before you trade in your current model, make sure other conditions aren't causing your problems. Low iron, anemia, very low blood pressure, edema in fingers, and certain medications can also cause problems in getting accurate blood glucose readings.

## Lancets

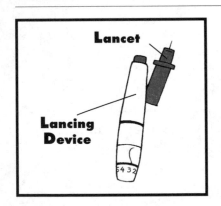

Many blood glucose meters come with a finger-sticking, or lancing, device and a few lancets. If this device works for you, fine. But if you want a different device or more than one, be aware that there are several kinds. Different lancets produce different sizes of blood drops. Make sure the device you are considering will help you get a drop of blood that is large enough for your meter. Finger-sticking devices often have two different caps or an adjustable tip that controls how deep the lancets poke your finger. Use the shallowest poke possible to draw blood. It hurts less and causes less scarring of your fingers. There is also a device that uses a tiny laser beam to create a small hole for blood sampling. If you have trouble with your dexterity, look for an automatic lancing device that resets easily with a simple push-pull movement.

Not all lancets fit all finger-sticking devices. Make sure that you can easily get replacement lancets to fit your device. Check the prices for the replacement lancets in any instrument you are considering purchasing. Lancets are sterile the first time only. Don't share lancets or lancing devices.

# Urine Test Strips

Along with monitoring your blood glucose, there are also times when you will need to test your urine for ketones. Glucose also shows up in your urine, and there are visual strips that can tell you if glucose levels in your urine are high. But they cannot measure levels that are low. Testing urine glucose is a very poor way to determine your blood glucose level.

### Test Strips for Urine Ketones

If you don't have enough insulin available, your body will burn fat instead of glucose. This can happen when your insulin dose

## Monitoring Ketones

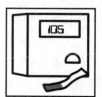

There are some times when you should always test for ketones:

- when your blood glucose readings are over 300 mg/dl
- when you are ill, especially when you have a high fever, bouts of vomiting, or diarrhea
- during pregnancy, daily before breakfast (fasting)
- during acute stress, whether it is physical (such as surgery) or psychological (such as a new job)
- when you are chronically tired
- when you have fruity breath, vomiting, breathing difficulties, or are having a hard time concentrating

## Fast Action for Ketones

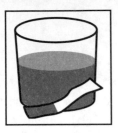

If you do have high ketones, along with high blood glucose levels, you need to lower them immediately. This can be done by

- taking additional insulin. Consult with your health care team in advance to know how much additional rapid- or short-acting insulin you may need.
- drinking plenty of water. This helps to prevent dehydration.
- avoiding exercise. Exercise just causes more fat-burning because there isn't any insulin. If you continue to exercise, you could counteract the effects of taking extra insulin.

isn't adequate or when your body works against the insulin with counterregulatory hormones, as during illness. This can also occur if you are severely restricting your carbohydrate intake. Some of the by-products of fat burning are ketones. Ketones are toxic to your body. It's important to detect them before they grow to large levels. The most common way to check ketones is with a urine test. Checking for urine ketones is important for people with diabetes, especially people with type 1 diabetes who do not make any insulin. People with type 2 diabetes usually produce some insulin and so are less likely to develop ketoacidosis. However, everyone with diabetes needs to know how and when to use ketone test strips. Test tablets are also available but are less convenient to use.

To test urine for ketones, you use a visually read strip. Ketone strips vary in how much time is needed between applying urine and getting the result—as little as 15 seconds or as long as 2 minutes. Read and follow the directions so you know how long to wait. Some ketone strips also measure glucose and have two test pads on each strip. You read the result by comparing the ketone pad with the ketone color chart.

The individually foil-wrapped ketone strips are the most expensive up front, but they last longer. Because you are unlikely to need to test ketones very often, they save you money in the long run. Ketone strips that come in a vial all spoil at the same time, probably about 6 months after you open it. However, each foil-wrapped strip has its own expiration date.

There are several reasons why you might have ketones in your urine:

- hyperglycemia or high blood glucose (high blood glucose levels are a sign that insulin is not available to let glucose into cells; your body breaks down fat because it can't use the glucose in the blood)
- illness
- lack of insulin
- effect of anti-insulin hormones
- too little food (this is called starvation ketosis and is usually seen when meals are very restricted in calories; pregnant women must make sure they are eating enough food to avoid starvation ketosis)
- hypoglycemia or low blood glucose (when no glucose is available, your body breaks down fat into glucose)

Unlike glucose levels, ketone levels aren't given in exact units like mg or dl. Instead, the side of the vial reads from zero and trace to small, moderate, and large. Some brands just score with + signs. Ask your health care team in advance what to do when you have moderate to large ketones. They may ask that you call right away or try taking additional insulin first. Be sure

## Making Mail Order Work for You

Purchasing your diabetes supplies, such as insulin and test strips, through a mail-order supplier can be one way to save money when buying in bulk. Here are some tips to help you use mail-order services wisely:

- If you live in a warm climate or order during the summer, ask how perishable items will be shipped. Insulin is sensitive to heat. Strips can spoil in excessive heat. Overnight shipping is best for these items.
- Find out prices by shopping around. Most mail-order firms have toll-free telephone numbers.
- When you start a new drug, whether it is insulin or an oral diabetes medication, buy it from a pharmacy. You may need a different dose—or you may stop taking the drug altogether.
- Don't buy large quantities of a drug until you find the safe, effective dose for you. This is especially true if the medication is new for you.
- Buy drugs you need now from the pharmacy. Use mail-order firms to buy drugs you use regularly.
- If you use Medicare to help you pay for supplies, note that prices shown in advertisements or quoted over the phone may differ from the amount that Medicare will reimburse for that item. You may need to pay the difference.
- Order your supplies far enough in advance that your current supply won't run out before the new ones arrive.
- Ask about generic drugs. Savings offered by mail-order firms come routinely from substituting generics for brand-name drugs.
- Inspect your prescription drugs carefully when they arrive. If they look different, call your supplier to double-check. Get the name of the manufacturer for your records.

## Making Mail Order Work for You (*Continued*)

- Always follow instructions when taking prescription drugs. If the instructions that arrive with your medications are different from those you remember, call your provider and ask which instructions to follow.
- Always keep copies of any orders you send through the mail. If you call in your order, be sure to write down when you placed the order and what you ordered.
- Inspect insulin vials carefully for signs of damage or crystallization on the inside of the vial. Call the mail-order firm immediately to report spoiled insulin.
- Check the expiration date on each item that arrives. If you'll need the item in 6 months, make sure it doesn't expire in 2 months. Send back all items with expiration dates that are just around the corner.

to talk to your provider about ketones during a regular visit, before an emergency develops. There is more information on hyperglycemia and ketosis in Chapter 5.

## Setting the Record Straight

One of the most important tools in your diabetes toolbox is also the most overlooked. The low-tech logbook may not look like much, but it will help you and your health care team understand your blood glucose levels and will alert you to any red flags that could signal a serious problem. Everyone gets a free logbook when buying a new meter. Many pharmacies don't carry logbooks because the meter manufacturers provide them to health care professionals instead. Ask your health care team if they can give you a logbook. You can also probably find log-books through most mail-order houses. Or call the toll-free number for your meter manufacturer to request more. You could also consider photocopying blank pages and compiling them in a loose-leaf notebook, or creating your own custom logbook.

You may want a lot of room to write in your logbook. Consider buying a spiral-bound notebook or using a loose-leaf notebook, where you can add pages as needed, to jot down extra notes. You may find it useful to have extra space to record different symptoms and situations that could be relevant to your health. Your logbook is an important tool for looking for patterns in your blood glucose control, so be sure that it is easy to use. Notebooks also offer lots of room to write for people whose fingers might be a little stiff.

## Odds and Ends

### Carrying Case

There are a few other items you may need to round out your tool kit. One is the carrying case for all your diabetes supplies. If you have tried to stuff your meter, pen or syringes and insulin, and other supplies into a purse or briefcase, you'll know how handy a special bag can be. These cases can help organize all your supplies and keep them in one convenient place. They can also insulate your insulin from hot or cold temperatures. Your carrying case doesn't necessarily have to be a top-of-the-line case. A fanny pack that holds your daily needed diabetes supplies can work, too.

### Glucose Tablets

In your carrying case—and in your purse, your car, your bathroom, and your nightstand—be sure to have some glucose

## Sample Logbook for Blood Sugar Record

| Day | Breakfast: Before/After | Lunch: Before/After | Dinner: Before/After | Bedtime | Other | Comments* |
|---|---|---|---|---|---|---|
| Sunday | | | | | | |
| Monday | | | | | | |
| Tuesday | | | | | | |
| Wednesday | | | | | | |
| Thursday | | | | | | |
| Friday | | | | | | |
| Saturday | | | | | | |

*Details about ketones, exercise, injection sites, problems, etc.

tablets or some other form of fast-acting carbohydrate on hand. Glucose tablets are probably the most handy. There may be times when your glucose level plummets and it is difficult to make it to the refrigerator for orange juice. Glucose tablets are easy to handle and they work within minutes. And you are less likely to overcompensate and eat too many glucose tablets because they don't seem like candy. Try a few different kinds of fruit-flavored tablets to find the one that tastes best to you. The tablets come with varying amounts of glucose. Check the label to see how much to take.

### Personal Identification

Don't forget to put some form of personal identification in your tool kit. This should identify you and your medical condition(s) in case you become unconscious or injured. The Medic Alert Foundation keeps updated medical information available on computer, 24 hours a day (see Resources). Other information cards, pendants, bracelets, and tags have all the necessary information printed right on them. Kid-sized, kid-colored, and designer IDs are also available.

## Shopping Around

Shopping for your diabetes tools may take a little patience. For example, if you are in the market for a new meter, you may have to first check your insurance or Medicare coverage. Otherwise, you may find what you think is the perfect meter for you, only to find that your insurance won't cover the cost. Many insurance companies follow Medicare guidelines for deciding what to reimburse. Currently, Medicare beneficiaries are covered for monthly glucose-testing supplies and one meter per year. Your insurance may cover the meter and the strips or just one of these.

## Stretching Your Diabetes Dollars

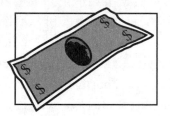

Living with diabetes can eat a major hole in your pocketbook. Here are a few money-saving tips to consider:

- Check blood glucose on a regular basis. Skipping tests may at first seem to save money. But in the long run, it could cost you more if your glucose is often out of range and you end up with acute or long-term complications.
- Think about using syringes more than once. There is no evidence that reusing syringes increases your chances for infection, if you follow proper precautions. Ask your health care team if it's safe for you and how to care for your syringes.
- Seek out rebates and trade-in discounts on meters.
- Take care of your equipment. Keep it clean and dry and keep it accessible.

Meters are usually deeply discounted by the manufacturer through rebates and coupons. The real investment is in the strips you buy on an ongoing basis. To get the latest information on the model you are interested in and any accessories it may require (such as strips and batteries), ask your diabetes educator or call the manufacturer's toll-free number and talk to someone in customer service.

If your insurance offers meters and strips through a mail-order program, you needn't worry about bargain hunting. However, you will need to get a prescription to be reimbursed for the meter and strips. You may also need to show a prescription for insulin and syringes to get reimbursed.

If your insurance doesn't cover the costs of supplies, check out the American Diabetes Association *Resource Guide*. You'll probably find a bargain, especially if you are shopping for strips. Most ads and mail-order houses offer better prices than you'll find at the local pharmacy. DME (Durable Medical Equipment) companies also offer a good variety of equipment at low prices. Some offer training as well. Pharmacies generally offer much smaller selections of equipment. However, if you have a good relationship with your pharmacist, you may ask him or her to order the machine you want. Although pharmacies can be more expensive, establishing a good working relationship with your pharmacist can save you a lot of running around over time. Pharmacists can often give you information on the ins and outs of many different products and models.

When dealing with mail-order houses, you have to pay extra attention to timing. Some will ship automatically. With others, you need to order your strips, insulin, and other equipment at least 2 weeks in advance of when you think you'll need them. Otherwise, you may find yourself high and dry without medication or test supplies. Also, if you are insured, dealing with a mail-order house may take additional time up front while the paperwork is processed. The company must confirm your insurance coverage before filling your first order.

Another shopping option is to visit a diabetes specialty store. To find one near you, call your local American Diabetes Association office (see Resources) or check in the phone book under "Medical Supplies" or "Diabetes." If you are lucky enough to have one nearby, you may be able to get many nonprescription items and diabetes information and support in one easy stop. Some pharmacies specialize in diabetes supplies and carry a large number of meters and other supplies. You may also find a selection of healthy foods, books, and information on local diabetes events and organizations. Many diabetes shops have a knowledgeable staff who can help you compare models, answer your questions, and provide training on complicated tools.

Most grocery store and chain pharmacies carry diabetes supplies. If your neighborhood store doesn't carry your brand of strips or meter, ask the pharmacist if a sister store does. Often stores in neighborhoods with many elderly people will carry more brands of supplies. Local pharmacists will know the products that they sell and will be able to spend time training you to use your purchase. This is a real, convenient advantage.

# Intensive Diabetes Management | 7

*It takes time and effort, but intensive diabetes management can increase your freedom and flexibility and help you avoid or delay long-term complications.*

When Katherine was diagnosed with diabetes, she was heartbroken. She had witnessed the devastation of the disease through her mother, who had lived with diabetes for 30 years. She stood by as her mother first lost her eyesight, then suffered a leg amputation, and finally succumbed to kidney failure. Katherine did not want to face the same ordeal. She learned from her diabetes educator that these complications were not always inevitable. There were steps she could take to greatly reduce her risk for these complications.

It always seemed obvious that keeping blood glucose levels as close to normal as possible would prevent diabetes complications. That's what researchers thought, but they couldn't prove it for sure. What if something else related to diabetes caused the complications? What if lowering blood glucose had no effect on complications?

But in recent years, two major research studies confirmed what many diabetes health professionals and people with diabetes had long suspected. The Diabetes Control and Complications Trial (DCCT) showed that by tightly managing blood glucose levels, people with type 1 diabetes could delay or even prevent many of the complications of diabetes. The results of another study, called the United Kingdom Prospective Diabetes Study (UKPDS), showed that tight blood glucose and blood pressure management can help people with type 2 diabetes delay or prevent the complications as well. These studies confirmed that it was the excess blood glucose that, after many years, caused people with diabetes to develop problems with their eyes, nerves, blood vessels, and kidneys.

The results of these two studies are very clear. The researchers in the DCCT found that after 10 years, intensive management reduced the risk of developing diabetic eye disease (retinopathy) by 76 percent. Among individuals who already had early signs of eye disease before entering the trial, intensive management slowed the progression of retinopathy by 54 percent. Tight blood glucose control also reduced the risk of kidney disease by 50 percent and that of nerve disease by 60 percent. Study volunteers, who ranged in age from 13 to 39, were too young to develop many heart-related problems, but were monitored for some of the signs of cardiovascular disease. The study found that those on intensive management had a 35 percent lower risk of developing high cholesterol levels, a major contributor to heart disease. Before the DCCT, many people with diabetes thought that complications would progress no matter what they did. After the DCCT, we know that way of thinking is wrong—keeping glucose levels close to nor-

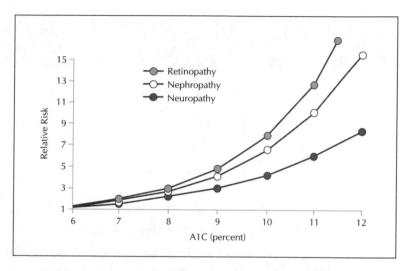

**Graph 1: The relationship of A1C levels to the risk of complications.**

mal does matter. The graph shows the relationship of A1C levels to complications as shown by the DCCT.

The other study—the UKPDS—showed that people who used an intensive program reduced their risk for microvascular complications by 25%, and if they lowered their blood pressure, they significantly reduced their risk of virtually all cardiovascular complications. That means far fewer strokes, heart attacks, and problems with atherosclerosis, as well as improved circulation to the legs and feet, which helps reduce problems with neuropathy.

The study found that for every 1 percent decrease in A1C, complications were reduced by 35 percent, heart attacks were reduced by 18 percent, and diabetes-related deaths were reduced by 25 percent. Tight blood pressure control reduced the risk of stroke by 44 percent and the risk of heart failure by 56 percent.

What do all these numbers mean? Intensive management of blood glucose and blood pressure can significantly reduce your risk of diabetes complications.

## Benefits of Intensive Diabetes Management Demonstrated by the DCCT

Keeping blood glucose levels close to normal reduces the risk of

- eye disease by 76 percent
- nerve disease by 60 percent
- kidney disease by 50 percent

Intensive diabetes management also has some drawbacks. It is more expensive and takes more time and effort. People in the DCCT using tight control had three times as many severe low blood sugar episodes than those on the standard treatment program. This happened because their overall blood glucose levels were much lower. And those practicing intensive management tended to gain more weight than those using a standard management plan. This is because they were no longer losing calories in the form of glucose in the urine. Taking more insulin made their bodies more efficient at capturing and storing calories. While these things are important to think about, it is also true that they are less likely to be problems with the insulins that are now available.

## Is Intensive Management Right for You?

You may already be reaching your glucose goals. Your A1C and blood pressure may be right where you want them to be. Or you may firmly believe that you are doing fine without intensifying your diabetes management. But even if you have your diabetes settled into a manageable routine, you may not like the idea of having your life dictated by your diabetes care or a schedule. So the idea of taking on intensive diabetes management, with even more blood glucose monitoring and more injections of insulin, may seem out of the question. But the truth is, intensive diabetes management may actually give you more freedom, not less.

If you take insulin, your schedule and activities are often dictated by when you took your last dose of insulin or when your next one is due. But the idea with intensive management is that, by monitoring frequently, you can make adjustments in your insulin dose to accommodate variety in your eating and activity patterns. Thus, by learning how to interpret your monitoring results and predict the effect your food and activities will have on your blood glucose level, you can learn to adjust your insulin doses to get greater flexibility in day-to-day living.

Here's a simple example of how it works.

To keep his blood glucose levels predictable, Jerry was used to eating the same thing for breakfast and lunch and injecting a certain dose of insulin before breakfast and another fixed dose of insulin before dinner. At dinner, he never knew what he might be having, so sometimes his blood glucose was really high in the morning, and sometimes he even had lows overnight. Jerry felt frustrated and guilty and sometimes avoided checking his blood glucose. He talked to his provider, who referred him to a diabetes education program. Jerry learned how food and insulin and exercise increased and decreased his blood glucose levels. He started taking four shots and testing four times a day instead of two. Over several weeks, Jerry learned to predict how much his blood glucose would go up when he ate certain foods. He also learned how much his blood glucose would go down if he added an extra unit or two of insulin, or when he rode his bicycle to work. After a few months, Jerry found he was able to eat at different times, or eat more or less food, and still get similar blood glucose readings because he increased or decreased his insulin dose to suit his carbohydrate intake. Jerry was able to add variety to his daily meals and lower his glucose levels.

Adopting an intensive management program does not happen overnight. It works better if you have the help and support of your family and your health care team. Intensive diabetes management takes commitment on your part. If you find that your current diabetes plan interferes with living the kind of life you would like, you may be more likely to stick with an intensive program. When you and your health care team decide to forge ahead, they will probably recommend that you attend classes or a series of training sessions to learn how to make adjustments in your diet, exercise, and insulin doses.

Intensive diabetes management can benefit almost any person with diabetes. For years, women with type 1 or type 2 diabetes who were planning a pregnancy and women who developed gestational diabetes have been advised to take an intensive approach to their diabetes. It is particularly important during pregnancy to keep glucose levels close to normal to avoid problems in the development and growth of the baby.

There are some people for whom intensive diabetes management is not safe. For instance, because tighter blood glucose levels bring a higher risk of severe hypoglycemia, intensive insulin therapy in children is risky. Severe hypoglycemia can interfere with normal brain development, particularly in very young children. Intensive diabetes management in children requires close supervision, usually from a diabetes specialist.

## Special Considerations for Intensive Diabetes Management

Aiming for near-normal blood glucose ranges may not be for you if you

- have a history of severe hypoglycemic episodes or hypo-glycemia unawareness;
- are younger than age 10, unless you have motivated and sup-portive parents and/or caregivers;
- are elderly, with other health problems or impairments;
- have cardiovascular disease, angina, or other medical condi-tions that can be aggravated by hypoglycemia;
- have severe complications of diabetes;
- have conditions such as debilitating arthritis or severe visual impairment that would functionally limit intensive management;
- have drug or alcohol abuse problems or are unable to make reasonable decisions about your everyday diabetes management;
- are unable or unwilling to carry out the tasks associated with intensive management.

Intensive diabetes management can be risky for the elderly because of the increased risk for hypoglycemia. Hypoglycemia may also make it harder to live alone or be independent. Some older people may find the potential benefits not worth the risk, particularly if they have other health problems or impairments. However, if you are an older person who believes that you will live long enough to reap the benefits (about 10 years) and are willing to take on this responsibility, then let your health care team know.

## No, Thanks, I'm Intense Enough Already

Even if you decide not to use an intensive diabetes management plan, there are still several simple things you can do to improve your blood glucose levels.

- Eat about the same amount and type of carbohydrate every day, at about the same time in relation to when you take your insulin or oral diabetes medication dose. Learn how to make adjustments from your health care team. For example, if your blood glucose check shows a level higher than your target range, take a small supplemental dose of rapid-acting or regular insulin, skip a snack, or if mealtime is coming up, eat less than usual. Getting extra exercise can also help sometimes. Increase your dose of rapid-acting or regular insulin (or plan to get some extra exercise) when you know you'll be eating more carbohydrates than usual. Take less insulin if you plan to eat less than usual. Learn how to make these adjustments from your health care team.
- If you feel like you're having low blood glucose, check. If you are low, eat 15 grams of carbohydrate, and recheck 10 to 15 minutes later. If you're still low, repeat: eat 15 grams of carbohydrate and recheck. This will keep you from having your blood glucose levels to go too high after a low. You may need less than 15 grams of carbohydrate to correct a low. Careful experimentation can help you find out what is best for you.

Intensive diabetes management may not be appropriate for people who are already experiencing severe complications of diabetes. Although intensive therapy can slow down the development of complications, there is no evidence to date that it can reverse the process.

Other health conditions can make intensive management unsafe. For example, individuals with coronary artery disease, irregular heart beats, cerebrovascular disease, angina, or other types of heart disease may not be suitable candidates for intensive therapy. Anyone taking medications, such as beta blockers, that may make it more difficult to detect hypoglycemia may be at higher risk when trying to achieve tight control.

## Education

The idea of embarking on an intensive diabetes management plan may seem a little overwhelming. There is a lot to remember. But keep in mind that it is an ongoing process. You can't learn it overnight and no one expects that of you. Your health care team is there to help you. You'll have many questions as you begin. How many units of insulin should I take if my blood glucose is a little high? How should I change what I eat at my next meal? It will require trial and error and the coordination and advice of your team members as you learn to make adjustments. Over a short period of time, you will gain the confidence to make these adjustments on your own.

Talk to your health care team members about the best way to approach intensive management. Maybe your local community hospital or health care team offers classes in intensive management. Or maybe your diabetes educator wants to arrange several one-on-one sessions to teach you what you need to know to make the program work for you. Whether you enroll in formal classes or arrange several individual sessions with your diabetes educator, check to see if the following subjects will be covered:

- nutritional guidelines and carbohydrate counting to determine the effect of food on blood glucose levels

- insulin action and dosage adjustment
- measuring the effects of exercise
- blood glucose and urine ketone monitoring and interpretation of the results
- strategies to help you make changes in your lifestyle and cope more effectively with diabetes

## Choosing Glucose Goals

The idea behind intensive diabetes management is to keep your blood glucose levels as close to normal as possible. If you decide that intensive management is for you, you will want to choose blood glucose goals as close to those of people without diabetes as is reasonable and safe for you. It's a group decision that you, your family, and your health care team need to make together.

For people without diabetes, blood glucose levels rarely go over 120 mg/dl, even after eating a meal. Their bodies take care of it for them. But when your body no longer does this for you, you need to take action to lower it: by injecting more insulin or compensating (with food or insulin) at the next mealtime. But 130 is not the magic number for everyone. Your target range may be a little higher (if you live alone) or lower (if you've just found out you're pregnant). What suits an otherwise healthy young adult with recently diagnosed type 1 diabetes may be very different from that for an elderly person with type 2 diabetes who has coronary artery disease or severe retinopathy. And an 11-year-old with working parents who spends lots of time alone may have different needs still. There are many factors to consider in setting your personal glucose goals:

- your age
- how long you've had diabetes
- the type of diabetes you have

- frequency and severity of hypoglycemia
- your lifestyle and occupation
- other medical conditions
- how much support you get from family and friends
- your personal motivation for diabetes self-management

One piece of information that came out of the DCCT is that even if you set goals that seem reasonable, they can be hard to reach. The DCCT goals for people in the intensive management group were to have near-normal blood glucose levels before and after meals and at bedtime. Most people just couldn't consistently reach these goals. No matter how hard you and your health care team work, it is difficult to keep blood glucose levels close to those found in people without diabetes.

The American Diabetes Association has established recommended targets for glucose levels (see the table below). These recommendations are based on research findings about preventing complications. You may choose these or different goals. But remember: The DCCT showed that any improvement in lowering blood glucose levels will definitely gain you real benefits.

Another way to measure blood glucose control is to measure A1C levels. In the DCCT, A1C measurements were taken to know how well people in the intensive treatment group were doing with overall control. Despite being unable to consistently

## Blood Glucose Goals

| | |
|---|---|
| Before meals _____ | 90 to 130 mg/dl |
| After meals _____ | less than 180 mg/dl |

reach the daily blood glucose goals, they lowered their A1C values dramatically. This improvement was seen after about 3–6 months of intensive management. Most had A1C values around 7 percent. This is a reasonable goal for most people with diabetes. The risk for nephropathy, retinopathy, and other complications increases as A1C goes up. The ADA recommends a target A1C value of <7 percent.

## Type 1 Diabetes

If you have type 1 diabetes, you will need to use multiple daily injections of rapid-acting or regular insulin or an insulin pump for intensive diabetes management. You may also find that combinations of rapid-acting or regular and glargine or NPH work for you. For more information on the insulin pump, see Chapter 4.

You will need to set a target range for your premeal blood glucose levels, say between 90 and 130 mg/dl. If your blood glucose levels fall below 70 mg/dl or rise above 130 mg/dl, then you'll need to take action to increase or decrease them. For example, if glucose levels are too low, you'll need to treat yourself for hypoglycemia, unless you're about to eat a meal. If levels are too high, you may need an extra dose of insulin. It will be the same routine when you check your blood glucose after mealtime. If your results are over 180 mg/dl, you'll need to take action. If your blood glucose is under 100 mg/dl before bedtime, you may need a little more food. You will need to talk with your provider about the best way for you to deal with high and low blood glucose levels. Supplemental doses of insulin are one way for you to deal with high blood glucose levels, but if you take too much insulin, you could be at risk for hypoglycemia. Your health care team can help you learn how to

**"Intensive diabetes management means I'll have more hypoglycemic reactions."**

This, unfortunately, turns out to be true. When you've worked out a plan that narrows your range of blood glucose highs and lows, you're always closer to low than you were on standard diabetes therapy. Your room for "error" becomes much narrower. This doesn't mean you need to avoid intensive management, however, unless hypoglycemic reactions would aggravate other health conditions.

You need to become an expert at telling when to pull out the meter and do a test and treat your hypoglycemia. The secret to keeping hypoglycemia from turning you away from intensive management is to prevent severe reactions. Act early, think clearly, and avoid letting your low level go so low that you need help to treat it.

Here's a sample chart for treating hypoglycemia. It's based on your blood glucose result. This chart gives an average: in general, each 5 grams of carbohydrate raises blood glucose about 15 mg/dl. After treating, your blood glucose goal is about 120 mg/dl. You'll need to figure out how much 5 grams of carbohydrate raises your blood glucose level.

| If your blood glucose is: | Eat this much carbohydrate: |
|---|---|
| Under 40 mg/dl | 30 grams |
| 40 to 50 mg/dl | 25 grams |
| 51 to 60 mg/dl | 20 grams |
| 61 to 70 mg/dl | 15 grams |

make adjustments based on patterns, your food intake, and activities and how to safely give supplemental doses of insulin.

Of course, the goals mentioned previously are guidelines only. Discuss your needs with your health care team to create a plan that will work for you. Your target glucose levels may change over time. For instance, you could find it harder and harder to detect hypoglycemia. This would call for increasing your target range and perhaps new training at recognizing your symptoms.

You'll probably want to check your blood glucose often: at least as often as you inject insulin (or take your bolus dose via a pump) and sometimes more. You could be monitoring seven times a day: before your three meals, after each meal, and before bedtime. You may even check at 3 a.m. once or twice a week. For instance, you will not want your blood glucose level to become too low during the night. But if you have experienced several severe hypoglycemic reactions, you may want to aim for a higher overnight blood glucose level. Every bit of testing gives you more knowledge of how your body reacts to food, exercise, and insulin (and stress or illness). Once you've settled into a comfortable routine, you may be able to do fewer tests. Remember that you are monitoring to get the information you need to make wise decisions as you manage your diabetes.

## Type 2 Diabetes

The blood glucose targets for a person with type 2 diabetes who wants to pursue intensive diabetes management are not much different from those for individuals with type 1 diabetes. Almost all people with diabetes can gain benefits from keeping blood glucose ranges close to normal. But the way someone with type 2 diabetes goes about reaching those targets may differ from someone with type 1 diabetes. It will still take a bit of trial and error to figure out what works best for you.

If you manage your diabetes with meal planning and exercise, adding an oral medication may help. If you already take oral medications, adding another pill or a once-a-day insulin injection may work. Ask your health care team whether it may be time for you to start insulin.

If you already take oral diabetes medications or insulin, you may need to take a more aggressive approach. Your therapy might even be similar to that of a person with type 1 diabetes who is pursuing intensive diabetes management. If you are on pills, you may need to switch to insulin. If you take insulin once or twice a day, you may need to increase to three or four shots a day.

Whatever methods you and your health care team choose for intensifying your diabetes management, you need to tailor your targets to your particular needs. For instance, you may want to watch out for weight gain that can accompany lowering your blood glucose levels. Adding an extra workout a week may be enough to counteract the fact that you're not losing as much glucose in your urine anymore. If you are just learning to treat low blood glucose levels, you'll want to make sure you're not adding more calories than you need when you have a reaction. Eating 15 grams of carbohydrate (see list on page 217) is usually enough. If you're still low after 10–15 minutes, repeat your treatment and test again.

## Pregnancy and Gestational Diabetes

Getting and keeping tight blood glucose control is especially important during pregnancy. If newly developed diabetes is left untreated, or if blood glucose levels are often out of range, several problems can develop for both mother and baby. However, keeping blood glucose levels near normal decreases the risks to mother and baby to the same level as women without diabetes. This is why intensive diabetes management is recommended for mothers-to-be with diabetes.

If you have diabetes, it's important to plan your pregnancy. Your blood glucose levels need to be as close to normal as possible before you get pregnant. Too much glucose in the blood in the first 2 months of pregnancy, while the baby is developing its nervous system, limbs, and organs, can cause birth defects. It also increases your risk of miscarriage. It's important to take care of your general health, too. Pregnant women with diabetes are more likely to develop high blood pressure, hypoglycemia, and a temporary worsening in the complications of diabetes, including retinopathy, if their blood glucose levels are not closely managed. Blood glucose goals for you are likely to be even lower than for people who are not pregnant. Tight premeal blood glucose levels for you may be 70 to 110 mg/dl. Ideal after-meal blood glucose levels might be less than 130 mg/dl.

Gestational diabetes shows itself a little more than halfway through the pregnancy. The baby is mostly developed and puts its energy into getting bigger. If you have too much glucose in your blood, the baby will take in the glucose, produce more insulin, and grow too big. Delivering a baby too large for its age is dangerous for baby and mother. For this reason, you will need a meal plan. About three-quarters of women with gestational diabetes manage their blood glucose levels with a meal plan. Regular exercise can also help to lower blood glucose levels.

Because you are aiming for a very tight range, your risk of hypoglycemia will increase. Make sure you can recognize early warning symptoms of low blood glucose. Check your blood glucose level often. When low, follow guidelines so that you can avoid overtreatment. Take 15 grams of carbohydrate (see the list on page 170), wait 10 to 15 minutes, and retest your blood. If you are still low, repeat this treatment. Try to avoid causing your blood glucose to go any higher than your target range.

Striving for these blood glucose targets requires extra effort and diligence. Although it is hard work, you are doing all that you can to ensure good health for yourself and your baby.

# Intensive Management Strategies

How do you go about keeping your blood glucose close to normal? Your tools are insulin and insulin delivery, oral medications, food, exercise, and blood glucose monitoring. Learning to use these old friends in new ways takes some practice.

## Insulin Plans

Intensive management means more than simply taking extra insulin. In fact, you may not increase the total amount of insulin you take at all. What does change is how and when you deliver it. You'll need to decide when to take it and how much to take to effectively cover your meals and your background (basal) glucose levels. You'll need to plan your insulin therapy to cover you throughout the day and night. The goal is to mimic the natural secretion of insulin from the pancreas as much as possible. As you recall, the pancreas continually secretes a low level of insulin at all times and secretes a higher level when there is more glucose in the blood, including after a meal. Therefore, your insulin plan needs to have low levels of insulin around at all or most times, with more available at meals. But just how do you do that? By taking several doses of rapid-acting or regular insulin or combinations of fast- and slower-acting insulins or by using an insulin pump.

If you decide not to use an insulin pump, your schedule will include three or more insulin doses each day. For example, you might take one injection before each meal and another before bed. You might want to inject an intermediate- or long-acting insulin at bedtime and a rapid-acting insulin before each meal. The insulin plans in Chapter 4 show different ways to do this. You will also have the opportunity to make adjustments during the day. If you are exercising after lunch, you might want to reduce the amount of your noontime insulin dose. If you are

## Elements of Intensive Management

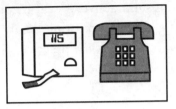

- checking blood glucose levels four or more times each day
- three or four daily insulin injections or an insulin pump
- adjusting insulin doses according to food intake, exercise, and blood glucose levels
- using a meal plan and exercising
- frequent contact with your health care team (once care routine is established)

going out to a fancy dinner where you know you'll be eating more than usual, you may want to take more insulin. Your diabetes educator can help you learn how to adjust your insulin doses.

You may want to try an insulin pump. The pump is usually worn on a belt clip or in a pocket and delivers insulin via tubing through the needle or catheter. With a pump, you keep a needle or catheter fixed in one position for a couple of days to provide insulin to your body continuously. Insulin pumps are programmed to deliver a steady supply of rapid- or short-acting insulin throughout the day. This is the basal infusion rate. You will program your basal infusion rate; it may change over the course of a day, delivering more when you need it (in the early morning hours when insulin resistance is high) or less at other times. When you need a burst of insulin to cover meals (the bolus infusion), you'll program the pump to deliver it. The amount may change depending on your blood glucose level and what you plan to eat. (For more about pumps, see Chapter 4.)

Your starting insulin doses for either injections or the pump will be based on your weight and current insulin program. For instance, for people with type 1 diabetes who are within 20 percent of their ideal body weight, the total daily insulin dose needed for intensive therapy is 0.5 to 1.0 units per kilogram of body weight. That means if you weigh 127 pounds (1 kilogram equals 2.2 pounds), you would take about 29 to 57 units of insulin each day. You would be at the high end of the range if you were insulin resistant and at the lower end of the range if you were very sensitive to insulin. About one-third to one-half of your total daily dose would provide your basal insulin level, and the rest would be used to cover meals. Most people start out with lower doses and gradually increase the amount of insulin until they reach their target.

Whichever formula or calculation you use, you will most likely have to make adjustments as you find the program that best suits you. You will probably have a plan for how to adjust your dose, but you will also need to be in close contact with your health care team. If you are pregnant, your total daily insulin dose will go up as you gain weight and develop more

## Insulin Distribution

Here is one formula that some people find helpful as a starting point for deciding how to distribute insulin throughout the day:

- 40 to 50 percent total insulin as the basal dose
- 15 to 25 percent before breakfast
- 15 percent before lunch
- 15 to 20 percent before supper
- 0 to 10 percent, as needed, to cover a bedtime snack

insulin resistance. Your insulin dose may even triple during the course of your pregnancy.

You will be able to make small adjustments throughout the day to accommodate your meals and activities. If monitoring shows that your blood glucose levels are too high, you need to take extra insulin or reduce the amount of carbohydrate in your next meal. Generally, 1 unit of insulin will lower blood glucose levels by about 25 to 100 mg/dl. You need to find out what is true for your body. You can also adjust your insulin intake to account for changes in meal patterns. In general, 1 unit of insulin will cover 10 to 15 grams of carbohydrate. You also need to find out if this is true for you.

It may be worth the effort. You will no longer have to keep a rigid schedule. The short-term benefits include, for example, going to a birthday party and eating cake (see the next section) or jogging an extra mile while keeping your blood glucose on track. Keeping complications at bay is the long-term benefit. Make sure to talk to your health care team about creating a starting plan and then making adjustments as your needs change.

## Food

The food you eat plays a big role in intensive diabetes management. In the past few years, the guidelines for food choices for people with diabetes have broadened to include more previously "forbidden" foods. This fits in well with intensive diabetes management, where you can adjust your therapy to suit your food preferences.

For example, a reasonable goal would be to derive 15 to 20 percent of all your calories from protein and less than 10 percent from saturated fat. The remaining calories can be divided between carbohydrates and monounsaturated fats. In addition, 20 to 35 grams per day of fiber and less than

2,400 milligrams of sodium per day are recommended. You and your dietitian will create a plan that works for you.

For more information on healthy eating, see Chapter 8.

**If You Use Insulin.** Work with your health care team, especially your dietitian, to create an eating plan:

- Start with a meal plan that takes into account your usual food intake. Your meal plan should have about the same number of calories, carbohydrates, and meal timing that you are already used to.
- Create an insulin schedule that follows your usual patterns of meals, exercise, and sleep.
- Time your insulin doses to match your meals. Your insulin should peak at the same time blood glucose levels from your meal are also peaking. By monitoring your blood glucose levels, you can adjust your insulin doses to suit your needs.
- Work with your health care team to explore "what if" situations and develop contingency plans that will guide you as you make adjustments in eating, exercise, and insulin patterns.

With these strategies in mind, you and your nutritional counselor can come up with a meal plan that uses basic carbohydrate counting as a system for quantifying food intake. You may find it easier at first to draw from a list of measured food exchanges. This will make it easier to match insulin doses to your carbohydrate intake. It will probably take a few months for you to get used to matching your food intake with your insulin dose to achieve your target blood glucose levels.

Once you have established insulin doses for different meals, you can practice predicting what insulin doses will match your food intake. It usually takes practice to estimate your insulin need in terms of the amount of carbohydrate you eat and adjust for changes in food intake and exercise. The next step is to learn to calculate and take extra or a corrective dose of rapid- or short-acting insulin when your blood glucose is higher than your target range. This is how you begin to fine-tune your insulin doses.

***Counting Carbohydrates.*** Counting carbohydrates gives you maximum variety in your eating plan. It is based on calculating your personal carbohydrate to insulin ratio. This gives you a good idea of how your body uses the insulin you inject to process the carbohydrate you eat. Your dietitian or diabetes educator can teach you to count carbohydrates.

The idea behind carbohydrate counting is to add up the grams of carbohydrates you eat in a meal and adjust the amount of insulin you take to handle the rise in blood glucose following a meal. With today's rapid-acting insulins, you can even take your insulin after your meal when you know exactly how many grams of carbohydrate you have eaten. This is especially useful for parents of young children who do not know in advance how much a child will eat at a meal.

Meet with your dietitian to learn how to count the carbohydrates in the foods you eat and adjust your insulin doses, to mimic the natural insulin release of a functioning pancreas. There are two basic methods for counting carbohydrates: counting carbohydrate choices and counting grams of carbohydrate. Counting carbohydrate choices is a little easier, but not as accurate. Counting grams of carbohydrate requires more effort but is more exact and may help you better achieve your blood glucose targets.

In general, if you are counting carbohydrate choices, you will use a meal plan that lists the serving size of one carbohydrate choice, also known as a carb choice. On average, carb choices contain 15 grams of carbohydrate. However, carb choices are based on averages, and there may be a significant difference between your estimate and the actual amount of carbohydrate you eat in a meal. Your dietitian can provide you with a list of carbohydrate choices for most of the foods you typically eat.

Counting grams of carbohydrates is a bit more work, but in the long run, will give you more flexibility in your meals and activities and help you better manage your blood glucose. For most packaged and processed foods, the number of grams in a serving is printed on the label. Some restaurants also provide dietary information. Most foods report the total grams of carbohydrate as well as the number of grams of dietary fiber. Because dietary fiber is included in the total grams of carbohydrate but is not digested into glucose, you will overestimate the carbohydrate content of high-fiber foods. When a food has 5 or more grams of fiber, you can subtract the number of grams of fiber from the number of grams of total carbohydrate to get a more accurate number of grams of carbohydrate that will be converted to glucose.

Once you know how many grams of carbohydrate you eat at each meal, you can then begin to make adjustments in the amount of insulin you take with each meal. In general, most adults with type 1 diabetes need 1 to 3 units of rapid- or short-acting insulin to handle 15 to 30 grams of carbohydrate. Most children need 1 unit for every 8 to 50 grams. If you count carbohydrate choices, figure on 1 unit of insulin for each carb choice (15 grams) as a starting point.

A good way to begin is with a fixed meal plan. And you will probably want to keep a detailed log of the food you eat, your activity level, your blood glucose readings, and the amount of insulin you take with each meal. Because everyone is different, you may need 1 unit for every 15 grams of carbohydrate, whereas someone else may need 1 unit of insulin for every 30 grams of carbohydrate.

Once you know how your body handles a given amount of insulin, you and your dietitian or nurse educator will meet and fine-tune your plan. Take into account any physical activities and how they affect your blood glucose levels, too.

However you decide to go about fine-tuning your insulin doses, remember that you still need to pay attention to your food choices. It's easy to get in the habit of eating fries and a shake and just taking more insulin. But even though you are counting carbohydrates, calories still count, too. Also check out *Carbohydrate Counting Made Easy*, a Fast Facts book from the American Diabetes Association.

It will take a while before you feel like you've mastered these food and insulin adjustments, but they can buy you greater flexibility in your activities and meals while keeping your blood glucose level where you want it.

*If You Are Pregnant.* One strategy for keeping blood glucose levels steady and low throughout the day is to distribute your total daily calories as follows:

- 10 to 15 percent of calories at breakfast
- 5 to 10 percent of calories at a mid-morning snack
- 20 to 30 percent of calories at lunch
- 5 to 10 percent calories at a mid-afternoon snack
- 30 to 40 percent of calories at dinner
- 5 to 10 percent of calories at a bedtime snack.

*If You Want to Lose Weight.* Intensive diabetes management sometimes causes weight gain. If this is a concern for you, the following strategies may help:

- Review your normal eating habits, including total calories, types of food, and how much fat and carbohydrate you eat, with your health care team, especially your dietitian.
- Distribute the food you eat throughout the day so that you don't eat too many calories or carbohydrates at one sitting. This can help even out glucose levels.
- Eat fewer calories each day. Your health care team can help you decide how many calories you need.
- If you're not exercising regularly, you can start. This will help counteract the better job your body is doing at capturing and storing glucose, as your glucose levels improve.
- Be careful not to overtreat the lows that are more common in intensive diabetes management. Follow the guidelines for doses of carbohydrates given on page 217 of this chapter.

## Coping

As you embark on an intensive approach to diabetes management, you may find that you need more support and encouragement in adjusting to the new routines. Sometimes you might just need someone to talk to, to discuss common problems, to air your concerns, or to just ask questions. Sometimes it will help to know that someone cares and understands what you are going through. You can look to several sources for the support and encouragement you will need. Your health care team, a special friend or family member, a religious organization, or a diabetes support group are all potential sources of support.

You may find that you want different kinds of support from different people. Friends and family may provide you with the encouragement you need to affirm your commitment to the intensive management. Maybe you need someone to reassure you—a cheerleader to help you stay on track. You may also need technical support—someone to answer your questions as they arise and reassure you that you are doing the right thing and making wise decisions. You might also need financial support or help with locating financial resources. Your health care team can help you in these areas. And you might just want someone to commiserate with. Look to support groups to find others who can listen and let you know that you're not alone. Support groups also give you the opportunity to help others, which can be therapeutic.

# Healthy Eating 8

*Food and blood glucose levels are intimately linked. Knowing what's in the food you eat—the calories, carbohydrates, protein, and fat—will make it easier for you to manage your blood glucose levels.*

Sharon was diagnosed with type 1 diabetes when she was 4 1/2 years old. Managing her diabetes at that age was a real challenge! After a few months, her parents had worked out a manageable blood testing and injection schedule, and Sharon didn't seem to mind too much. The bigger problem was with food. Getting any 4-year-old to eat healthy foods is hard enough. How would they ever manage a diabetes diet? And soon her 5th birthday would be coming up. Sharon's parents were concerned that she would forever be missing out on many of the joys of childhood—birthday parties, holiday dinners, and baking cookies—which all seemed to work against her meal plan.

Adam had always had a problem keeping his weight where he wanted it. And since he retired last year, he'd gained a few more pounds. Now he and Sarah were about to celebrate their 40th wedding anniversary with a Caribbean cruise. But last month he was diagnosed with type 2 diabetes. His diabetes care provider thought he could manage it through diet. But how could he ever stick to a diet while on a cruise? Should he call it off?

Nancy was thoroughly enjoying her second pregnancy. She exercised every day—walking or swimming—and ate a fairly balanced diet. She did give in to temptation and had some ice cream every afternoon, but it didn't seem to cause any problems. The baby was active and gaining weight at a steady pace, and she was right on target in her weight gain. But a routine glucose test during her 24th week showed that she had gestational diabetes. Would the baby be all right? She had already given up coffee and alcohol. Now she would have to give up the ice cream. Could she stand 3 months without any sort of special treat?

For many people with diabetes, food is the biggest struggle. The millions of us who have ever tried a "diet" know how hard it is to change how we eat. Diabetes is filled with food myths, starting with what causes diabetes. Have you ever been told that eating too much sugar gives you diabetes? (See Chapter 1, page 10, to dispel this myth.) And the good-hearted people in your life may often remind you that you're not supposed to eat sugar (also untrue; see the Diabetes: Myth or Fact in this chapter on page 240). Most people need help knowing what's true and what's not about diabetes and food. Your time and money will be well spent if you decide to get some education from a registered dietitian or a certified diabetes educator.

The truth is, healthy eating for a person with diabetes is no different from healthy eating for a person without diabetes. It's a matter of eating a wide variety of foods and a balanced amount of carbohydrates, proteins, and fat. It doesn't mean you have to give up all sugars or special treats. You just have to make sure you account for the carbohydrate, fat, and calories in your total meal plan for the day. Nancy may be able to have ice cream, Arthur can go on a cruise, and Sharon can attend birthday parties and even have cake like the other children. Ask your diabetes care provider, dietitian, or diabetes educator for guidance. They may suggest you make up for special treats by eating less of something else, exercising a little longer, or taking an added amount of insulin.

People without diabetes may not notice the immediate effects of choosing an extra doughnut for breakfast. Their bodies balance the extra carbohydrates by putting out more insulin. But if you have diabetes, you have to do the balancing act your body used to do for you. You need to make sure that your calorie and carbohydrate intake is balanced with your insulin doses, oral medication, and physical activity to keep your blood glucose levels on target. And, by eating more nutritious meals, you may improve your overall health and lower your risk for heart disease, some cancers, and hypertension.

## What's in a Healthy Meal Plan?

Many people find that it helps not to think of their meal plan as a "diet." After all, no one could "follow a diet" for the rest of their lives. If you are on a diet, it's easy to go off your diet. And once off, it's even easier to stay off. "Well, I've already blown my diet for today, so another slice of cheesecake won't hurt," you might think. But that will only make matters worse. Instead, think of your meal plan as a new way of eating. But in planning for that new way of life, make sure you work with your dietitian to develop a plan you can stick with. If your goal is to lose pounds, a low-calorie diet may look good on paper, but if you can't use it, it won't do any good.

In working out your nutrition plan, your dietitian or diabetes educator can work with you to achieve your goals. If you have type 2 diabetes and are overweight, maybe you want to shed a few pounds. Or maybe you want to manage your blood glucose levels through careful meal planning. If you have type 1 diabetes, you may want to learn to balance food intake with insulin. Or you may want to find out how your diet fits in with intensive management.

Once you decide on your weight, activity, and blood glucose goals (see Chapter 2), you need to work out a meal plan. Tell your dietitian about foods you absolutely can't stand, foods you can't do without, family food traditions, your schedule, how you like to cook, and how often you eat away from home. Your nutrition counselor can help you make a plan that will work for you and help you reach your goals. Just as finding the right treatment plan takes time and experience, so does finding the right meal plan.

Just what is involved in devising a healthy meal plan? A helpful food plan will make it easier, not harder, to manage blood glucose levels. Your eating plan should

- include foods you like and that are important for you;
- take your daily activities and schedule into account;
- be flexible;
- help you keep your blood glucose levels within your target range;
- help you reach and maintain a healthy weight;
- help prevent diseases and conditions, such as heart disease, high blood pressure, and cancer, which are linked to diet.

# Variety through Food Groups

The best approach to healthy eating is to eat a wide variety of foods. This goes for everyone, whether you have type 1, type 2, or gestational diabetes—and even if you don't have diabetes. No single food group can provide you with all the nutrients your body needs. Your body requires nutrients to repair and replace proteins, tissues, and cells throughout your body and to keep you rolling along. Your body needs three important nutrients to do this: protein, carbohydrate, and fat, as well as vitamins and minerals. Various combinations of these nutrients are found in different foods. So, by eating a variety of foods, you are sure to get all the nutrients you need. This is much better than taking vitamin supplements, because nature combines the needed nutrients in food in a way that your body can best use them.

Where can you find the nutrients you need? Healthy sources of carbohydrates (starches and sugars) include cereals, whole grains, pasta, bread, fruit, vegetables, legumes, and milk products. Protein can be found in meat, milk products, poultry, eggs, and fish. There is also a smaller amount of protein in grains, bread, nuts, and vegetables. You can find fat in meat, milk products, oils, and nuts.

Just about all foods provide your body with energy. The amount of energy they provide is measured in calories. Any foods that are not used as energy are stored as fat in your body. The trick is to try to balance the total number of calories you take in with the total number you burn up. Carbohydrates and proteins provide about the same amount of energy—4 calories per gram. Fats provide more than twice that amount—9 calories per gram. So if you are trying to lose or maintain your weight, proteins and carbohydrates give you fewer calories per bite than high-fat foods. A high-fat diet can also put you at greater risk for developing heart disease and certain cancers.

Think about the different food groups when you are planning your meals.

- *Fats and sweets:* Eat small amounts of these foods, and choose healthier, unsaturated fats when possible. Limit foods with saturated and trans fats.

- *Beans, meat, eggs, and dairy products:* Eat slightly more of these foods, but choose lower-fat versions.

- *Vegetables, fruits, cereals, grains, pastas, and breads:* Choose most of your foods from the whole-grain carbohydrate, fruit, and vegetables groups. These foods are loaded with nutrition, providing easily used energy, fiber, vitamins, and minerals. They also tend to be lower in calories than foods in the other groups.

## Carbohydrates

Carbohydrates include sugars, such as sucrose, fructose, and lactose, and large, complex molecules, such as starch. In the body, most carbohydrates get broken down into glucose, a sugar that is the body's main source of energy. Starches are made of many glucose molecules linked together. Sugars have only one or two molecules, of which one may be glucose.

Contrary to popular belief, whether a carbohydrate is a sugar or a starch has no effect on how fast glucose gets into the blood. Here are some things that do matter:

- how much carbohydrate you eat at a meal
- the way the food is prepared
- the combination of foods eaten at a particular sitting

For example, if a cookie made with sugar has 12 grams of carbohydrate and a cookie made with an artificial sweetener has 12 grams of carbohydrate, the effect on the blood glucose

## The Carbohydrate–Blood Glucose Connection

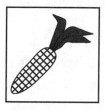 The lion's share of the glucose in your blood after a meal comes from the carbohydrate in your food. As the carbohydrate is broken down into glucose and absorbed, the amount of glucose in your blood goes up.

Different kinds of foods produce different amounts of blood glucose. There are several reasons for this:

- First, some foods contain more carbohydrates per serving than others. One popcorn cake has 8 grams of carbohydrate, 1/2 cup of kernel corn has 11 grams of carbohydrate, and 1/2 cup of creamed corn has 21 grams of carbohydrate. The more carbohydrate you eat at a meal, the higher your blood glucose level goes.
- Second is how fast the glucose is freed from the food. Carbohydrates come in several forms that take various amounts of time to break down. Food that stays in bigger pieces, like kernels of corn, breaks down more slowly than smaller pieces, like the bits in creamed corn. Cooked food digests faster than raw food. Food that contains liquid (the creamed corn) digests more quickly than dry food (the popcorn cake). Food that digests more slowly will release the carbohydrate into the blood more slowly. Your blood levels of glucose may not rise as high.
- Finally, combination foods, those that contain carbohydrates plus other nutrients such as fat, take longer to digest. This is why ice cream or a candy bar doesn't work well to treat low blood glucose. Your glucose levels may not rise until later because of the fat in these foods.

will be similar. Fat slows down the absorption of food. Therefore, adding fat to a carbohydrate food during preparation or at the table will slow digestion of the carbohydrate and delay the effect on blood glucose.

By measuring blood glucose levels 1 and 2 hours after your meals, you can get a feel for how different foods and patterns of eating affect your blood glucose levels. You most likely will begin to think about your total carbohydrate intake and how it changes your blood glucose levels. If you plan to eat a certain amount of carbohydrates each day or at a particular meal, you may find that if you eat too many sugary foods, you'll only get to eat a few of the more nutritious—and often more filling—starchy foods.

Calorie-free sugar substitutes do not raise blood glucose levels because they don't contain any carbohydrates. These include artificial sweeteners such as aspartame (Nutrasweet), acesulfame-K, sucralose (Splenda), and saccharin. Some sugar alcohols, which serve as sugar substitutes, have calories and are absorbed into the blood. These include sorbitol, mannitol, and xylitol. They are usually absorbed more slowly than glucose and usually cause a smaller rise in blood glucose levels than glucose or sucrose. But beware. If you eat these sweeteners in large amounts (more than 20 to 50 grams, or 2/3 to 1 2/3 ounces in a day), you may experience intestinal distress and diarrhea. Erythritol is a sugar alcohol that has fewer calories and fewer digestive side effects.

Get in the habit of reading the labels of all the foods you eat. You may be surprised. Many foods that have low-calorie sweeteners in them, such as diet desserts, often contain starches, other sugars, fats, and proteins. These substances contribute calories and can cause blood glucose levels to rise.

Also watch out for low-fat and no-fat items. Often, these products have ingredients added that can affect blood glucose levels. Many of these ingredients are modified forms of carbohydrate that are used as emulsifiers or bulking agents.

TIP

Artificial sweeteners give you the sweet taste of sugar without its calories and without raising your blood glucose levels. One packet gives the same sweetness as two teaspoons of table sugar. Artificial sweeteners are okay for everyone, young or old, except that pregnant or breastfeeding women should not use saccharin and people with phenylketonuria should not use aspartame.

For example, maltodextrin and polydextrose can be found in products such as sugar-free, nonfat yogurt or low-fat pudding or ice cream. Maltodextrin is digested like a carbohydrate and provides 4 calories per gram. Polydextrose for the most part passes through the body, so it only has 1 calorie per gram. Maltodextrins, because they are absorbed, have some effect on blood glucose level, whereas polydextrose has very little effect. You should be aware that even if a product is labeled as low calorie, low sugar, or sugar free, it may contain substances that raise glucose in the blood. It can be difficult to understand what some of the ingredients are. Ask your dietitian what ingredients to look for.

## Protein

Proteins are used as replacement parts in the body. They are not used for energy unless there are not enough carbohydrates and fats present. Eating protein is an important part of any healthy diet. However, many Americans eat more protein than they need. People who have kidney problems or nephropathy may be advised to limit the amount of protein they eat.

Meat, poultry, milk products, and eggs are all good sources of high-quality protein, but they also come with cholesterol and saturated fat. Select low-fat milk products and lean cuts of meat and poultry. Seafood is a good source of protein, and most kinds of seafood are lower in saturated fat and cholesterol than meat and contain valuable omega-3 fats.

FACT OR MYTH?

"When I found out I had type 2 diabetes, I said 'no' to sugar. No more sugar in my tea; no more cakes, cookies, or pies; and no more jelly on my toast. I even switched from my favorite brand of peanut butter because it had sugar in it."

These efforts have most likely made for a healthier meal plan. But you probably didn't have to go to such extreme measures.

Sugar has long had a bad reputation, especially among people with diabetes. People used to think that eating sugar would cause blood glucose levels to rise much more rapidly than eating other types of carbohydrates, such as bread or potatoes. So although bread and potatoes were okay to eat, pure sugar or sugar-laden treats were considered taboo.

It turns out that sugar's bad rap is not entirely deserved. Researchers are now finding that the extent to which blood glucose rises after eating carbohydrates is due to both the total amount of carbohydrate (all sources) and the type of carbohydrate. What also seems to matter in how quickly your blood glucose levels rise is the other foods you eat in combination with carbohydrates and how the food is cooked. Foods that include fat are digested much more slowly.

Foods that contain sugar can be part of your diabetes meal plan. You need to account for the calories and carbohydrate content of the sugar you eat, and often note the effects on your overall blood glucose levels. But you still need to count sugar as a carbohydrate, and it has little nutritional value. If you include lots of sugary items in your diet, you won't be able to eat as much of the

**FACT OR MYTH?** (*Continued*)

nutrient-rich carbohydrates such as grains and cereals that your body needs to keep you healthy.

Your dietitian can help you learn how to count sugar in your meal plan. For example, if you plan on having a piece of cake for dessert, you might want to skip the roll you normally have at dinnertime. Your dietitian or provider can also help you decide whether you need to adjust your insulin dose to deal with extra carbohydrates in your meal plan.

You can also find protein in legumes, grains, and vegetables. Nuts are laden with fat, but most nuts do not contain saturated fat (coconut is an exception). Vegetables, grains, and legumes are low in fat, contain no cholesterol, and have other nutrients as well. (Cholesterol is only found in animal products.)

For example, a 1/3 cup serving of cooked kidney beans has 3 grams of protein. So does 1/2 cup of corn. Both of these contain 15 grams of carbohydrate and count as 1 carbohydrate choice or 1 starch exchange. One-half cup of cooked non-starchy vegetables, such as carrots, broccoli, or zucchini, gives you 5 grams of carbohydrate and 2 grams of protein and counts as 1 vegetable exchange.

## Fats and Cholesterol

Everyone needs some fat in their diet to make sure their bodies function properly. Fats are used to rebuild the membranes that protect the cells in your body and to help the cells in your body send signals. Fats are also stored and used as energy reserves. But

## Skinny Meat

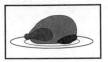

There are several ways you can reduce the fat in meat:

- Broil, roast, grill, steam, or poach instead of frying.
- Cut off all visible fat before or after cooking and remove the skin from chicken and turkey.
- Chill meat broth and drippings so the fat rises and solidifies. Then it can be skimmed off the top before serving or making gravy. You can also use this method to reduce the fat in canned or homemade broths and soups.
- Buy lean cuts of meat. Ask your butcher to tenderize them through mechanical means rather than with chemical additives.
- Try quick-cooking methods such as stir-frying meat that you have marinated using tiny amounts of olive or canola oil or dressing with lots of seasoning to enhance juiciness and flavor.

too much fat can clog up blood vessels and increase your chances of developing heart disease and stroke. Many Americans eat too much fat. For healthy living, you are better off trying to limit the amount of fat, especially saturated fat and trans fatty acids.

Cholesterol is a kind of lipid substance that your body makes. It is used to make and repair the cell membranes in your body. It is also used to make many of the steroid hormones such as estrogen and testosterone that your body needs. But too much cholesterol in the blood can clog your arteries and cause heart disease and stroke. In addition to the cholesterol your body makes on its own, the cholesterol and saturated fats that you eat can raise blood cholesterol levels.

Harvey was at risk for a heart attack. He already knew he had type 2 diabetes. He was about 50 pounds overweight and was doing his best to watch his carbohydrate intake. But, when he visited his provider for a checkup last year, he found that his cholesterol level had skyrocketed.

He decided to cut down on the cholesterol in his diet by avoiding eggs and not eating red meats. But, his cholesterol levels were about the same. As his dietitian explained, eating less cholesterol is one step to reducing blood cholesterol but is not beneficial if the saturated fats and trans fatty acids in the diet are not also reduced. Your body makes cholesterol from the saturated and trans fats in your diet. She recommended switching to low-fat dairy products and leaner cuts of meat to reduce Harvey's intake of cholesterol and saturated fat. After several months of using skim milk and low-fat cheeses instead of the high-fat varieties he was used to, Harvey saw his cholesterol levels start to come down.

How do you know how much fat is in the food you eat? Sometimes it can be difficult, especially when you are eating out. For foods you buy and prepare yourself, check the food labels. The Nutrition Facts label tells you how much fat, saturated fat, and calories from fat are in one serving. If you are cooking a meal or dish with lots of ingredients, try to add up the fat and calories from each ingredient and divide by the number of servings. If you are eating out, many restaurants, particularly chain and fast food restaurants, now provide nutritional information on request. If you are uncertain about any foods, ask your dietitian for an estimate. At the end of the day, add up all the calories from fat from the labels on the foods you've eaten and any other hidden fats in foods without labels. This

## Figuring Out Fat

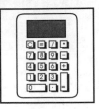

Many people with diabetes have high cholesterol levels. If you need to limit your fat and cholesterol intake, try not to eat more than 300 milligrams of cholesterol a day. If your LDL cholesterol is over 100 mg/dl, you may benefit by reducing your cholesterol intake to less than 200 milligrams per day. Less than 30 percent of your total calories each day should come from fat (with less than 10 percent from saturated fats). If you find that you've eaten too much fat or cholesterol in one day, eat less for the next couple of days.

Here's an easy way to figure out how much fat to eat each day. First, decide on the number of calories you eat in a day. Let's say you eat 1,800 calories a day. Drop the last number, so 1,800 becomes 180. Now divide by 3. The answer, which is 60, is the number of grams of fat you can eat each day and still end up eating less than 30 percent of your total calories from fat.

will give you the total of daily calories from fat. Divide this by the total calories you've eaten for the day and multiply by 100. This will give you the percent of total calories from fat.

***Hidden Fat.*** Be careful when you find cookies marked as "sugar free" or other desserts marketed specifically for people with diabetes. They may be sugar free, but more than 60 percent of their calories can come from fat. You will find saturated fat in all animal products such as butter, whole milk, half-and-half, and meat fat. The vegetable products high in saturated fats and trans fatty acids are palm oil, palm kernel oil, cocoa butter

## Types of Fat

Spend your fat calories wisely. Opt for fats that are poly- or monounsaturated, and avoid saturated and trans fats. All fats have the same number of calories.

| Saturated fats (avoid these): | Trans fats (avoid these): | Polyunsaturated fats: | Monounsaturated fats: | Omega-3 and omega-6 fats: |
|---|---|---|---|---|
| • bacon and bacon grease | • stick margarine | • corn oil | • avocados | • fish oil |
| • butter | • shortening | • cottonseed oil | • canola oil | • flaxseed oil |
| • cocoa butter (chocolate) | • fast-food french fries | • margarine | • olive oil | • soybean oil |
| • coconut oil | • processed snack foods (crackers and chips) | • mayonnaise | • nuts— almonds, cashews, hazelnuts, macadamias, peanuts, and pistachios | • tuna |
| • cream cheese | | • safflower oil | | • bluefish |
| • lard | • processed baked goods (muffins, cookies, and cakes) | • salad dressings | | • lake trout |
| • meat fat | | • soybean oil | | • sardines |
| • palm oil | | • sunflower oil | | |
| • solid shortening | • any product containing hydrogenated oil | | • peanut butter | |
| • sour cream | | | | |

(chocolate), coconut oil, solid shortening, and partially hydro-genated oils. Often these fats are found in mixes for pancakes, biscuits, cookies, crackers, cakes, and some snack chips.

***Preferred Fats.*** Not all fats are created equal. To keep your heart and blood vessels healthy, choose fats that are not saturated. Unsaturated fats (monounsaturated and polyunsaturated) are found mostly in plant foods, such as nuts and olives. They are usually liquid at room temperature, as opposed to saturated

## Cutting Down on Fat and Cholesterol

The following simple steps can help keep dietary fat and choles-terol in check:

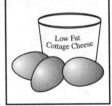

- Choose lean cuts of meat. Look for descriptions such as loin, round, lean, choice, and select.
- Remove visible fat from meats and skin from poultry, preferably before cooking.
- Choose fish and skinless poultry and lean meats.
- Try to limit your portions of lean meat, fish, or poultry to 3 ounces per meal—about the size of a deck of cards. One half of a skinless, boneless chicken breast is about 3 ounces of meat.
- Avoid fried foods.
- Limit the number of eggs you eat to four per week.
- Use a nonfat cooking spray on pans and cooking utensils to prevent sticking.
- Select reduced-fat or fat-free dairy products, such as salad dressings, baked goods, luncheon meats, soups, and dairy products.

fats, which are usually solid at room temperature. Corn, cottonseed, sunflower, safflower, and soybean oils are all polyunsaturated, whereas olive and canola oils are monounsaturated. It is recommended that people with diabetes decrease saturated fat intake to less than 10 percent of calories and eliminate trans fats. Select the rest of your fats from food with mono- or polyunsaturated fats. Omega-3 and omega-6 fats are found in fish oil and flaxseed and soybean oils. Tuna, bluefish, lake trout, and sardines are all high in omega-3 fats. These lower triglycerides and help protect your heart. Three servings per week are recommended. Choose margarine that has a liquid oil, such as olive oil or soybean oil, as its first ingredient rather than a partially hydrogenated oil or trans fat. Hydrogenated margarine has 0.6 grams of saturated fat per teaspoon and butter has 2.5 grams per teaspoon.

Trans fats are produced when liquid oil is made into a solid fat through a process called hydrogenation. Trans fats act like saturated fats and can raise your cholesterol level. Beginning in 2006, trans fat will be listed in product nutrition labels, making it easier to identify them. You can also find out which foods contain trans fats by reading the ingredient list on food labels. Look for phrases like hydrogenated oil or partially hydrogenated oil and avoid foods that have these ingredients. Trans fats show up in many processed snack foods, such as crackers and chips, and in processed baked goods, such as muffins, cakes, and cookies. Fast-food items such as french fries may contain trans fats.

## Vitamins and Minerals

People with diabetes have the same requirements for vitamins and minerals as people without diabetes. If you are eating a variety of foods, rich in vegetables, fruits, cereals, and grains, then you are most likely getting all the vitamins and minerals you need. The one exception may be the need for calcium to prevent osteoporosis. Large doses of micronutrients have not been shown to help diabetes or blood glucose levels. In fact, large doses of some vitamins can be harmful. If you think you may not be getting all the vitamins and minerals you need, check with your dietitian before you take any vitamin or herbal supplements. A few changes in your food choices may correct the nutritional deficiency.

If you are thinking about becoming pregnant or are pregnant, you have slightly different nutritional needs. You may need a prenatal vitamin or a multivitamin. Folate is generally recommended during pregnancy. Check with your dietitian or doctor about your needs (see the section on Medical Nutrition Therapy).

## Salt

Many people with diabetes, especially those with type 2 diabetes, may also have high blood pressure. High blood pressure can increase the risk of heart disease and stroke. And for some people, too much dietary salt can increase blood pressure. So, if you tend to have high blood pressure, you may try reducing your salt intake.

But what does that mean? Just stop shaking table salt on your food? That's part of it, but it may sometimes be difficult to figure out where all the salt in your diet is coming from. Many foods contain salt or another ingredient high in sodium, the element in salt that affects blood pressure. Sometimes it's rather obvious, because the foods taste salty, such as pickles and bacon. But there can be hidden salt in many foods, such as cheeses, salad dressings, cold cuts, canned soups, and fast foods. Even some peanut butters contain added salt. Take the salt shaker off the table, read labels to get an idea of salt or sodium content, and try other flavorings such as herbs and spices to make your food tastier. Remember, a little salt goes a long way.

FACT OR MYTH?

## "People with diabetes can't drink alcoholic beverages."

Not true. If your blood glucose levels are on target, it is unlikely that an occasional alcoholic drink at mealtime will harm you. In fact, a recent study published in *JAMA* showed that light to moderate alcohol intake is associated with reduced risk of death due to coronary heart disease for people with type 2 diabetes. The key is to drink moderately. Moderate drinking is defined as no more than one drink a day for women and two drinks a day for men. One drink is 12 ounces of regular beer, 5 ounces of wine, or 1 1/2 ounces of 80 proof distilled spirits. Remember these tips:

- Alcohol contains calories, almost as many per gram as fat. If weight loss is one of your goals, then you need to think about the extra calories from alcohol. Generally, alcohol is substituted for fat calories, with one drink equal to 2 fat exchanges or 90 calories.
- Alcohol can affect the blood glucose level, most often causing a very low blood sugar when consumed on an empty stomach. To prevent hypoglycemia, drink alcohol only with food if you use sulfonylureas or insulin.
- The signs of hypoglycemia (no matter what the cause) are very similar to the signs of inebriation. There is the risk that people will think you are intoxicated if they smell alcohol on your breath. They may not consider the possibility that you have a low blood sugar and need help quickly.
- Some people have hypoglycemia unawareness, a lack of symptoms of low blood sugar. Drinking alcohol increases their risk for hypoglycemia.
- Some medications, including some diabetes medications, require limits on alcohol use.

*(Continued)*

**FACT OR MYTH?** *(Continued)*

- If you have health problems such as pancreatitis, high triglyc- eride levels, gastric problems, neuropathy, kidney disease, or certain types of heart disease, you may be advised to abstain from alcohol.
- Do not drink and drive is sound advice for everyone. But because of the added risk for hypoglycemia from alcohol, it is especially true for people with diabetes.

Alcohol can affect your thought processes and inhibitions. It's easy to overeat when you are drinking. In addition, you need to be able to think clearly enough to monitor your blood glucose levels and to know what to do should they drop too low. If you are drinking, make sure to tell a friend what to do in the event of low blood glucose. Your friend should be prepared to take action even if you are not able to cooperate.

## Medical Nutrition Therapy: Your Meal Plan

Keep in mind that a healthy meal plan for you is just a healthy meal plan. You don't have to worry about following some strange diet involving weird foods that no one else in your fam- ily will want to touch. You will be developing a healthy living strategy that will benefit all the members of your household. Often, family members will not even realize that they are eat- ing a "diabetes meal plan."

Although your entire household will probably be part of your new eating strategy, you will most likely be the one setting the nutritional goals. Your provider and dietitian may recom- mend certain goals, but it is up to you to choose the ones that are meaningful and realistic for you. The more aware you are of your goals, the more your nutritional plan will reflect your needs, tastes, preferences, and lifestyle—and the more likely you are to succeed.

After first consulting with your diabetes care provider, you will most likely set up a visit with your dietitian to develop your mealtime strategy. You may feel that you don't really need a dietitian. Maybe you've seen sample meal plans recommended for people with diabetes that look easy enough to use. But remember, your meal plan is not a short-term diet that you can follow for a few weeks. You have developed a new way of eating that will stay with you throughout your life. Your dietitian or diabetes educator can help you tailor a meal plan to suit your tastes. And as you reach your goals or lifestyle changes occur, you can remodel your meal plan to suit these changes. Even if you are an old hand at planning meals, products change, your life and health needs change, and you change. As these events occur, your dietary goals will change, and most likely you will need a new plan.

A dietitian can help you learn any of these approaches to managing your food:

- counting calories
- counting fat grams
- counting carbohydrates
- counting sodium milligrams
- counting food exchanges
- changing your eating habits
- meeting specific nutritional goals (for instance, keeping protein intake low or eating vegetarian)

A dietitian with experience in diabetes care can help you develop new ways to look at food. You might want to get a better sense of matching your carbohydrate intake to your insulin doses to keep your glucose in balance. Or maybe you'd like to know how to manage your blood glucose using a vegetarian diet. Or perhaps you would like to lose weight. Your dietitian can help you resolve many issues:

- how many calories you need to eat each day
- how many grams of carbohydrates to eat each day and keep your blood glucose levels within your target range
- how many grams of fat to eat if you want to keep your fat intake to less than 30 percent (including only 10 percent saturated fat) of calories
- new ideas for breakfast, lunch, dinner, and snacks
- how to adjust your meals (or medications) for exercise
- foods to have on hand to treat hypoglycemia
- how to manage your diabetes when you travel across time zones
- how to handle changes in eating on sick days

To get started, or to try a new approach, you may want to try out some meals that are already measured and counted for you. These can be found in the ADA's *Month of Meals* series of books. At first, trying to figure out how to match your food choices to these guidelines may seem overwhelming. But try to keep in mind that developing a workable meal plan takes time and a little trial and error.

## Shopping Wisely

Sorting out all the various food claims as you make your way through the grocery aisles may at first require a little detective work. What do they mean by low fat? Is this a food that I can easily accommodate in my meal plan, or is it going to be loaded with lots of extras (like added sugars that will throw my carbohydrate count out of whack)? Once you know your daily plan for calories, fat, saturated fat, cholesterol, and carbohydrate, as well as fiber and sodium, you will find information about all of these nutrients on every food label. Reading food labels may seem daunting at first, but your dietitian can help you understand what to be on the lookout for.

As you shop, the easiest way to compare packaged foods is to look at the Nutrition Facts label. As shown in the sample label from a can of chili with beans, you'll find the serving size, the number of calories per serving, and the calories from fat. (Pay special attention to the serving size. A bag of potato chips may not seem all that bad in terms of calories and fat content until you realize that the bag actually contains three and a half servings, not one.) Below this information and on the left are the actual number of calories, grams of fat, cholesterol, sodium,

# Nutrition Facts

**Serving Size** 1 cup (253g)
**Servings Per Container** 2

**Amount Per Serving**

**Calories** 260   **Calories from Fat** 72

|  | % Daily Values |
|---|---|
| **Total Fat** 8g | 13% |
| Saturated Fat 3g | 17% |
| Trans Fat 0.5g | |
| **Cholesterol** 130mg | 44% |
| **Sodium** 1,010mg | 42% |
| **Total Carbohydrate** 22g | 7% |
| Dietary Fiber 9g | 36% |
| Sugars 4g | |
| **Protein** 25g | |

carbohydrate, and protein in one serving. On the right, you will find the % Daily Value. The % Daily Value tells you how much of the total daily intake you use up when you eat one serving of this food. These numbers assume that you are eating 2,000 calories each day. The actual percentages may be higher or lower depending on how many calories you need. If you are eating less than 2,000 calories, you will be using up a greater percentage of your daily intake. If you are eating more than 2,000 calories each day, you will actually be using up a lower percentage of your daily intake for each serving as listed.

The chili label on page 253 shows that if you are on a 2,000-calories-a-day meal plan, a cup of chili gives you 8 grams of fat (3 grams are saturated fat), 72 calories from fat, and 13 percent of your recommended fat allowance for the day.

Eating the whole can (two servings) would give you 144 calories from fat or 26 percent of your daily fat limit. Is this too high? Should you avoid this chili? The answer depends on what you eat with the chili and at other meals during the day. Even 2 cups of chili as an entree for your evening meal would not be out of line if you accompanied it with a salad with reduced-fat or fat-free dressing, a whole-grain roll or bread, and fruit or fat-free frozen yogurt for dessert. Most important is that you do not garnish the chili with high-fat foods such as cheddar cheese and sour cream or eat it with tortilla chips or cornbread. With careful planning, the chili meal can be kept under 30 percent of your daily fat calorie allowance.

Along with fat, you also need to consider the carbohydrate content of foods. One serving of this chili provides 22 grams of carbohydrate or 7 percent of the total carbohydrate you are try-ing to eat each day. Under the heading "Total Carbohydrate" is 4 grams of sugars. These include both the sugar naturally present in the tomatoes, as well as the added sucrose. All sugars—whether added or naturally present—are listed in the

Nutrition Facts. This means that the lactose in yogurt and the fructose in fruit juice show up as sugars on the labels, even though they occur naturally. Naturally occurring sugars have the same effect on blood glucose as other sugars.

The chili does not provide much of your daily quota for carbohydrates. Even if you eat 2 cups of chili, you have only 14 percent of the recommended intake. The low-fat choices of salad, whole-grain bread, and fruit or frozen yogurt suggested above help. They are rich sources of carbohydrate, providing 35 grams and another 12 percent, bringing the total carbohydrate in the meal to 26 percent of the recommended daily intake.

**Health Claims.** Food manufacturers can only make health claims on food labels that are supported by scientific research. These claims suggest a relationship between potentially harmful or helpful items or ingredients and a particular disease or condition. Some valid claims include links between the following:

- calcium and osteoporosis
- fiber-containing grain products, fruits, and vegetables, and cancer
- fruits and vegetables and cancer
- fruits, vegetables, and grain products that contain fiber—particularly soluble fiber—and the risk of coronary heart disease
- fat and cancer
- saturated fat and cholesterol and coronary artery disease
- sodium and hypertension
- folate and neural tube defects
- olive oil and coronary heart disease

**Other Claims.** Manufacturers also make claims about the nutritional value of their products. Sometimes it can be a little confus-

ing. What's the difference between low-calorie or "lite"? What is
"natural"? Here's what some of those claims really mean:

- **Calorie-free** means that the product has less than 5 calories
  per serving or other designated amount (make sure to note
  the size of the serving).
- **Low calorie** means 40 calories or less per serving.
- **Light** or **lite** means that the food has one-third less
  calories or 50 percent less fat than the foods it is being
  compared with, usually the full-calorie version of the
  same food.
- **Less** and **reduced** (as in fat or sugar) mean that the food is
  at least 25 percent lower in calories or other ingredients
  compared to the full-calorie or nonreduced version. When
  these words are used on a label, the actual percentages
  must also be included, for example, "50 percent less salt"
  or "fat reduced by 25 percent."
- **Cholesterol free** means that the food must contain less than
  2 milligrams of cholesterol and 2 grams or less of saturated
  fat per serving. For example, although vegetable oils contain no cholesterol, they are 100 percent fat. Vegetable oils
  are still preferable to butter or lard because they have less
  saturated fat. But a tablespoon of vegetable oil still has
  about 14 grams of fat and the same 126 calories found in a
  tablespoon of butter or cream.
- **Low cholesterol** indicates that a given serving contains
  20 milligrams or less of cholesterol and 2 grams or less of
  saturated fat per serving.
- **Low fat** means that a food must have 3 grams or less of fat
  per serving.
- **Fat free** means that a food has less than 0.5 grams of fat per
  serving.

- **Low saturated fat** means that a food has 1 gram or less of saturated fat per serving and not more than 15 percent of its calories from saturated fat.
- **Low-sodium** foods contain 140 milligrams or less of sodium per serving and per 100 grams of food. Ordinary table salt (sodium chloride) is not the only source of sodium. It is also found in monosodium glutamate (MSG), sodium bicarbonate (baking soda), and sodium nitrate and occurs naturally in some foods.
- **Very low sodium** means that a food contains 35 milligrams or less of sodium per serving and per 100 grams of food.
- **Sodium-free** or salt-free items have less than 5 milligrams of sodium per serving.
- **Light in salt** means that the food has 50 percent less sodium than the regular version.
- **Sugar free** means that the item has less than 0.5 grams of sugar per serving.
- **Dietetic** has no standard meaning. It indicates only that something has been changed or replaced. It could contain less sugar, less salt, less fat, or less cholesterol than the regular version of the same product. For example, if you look at a package of "dietetic" cookies, you might find that they are low in sodium but are not as low in calories or sugar as you might be led to believe.
- **Natural** has no specific meaning except for meat and poultry products. Here it means that no chemical preservatives, hormones, or similar substances have been added. On other food labels, the word "natural" is not restricted to any particular meaning by government regulation.
- **Fresh** can only be used to describe raw food that has not been frozen, heat-processed, or preserved in some other way.

TIP

Cooked oatmeal is an inexpensive, healthy cereal.

*Healthy Food Shopping.* Here are some tips for buying foods that will fit in with your healthy meal plan. Try to choose foods that are rich in vitamins, minerals, and fiber and low in fat and cholesterol. Keep in mind that the ingredients list on all food labels is in order of greatest amount by weight. That is, those ingredients that make up the largest percentage of the product are listed first and those that make up a smaller percentage of the total are listed last.

- **Bread.** Look for low-fat varieties that list whole grains as the first ingredient on the label.
- **Cereal.** Choose brands that list whole grains first on the label and contain (per serving):
  - 3 or more grams of dietary fiber
  - 1 gram or less of fat
  - 5 grams or less of sugar
- **Crackers and snack foods.** Look for whole grains listed first on the label and 2 grams or less of fat per serving (5 to 12 crackers). Consider pretzels or plain popcorn (air-popped, with no cheese or butter, 2 grams of fat or less per serving) as low-fat snacks. Check sodium content per serving. Try to keep it under 400 milligrams per serving.
- **Rice, pasta, and whole grains.** Choose converted, brown, or wild rice of any type. Look for unfilled fresh or dried pasta, preferably made with whole-grain flours. Try to avoid pastas that also contain eggs and fat.

TIP

Try using nonstick vegetable cooking spray for cooking, and cut back on oil. Use seasonings and condiments that add flavor but not calories to your meals. Try the good taste of fresh herbs for added flavor.

**TIP**

Ask your butcher to cut 4-ounce servings of raw meat. On cooking, it will shrink to a 3-ounce serving size.

- **Frozen desserts.** Choose varieties that contain 3 grams or less of fat per 4-ounce serving (1/2 cup). Look for low-fat frozen yogurt or low- or fat-free ice cream. Try frozen fruit juice bars with fewer than 70 calories per bar. Avoid foods made with cream of coconut, coconut milk, or coconut or palm oil, which are high in saturated fat or contain trans fatty acids.

- **Milk.** Choose:
  - Fat-free or 1 percent milk—they're lower in fat
  - Buttermilk made from low-fat milk
  - Low-fat and fat-free yogurt, artificially sweetened or unsweetened

- **Cheese.** Look for fat-free and reduced-fat cheeses with 6 grams of fat per ounce or less. Try:
  - Fat-free mozzarella and low-fat Farmer's cheeses
  - Fat-free or low-fat ricotta cheese
  - Fat-free or 1 percent fat cottage cheese

- **Red meat.** Beef, veal, and pork are labeled by animal, body part, and type of cut: for example, "pork loin chops." Meat is graded based on its fat content. Prime is highest in fat and Choice, or Select, is lowest in fat. Choose lower-fat grades of meat, such as Select, and lean body parts, such as beef round or sirloin, pork tenderloin, and lamb leg.

**TIP**

Look for ground turkey that is less than 7 to 8 percent fat by weight (36 percent or less of its calories from fat). Often the fatty skin is ground in with the meat, giving it a higher fat content.

- **Luncheon meat.** Look for lean or 95 percent fat-free meats (by weight) with:
  - 30 to 55 calories per ounce
  - 3 grams of fat or less per ounce

- **Poultry.** Breast meat is the leanest of all. Removing the skin before cooking cuts fat by 50 to 75 percent and cholesterol by 12 percent. When turkey or chicken is used to make salami, bologna, hot dogs, and bacon, they can be high in fat. Look for those that are 30 percent fat or less.
- **Seafood.** Supermarkets offer a wide variety of seafood. Buy fresh fish or shellfish. Look for clear eyes, red gills, shiny skin, and no "fishy" smell. Shrimp is usually shipped frozen to preserve freshness. Choose canned fish packed in water or with the oil rinsed off. Look for low-sodium products.
- **Vegetables.** Fresh and frozen vegetables are the most nutritious per bite. Drain and rinse canned vegetables to reduce sodium content.
- **Fruit and fruit juice.** Choose fresh, frozen, or dried fruit, preferably without added sugar. Look for 100 percent pure fruit juice. Fruit juices made from concentrate can come fresh, canned, bottled, or frozen. Check labels of brands that say "made with 100 percent juice." These drinks may list other ingredients. Look for "no sugar added," although the natural sugar in fruit juice will raise your blood glucose. Check the Nutrition Facts label.
- **Margarine and oil.** Choose:
  - Olive, canola, soybean, safflower, sesame, sunflower, or corn oils
  - Brands with liquid oil listed first on the label
  - Brands that contain 1 gram or less of saturated fat per serving (usually 1 tablespoon) and no trans fatty acids.
- **Salad dressings.** Try reduced-calorie and fat-free types. Include the carbohydrates in your meal plan.
- **Sour cream and cream cheese.** Try fat-free or light sour cream or cream cheese. As an alternative to sour cream, consider using fat-free or low-fat yogurt, either plain or flavored with chives, herbs, and spices.

TIP

Some fat-free cookies have more calories than the original recipe because of added sugar. Avoid palm, coconut, and hydrogenated oils.

- **Soup.** Choose low-sodium, reduced-fat varieties. In preparing cream soups, use fat-free or low-fat milk or water.
- **Cookies and cakes.** Choose brands that contain 3 grams or less of fat per 100 calories. Angel food cake is made without fat and has no cholesterol. Other cakes can be made without cholesterol by using egg substitutes but usually not without fat. Some substitute applesauce or nonfat yogurt for oil. Many cake mixes now include directions for low-fat and low-cholesterol variations.

## Eating Out

Going out to eat is a part of today's lifestyle, and there is no reason to avoid it just because you have diabetes. However, as for anyone, it is important that you know what you are eating. You may want to consider calling restaurants in advance to ask about menu options. When you do dine out, keep the following in mind:

- If you don't know the ingredients in a dish or the serving size, don't be afraid to ask.
- Try to eat portions similar to what you would eat at home. Don't feel a need to clean your plate just to get your money's worth. Some restaurants allow you to order smaller portions at reduced prices. If larger portions are served, put the extra in a "doggy bag" even before you begin to eat. Or share your meal with your dining companions. If you are dining with a family member or a

good friend, one person can order a salad and the other can
order an entrée and you can share.

■ Ask that no butter or salt be used in preparing your meal.

■ Ask that sauces, gravy, salad dressings, sour cream,
and butter be served on the side or left off altogether.

■ Choose broiled, baked, poached, or grilled meats and fish
rather than fried. If food is breaded, peel off the outer coating to get rid of the extra fat.

■ Try asking for substitutions, such as low-fat cottage cheese,
baked potato, or even a double portion of vegetables
instead of French fries.

■ Ask for low-calorie items, such as low-calorie salad dressings or broiled, steamed, or poached fish, instead of fried,
even if they are not listed on the menu.

■ **Plan ahead.** Ask your health care team for guidelines on
adjusting your insulin dose to account for changes in your
meal plan.

## Problem Solving

Without a doubt, special circumstances are likely to come up
from time to time. Disruptions in your schedule, holidays, and
parties are inevitable. Here are some tips to help you deal with
those situations.

> **TIP**
>
> Instead of eating until
> you are full, eat until
> you are no longer
> hungry.

*Eating Later than Usual.* If you can't
change the timing of your insulin dose, eat
a piece of fruit or a starchy, low-fat snack
from that meal at your usual mealtime.
Even if you are not taking insulin, you
may need a snack if your meal is later than
usual. Just make sure to account for it
in your overall daily tally. Always carry

## Traveling

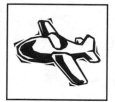 Problems often arise while you're traveling, even with the best-laid plans. What if your train breaks down or your meal service is delayed on your flight? Use these hints for smoother travels:

- Don't take your mealtime insulin unless you are sure that you can follow it with food.
- Carry an emergency snack pack that contains a nutritious and somewhat substantial snack, for example, crackers and cheese or peanut butter, granola bars, peanut butter, or dried fruit and nuts. Also carry some form of quick-acting glucose (hard candy or glucose tablets) in case of low blood sugar.
- If you are changing time zones, talk to your health care team about adjusting the timing of your meals, exercise, and insulin doses.
- Consider intensive diabetes management if you want to vary your mealtimes on a daily basis. This could be in order if you do a lot of traveling or your schedule is unpredictable.
- When you're on the move, keep your medications or insulin, as well as injecting and glucose testing supplies, with you at all times.

snacks with you. You never know when you might get stuck in traffic or delayed at work. If you plan to go out for brunch, eat an early-morning snack. Then, use your lunchtime meal plan and what is left of your usual breakfast plan. If dinner is to be very late, have your bedtime snack at your normal dinnertime. If you are taking insulin, you will need to adjust your rapid- or short-acting dose to account for these changes. If you are not sure how to do this, talk to your health care team.

***Eating More Often than Usual.*** At holidays, it may seem like you're around food all day long. Try dividing your total food for the day into snack-size meals. Then you can spread the food out a little more than usual without going over your usual amounts.

***Eating More Food than Usual.*** Sometimes going to parties, having friends visit, or just dining out may tempt you to overeat. And you are bound to eat a little more than you planned on occasion. Overeating may make you feel guilty or as if you are "cheating." It may help to remember that it is about making choices. Plan ahead what you want to do. If you decide to eat more than usual, think about using your other blood glucose management tools. Do a little more exercise than usual either before or after the event. Regardless of what you decide, think afterward if you made the right choice. Ask yourself if the benefit was worth what you gave up. You are the only one who can decide that for yourself.

## Eating Disorders

Eating disorders occur among people with diabetes just as they do in the general population. Some researchers believe that individuals with diabetes may have an increased risk for eating disorders because they have to pay more attention to what they are eating. Unfortunately, in our society, the self-worth of many people comes from having a "perfect" body. Some people resort to extreme measures to get or stay thin.

There are two main eating disorders: anorexia nervosa and bulimia. Each has a distinct set of warning signs. People with anorexia refrain from eating in order to stay thin. Their perception of their body is often out of tune with reality. Even very thin women sometimes perceive themselves as being overweight. People with bulimia will often eat normal or even excessive amounts of food and then purge the food by inducing vomiting or taking laxatives. Over time, bulimia can cause problems with the esophagus, as well as many dental problems. Both disorders stress the body and deny it the necessary nutrients.

People with diabetes and eating disorders are likely to have more episodes of ketoacidosis (type 1 diabetes) and hypoglycemia, and their A1C levels tend to be higher. And because their blood glucose is often out of range, the risk for diabetes complications is also greater.

A disorder similar to these eating disorders has been found in people with diabetes who use insulin. They intentionally reduce or omit insulin doses in an attempt to lose glucose and calories in the urine. As in other eating disorders, people who omit insulin for weight loss have more episodes of ketoacidosis and problems managing their glucose levels.

If you have an eating disorder or are omitting insulin for weight control, professional help is available. Eating disorders are serious and can lead to acute complications and even death. Please talk to someone with whom you feel comfortable discussing your feelings. Ask your provider to recommend a mental health counselor who can work with the other members of your health care team. Your entire team will work with you and your family to help you understand your disorder and how to treat it. It may help you to join a support group. Talking to others who have similar problems can help you feel understood.

## Losing Weight

People with type 2 diabetes are more likely to be overweight and are likely to benefit from weight loss. If you are overweight, losing weight is one of the single greatest steps you can take to lower your blood glucose levels. Often people with type 2 diabetes who initially take insulin or oral medications find that once they lose weight, they can manage their blood glucose through diet alone. But anyone can, from time to time, need to lose weight—even people with type 1 diabetes. The exception to this is women during pregnancy, a time when losing weight is probably not safe for the growing baby.

If you are beginning to use a healthy eating plan, you are probably already on your way to losing weight. Talk to your dietitian about your weight loss goals and set up a realistic plan for achieving those goals. But don't try to lose too much weight too quickly. You want to develop a new way of eating that you can continue with throughout your life.

**Are You Obese?** More than 75 percent of all people with type 2 diabetes either are or were obese at one time or another. But what is obesity? In medical terms, obesity refers to anyone with a body mass index (BMI) of 30 or above. Anyone with a BMI of 25–29 is considered overweight. But what is a healthy weight for you? A BMI chart can help you determine what weight is healthy for you (see page 5 in Chapter 1). BMI takes your height into account and is a good estimate of percent body fat.

Because muscle weighs more than fat, someone who has a lot of muscle can have a high BMI but be at a healthy weight. And the same weight of muscle and fat can have very different health consequences. Muscle earns its keep by burning calories, but fat is stored energy. It accumulates when your food intake exceeds the amount of energy your body uses for growth, repair, and physical activity. Older adults can have a healthy weight on a BMI chart but not have adequate muscle for good health. The BMI chart does not apply to children, adolescents, or pregnant women.

*The Body Fat–Insulin Resistance Connection.* Extra food that your body doesn't need is stored in fat cells as triglycerides. The size and number of fat cells increases with increased body fat. Having too much fat, especially on the upper body, decreases your body's ability to use insulin. This is called insulin resistance. Being overweight and overfat also strains your pancreas, and it has a harder time making the insulin your body needs. So, by getting rid of excess body fat, you can improve your sensitivity to insulin. This will help you lower your blood glucose level. See Chapter 5 for more about strategies for managing your blood glucose.

*Managing Your Weight.* The best approach to weight is a combination of exercise and a healthy diet. No one plan works for everyone. Some people find it easier to restrict their calories. Some find it easier to exercise harder. Whatever your approach, a cornerstone will be to develop a lifetime plan of healthy eating and regular exercise. It helps to have some people to cheer you on: your family and friends, your dietitian, and your health care provider. A steady loss of 1 pound per week or less is a safe and effective means to reach your goal. Talk to your dietitian about possible approaches. These can include one or more of the following:

- a nutritionally sound, calorie-restricted, low-fat meal plan designed to achieve gradual weight loss over several months
- decreasing portion sizes or eliminating certain foods
- setting behavioral goals

The most important thing you can do to lose weight is to choose weekly or monthly goals and short-term strategies to reach those goals. You will be more likely to succeed if you take one step and one day at a time.

If you use insulin or an oral diabetes medication to manage your diabetes, you need to monitor your blood glucose levels as you lose weight. You may be able to reduce the dose of your medication as weight loss lowers your glucose levels. If you have episodes of hypoglycemia, you will need to treat them with food, and this adds calories and can slow down your weight loss. Call a member of your health care team if you start to have more frequent low blood glucose reactions so they can advise you on decreasing your insulin or oral diabetes medication dose.

Creating a healthy weight loss plan is not much different than a healthy eating plan for someone who doesn't need to lose weight. You will need to eat fewer calories than you are used to. You will still want to eat a variety of foods and include a lot of fruits, vegetables, and grains. But you won't necessarily have to eat less food. One way to lose weight is to cut down on the fat in your diet. Each gram of fat in your diet provides twice as many calories as a gram of protein or carbohydrate. To get started, think about substituting some of the fat in your diet with these low-fat, nutrient-rich foods:

- **Bread.** Bread, especially whole-grain varieties, is filling, low fat, and nutritious. Good, fresh bread doesn't need any topping. Stick with whole-grain breads, English muffins, bagels, and pita bread. Steer clear of muffins and crackers, which often have a lot of added fat.
- **Pasta.** Like bread, pasta is filling, versatile, and nutritious. Whether you make your own or buy prepared noodles, avoid those made with eggs and added fat. Keep track of your portion sizes. You can make a good-tasting pasta with semolina flour and water.
- **Other grains.** Try wheat, rice, bulgur, millet, couscous, and barley. Or get adventurous and go for quinoa and

amaranth. They can be used as additives in soups and casseroles, topped with vegetables, or eaten as dishes in their own right.

- **Beans.** Beans are high-fiber, low-fat protein sources that can be used in soups and casseroles, combined with rice, used as a salad topping, or eaten by themselves.
- **Potatoes.** The potato has lots of fiber and vitamins and no fat. Try topping a baked potato with a tablespoon of fat-free yogurt or sour cream or low-fat cottage cheese. Sprinkle with herbs for added flavor. Steamed vegetables or salsa make great toppings for a baked potato. Butter or sour cream can add significantly to the calorie level.
- **Dark, leafy vegetables.** Spinach, chicory, sorrel, Swiss chard, and even dandelion and turnip greens are rich in vitamins with no fat. The darker the color, the more vitamins the vegetable usually has.
- **Cruciferous vegetables.** Broccoli, cabbage, bok choy, Brussels sprouts, cauliflower, and kale are rich in vitamins and high in antioxidants, substances that may protect against heart disease and certain cancers.
- **Fruits.** Most fruits, especially those high in vitamin C, such as grapefruit, oranges, and papayas, are low in calories and fat and high in fiber. Skip avocados—they're full of fat. Ask your pharmacist or doctor about eating grapefruit and Seville oranges. They interfere with drugs such as statins, calcium channel blockers, birth control pills, transplant medications, and some heart medications.
- **Fat-free milk.** Fat-free milk and products made from fat-free milk have most of the fat removed, making it a good low-fat protein source.

As you plan your weight loss program, think ahead to keeping your new weight. Many people are successful in losing weight but have a hard time keeping it off. What are the strategies used by people who take it off and keep it off? Studies show that exercise is an important part of both taking the pounds off and keeping them off. People who keep lost weight off say that daily exercise is an essential part of their lifestyle. They also report eating more fruits and vegetables than before, a healthy habit they hung on to even after they went off their "diet."

## Pregnancy

Whether you have diabetes before pregnancy or develop gestational diabetes during pregnancy, you will want to pay special attention to the food you eat. Eating healthy during pregnancy really isn't all that different from a healthy diet for anyone. However, you will find that you and your growing baby require more nutrients than you did before your pregnancy. For example, you will need more protein, calcium, iron, and vitamins while you are pregnant. Your appetite may increase, especially in the last months of pregnancy.

It is important to talk to your provider and dietitian before you decide to become pregnant, because good nutrition starts even before conception. For instance, your provider or dietitian will advise you to take folate as a precaution against neural tube defects, which can occur early in the baby's development. Having near-normal blood glucose levels before conceiving is another safeguard against birth defects. If you are overweight, a calorie-restricted diet may be recommended before you conceive.

Once you are pregnant, your dietitian, your diabetes care provider, and your obstetrician can assess your dietary needs and work with you to develop a meal plan that you can use throughout your pregnancy. You will need to take into account

## Portion Control: Another Step toward Weight Loss

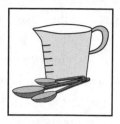

- Invest in a set of measuring cups and spoons and a food scale that weighs food in ounces or grams.
- Serve yourself your usual portion. Now measure it. Is it more or less than you expected?
- Weigh a piece of bread or a bagel. One serving of bread is one ounce. How does yours compare?
- Try dividing and weighing portions of different meats and seafoods before cooking. One serving of meat is four ounces raw (three ounces after cooking).
- Practicing portion control at home will help you estimate how much of your meal to set aside for a doggy bag when eating out.

your overall health and nutritional status. Here's what you'll need to know:

- how many calories you need to eat each day
- whether you will need a prenatal vitamin supplement
- how to divide your daily calories and carbohydrates between meals and snacks
- goals for your blood sugar readings throughout the day

Your dietitian and other members of your health care team can also help you ease into making lower-fat food choices if controlling weight gain is one of your goals. If you are suffering from nausea, your dietitian can teach you how to incorporate snacks at certain times. If you are taking insulin, you will

**TIP**

You may be advised to eat a small breakfast because blood glucose is more likely to be high first thing in the morning.

also need to learn how to adjust your insulin doses to match the changes in your diet. As your pregnancy proceeds, insulin resistance increases, and you'll need more insulin. Ask your dietitian and doctor about the use of caffeine, alcohol, and artificial sweeteners during pregnancy. Unless you have special needs, it is safe to use the artificial sweeteners aspartame and acesulfame-K during pregnancy. You need to avoid saccharin during pregnancy and when breastfeeding. Alcohol is generally not recommended for anyone during pregnancy and can increase the risk of hypoglycemia among women with diabetes.

# Keeping Fit 9

*A healthy, active lifestyle is a lifetime plan. Get off on the right foot by starting with a thorough preexercise exam and fitness testing. Then set a goal, make a plan, and go for it.*

Larry was a self-described couch potato. He worked 10 to 12 hours a day, and the last thing he wanted to do when he got home was to go jogging. All he wanted to do was sit down with a nice cold beer and relax. But since he was diagnosed with type 2 diabetes 3 years ago, he had been trying to start an exercise program. But how would he ever find the time?

Charlotte was in the middle of training for her first marathon. She had run track in high school but wanted to do a marathon before starting college in the fall. But in the middle of her fourth week of training, she was diagnosed with type 1 diabetes. Would she be able to do the marathon? Would she even be allowed to run at all?

Diabetes or no diabetes, regular physical activity improves your overall health and helps protect you against heart disease. It can increase your energy level and help you lose weight or stay at the same weight. And because exercise clears glucose from the blood, it fits nicely into a diabetes care program. The benefits of regular exercise sound almost too good to be true. But this is one miracle cure that really lives up to its advertising. And the more researchers study the benefits of regular exercise, the better the news gets.

One great benefit of regular exercise, especially aerobic exercise, is that it improves your heart, lungs, and blood vessels (your cardiovascular system) and protects against heart disease and stroke. It does this by strengthening your heart and circulatory system. This is important for anyone, but especially for people with diabetes, who are at greater risk for develop-

## Exercise Will Do You Good

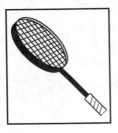

Your individual response to regular exercise may include any of the following:

- improvements in your sense of well-being, energy level, and quality of life
- lower blood glucose levels
- improvement in insulin sensitivity
- lower A1C levels
- decreased triglyceride levels
- increased HDL (good) cholesterol
- improvements in mild to moderate hypertension
- burning more calories
- conditioning of the cardiovascular system
- increased strength and flexibility

ing hardening of the arteries (arteriosclerosis) and other types of cardiovascular disease. Active movement, the kind that makes you breathe a little deeper and gets your heart pumping, improves the flow of blood through your blood vessels. Exercise helps to decrease blood cholesterol and increase levels of "good" high-density lipoprotein (HDL) cholesterol in the blood. Not only that, exercise removes glucose from your blood, both while you are exercising and for several hours afterward. For people who treat their diabetes with insulin, this could mean that you can use less insulin or eat more on the days you work out. For people with type 2 diabetes, a regular exercise program combined with a healthy diet could mean that you can manage your blood glucose without the use of insulin or oral agents or that you can get by with less medication.

Regular exercise can help you to look and feel better, physically and emotionally. It can help you lose weight and body fat and increase muscle tone and strength. For women, exercise, especially weight-bearing activities, can help preserve bone mass and prevent osteoporosis. It is a good way to handle stress as well.

## Before You Begin

You may be an old hand at fitness like Charlotte who's just been diagnosed with diabetes. Or perhaps you have been living with diabetes for a while like Larry and want to start an exercise program or make changes in your existing program. The first step is to choose the type of exercise you will do. Be sure to pick something you will enjoy and can do regularly. Think creatively: for example, maybe you find walking boring but love to dance. Don't try to force yourself to walk. Plan a time each day to put on some music that gets you moving and dance.

Be sure your plan takes into account different situations. For example, if it is too hot or too cold, consider walking at a local mall or around your house. One approach to exercise is the lifetime activity model, where you accumulate a daily total of 30 minutes of moderately intense activity. Another approach is to walk each day for a set number of steps or length of time. The third is a planned aerobic program. Types of exercises can include aerobics classes or videotapes, swimming, dancing, jogging, or cycling.

No matter what type of exercise you choose, a visit with your health care team is in order. If you haven't done so recently, you should have a complete history and physical examination. You will also want to talk to your team about adjusting your eating plan and your insulin or oral diabetes medication to keep your blood glucose levels on target. And you may want to talk to your diabetes care provider, an exercise physiologist, or your diabetes educator about finding an activity that's right for you.

You will want to make sure that you don't have health problems that may keep you from exercising safely. If you are going to begin a regular exercise program, you need to be tested for evidence of retinopathy and cardiac disease and any problems with kidney or nerve function. If you have any of these problems, it doesn't necessarily mean you can't exercise. But these complications need to be considered, and perhaps treated, before you start working out regularly. For instance, you may need laser surgery to stop the advance of retinopathy. Even after laser surgery, you may be advised to avoid certain activities or to take certain precautions. Talk with your provider and ophthalmologist about what activities are safest for you.

By the time you've finished talking with your health care team about your exercise plans and the results of your exercise tests are in, you should be able to answer these questions:

## Do I Need an Exercise Specialist?

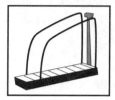 If you are about to begin a moderate- to high-intensity exercise program, you may need a graded exercise test. If your provider doesn't perform exercise testing, you'll need a referral to a doctor, an exercise physiologist, or a wellness program that does.

If you are over 35, have heart disease or cardiovascular risk factors, or have microvascular complications, peripheral vascular disease, or autonomic neuropathy, you'll need a treadmill stress test that includes an electrocardiogram. This will test how a workout affects your heart activity and blood pressure. It can also help detect "silent" heart disease. You will be asked to walk on a treadmill while your blood pressure and heart function are monitored.

Exercise physiologists—people trained to study the effects of physical activity on the body—do a variety of tests to determine your fitness level. In addition to a treadmill stress test to find out how much exercise you can safely do, they'll measure your strength, flexibility, and endurance and the percent body fat. Together with your provider, you and the exercise physiologist can create an exercise plan.

Many hospitals and universities have wellness programs for people with diabetes or rehabilitation programs for people who've had heart surgery or a stroke. These programs offer stress tests by exercise physiologists and a full range of exercise options to get you started in a medically supervised environment.

- How can I safely exercise? What times of the day are best for me?
- How long should my exercise sessions be?
- How hard can I safely exercise?

- Is it more effective to stick to the same routine each time, or can I vary the length and intensity of my workouts?
- How can I monitor how hard I exercise? Should I count my heart rate? What's my target heart rate? How often should I monitor?
- Are there any types of exercise I should avoid?
- Are there symptoms (for hypoglycemia or heart disease) that I should watch out for?
- Are there special precautions I should take?
- Do I need to take less insulin or change my injection site before I exercise?
- Do I need to modify my meal plan?
- Will oral agents affect me differently if I exercise?

## Exercising Safely

The best rule of thumb for a safe workout is to listen to your body. You should not have too much fatigue, pain, or shortness of breath. Doing too much too fast can lead to injuries or even life-threatening situations. And if you are injured, this could prevent you from doing anything at all. But how much is too much?

If you decide to do an aerobic activity program, plan your workout sessions to include 5 to 10 minutes of warm-up exercises and gentle stretching. Follow this with at least 20 to 30 minutes of aerobic activity. The aerobic activity should rev you up and get your heart pumping and blood flowing but should not be so intense as to cause shortness of breath, weakness, or intense pain. One easy guideline to remember is that, during your workout, you should still be able to carry on a conversation with your workout partner. Follow the aerobic activity with 5 to 10 minutes of cool-down exercises and stretching. Regular aerobic exercise, which keeps your body moving,

FACT OR MYTH?

**"You know I can't overdo it. I have diabetes. Exercise might make my complications worse."**

There are circumstances where diabetes complications might affect your choice of activity:

- If you have peripheral neuropathy and numb feet, you may need to limit weight-bearing exercise such as jogging. Riding a stationary bike or walking may be a safe alternative, but you will need to take extra care to protect your feet.

- If you have autonomic neuropathy that affects your heart rate and blood pressure control, you may need to avoid certain aerobic activities.

- If you exercise with untreated proliferative retinopathy and without the guidance of your ophthalmologist and provider, you are threatening your vision. Straining, jarring, or movements such as weight lifting may cause additional damage.

- If you have hypertension or heart disease, avoid exercises that involve pushing against an immovable object (such as a wall) or isometric exercises, where you keep your muscles contracted. Talk to your provider about exercises that are safe for you. Walking and swimming are often safe options.

- If you are on dialysis, you can benefit from a gradually progressing exercise program.

- If you've had an organ transplant, exercise can be helpful. Anti-rejection drugs often cause weight gain and muscle wasting. Try aerobic and strength training once you are given the okay and are ready.

benefits your heart, lungs, and muscles. It is the best way to burn calories and get rid of fat. Stretching increases your flexibility. To see improvement, you'll need to work out at least three to four times per week. You might want to alternate days of aerobic activity with days set aside for strengthening activities for muscle toning. For more intense workouts, you might want to alternate resting days and workout days. But some people find it easier to manage their blood glucose levels if they keep a similar exercise routine each day.

### Warm-Up Phase

Always warm up for 5 to 10 minutes before any physical activity. Move slowly at first, using low-intensity, easy movements. Once your muscles are warm, gentle stretching for 5 to 10 minutes is recommended—but no bouncing. Warming up before you stretch or exercise reduces your risk for muscle pulls and other injuries. For example, if you choose a walking program, walk at an easy or comfortable pace for about 5 to 10 minutes, then stop and do some stretching. Resume walking, and gradually increase the pace. Continue to increase the intensity of the workout until you reach the aerobic phase. For a running program, you could also start out by walking, then stretching. Then try a brisk walk or an easy jog to take you into the aerobic phase.

### Aerobic Phase

During the aerobic phase, you rev up, keep your body moving, and get your heart pumping. Your muscles will require more oxygen during this phase. Your heart beats faster and your lungs breathe deeper to deliver the oxygen through your small blood vessels to the muscles that need it. During this phase, you should be at your target heart rate. Stop every 10 to 15 minutes and count your pulse for 6 seconds and then add a zero. This tells you beats per minute and helps you keep in your target range.

If you are starting a new exercise program, you may not be able to sustain aerobic activity for very long. That's okay. Try

## What's My Target?

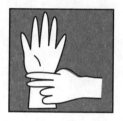

The calculation below shows you how to determine your target heart rate range, based on your age. This calculation does not work for people with autonomic neuropathy that affects their heart rate or people who take medications that affect their heart rate. Your provider or exercise physiologist can advise you on the target zone that is safe for you. An exercise stress test can help determine this.

1. Measure your heart rate while at rest. To do this, count the number of beats your heart makes in 1 full minute the first thing in the morning, before you get out of bed. Begin counting the first beat as zero. This is your resting heart rate (HRrest).
2. Determine your maximum heart rate (HRmax) by subtracting your age from 220: 220 – age = HRmax.
3. Subtract your resting heart rate from your maximum heart rate to determine your maximum heart rate reserve (HRmax reserve). HRmax – HRrest = HRmax reserve.
4. Multiply HRmax reserve by 0.5 and 0.7 to determine 50% and 70% of your heart rate reserve. When added to your resting

*(Continued)*

## What's My Target? (*Continued*)

heart rate, this gives you the lower and upper limits of your heart rate during an aerobic workout. For example, if you are 40 years old, your maximum heart rate is 180 (220 − 40 = 180). If your resting heart rate is 75, you would have a heart rate target range of 128 to 149 (see below), to be working at 50 to 70% of your aerobic capacity.

**Example:**

|  | Lower Limit | Upper Limit |
|---|---|---|
| HRmax − HRrest | 180<br>− 75 | 180<br>− 75 |
| HRmax reserve<br>3% intensity | 105<br>× 0.5 | 105<br>× 0.7 |
| %HRreserve<br>+ HRrest | 53<br>+ 75 | 74<br>+ 75 |
| Target HR | 128 | 149 |

**Be careful! This calculation does not take into account any of your specific health conditions or medications. Check that your provider agrees that the target heart rate you've calculated is safe for you.**

5 to 10 minutes at first, and gradually increase the aerobic phase. Eventually, you will be able to go the full 20 to 30 minutes. Just listen to your body and slow down when you need to. If you know you don't have to do the full 20 to 30 minutes at first, it can be less daunting. And an easy workout is better than

none at all. Sometimes once you get going, you will feel better and will go the whole way. However, if you start an aerobic workout and feel increasingly worse, slow down. If you think you are having a low blood glucose reaction, stop and check your blood glucose. If this is not possible, treat your symptoms and check your blood glucose as soon as you can.

## Cool-Down Phase

Never stop exercising abruptly, no matter how tired you are. This reduces your risk of soreness and muscle cramps. Keep your legs and arms moving at a relaxed pace. Walk around, step side to side, walk in place, or try some easy kicks for 5 to 10 minutes. Avoid bending over so that your head is below the level of your heart until you have cooled down. This "cool-down" allows your heart rate and breathing to slow gradually as your movement slows. Afterward, stretch out your muscles again while they are warm. You will be able to stretch much more freely than in the warm-up phase.

## Keeping Pace

In her book, *Women's Running*, Dr. Joan Ullyot described her husband's reaction to her new-found interest in running. She was a self-described "cream puff" before she decided to take up running in her 30s. After a few weeks, she came in from a particularly exhilarating run and told her husband, an avid runner and long-time marathoner, how much she enjoyed it. "You enjoy it?" her husband asked. "Then you must be doing something wrong!"

Unfortunately, too many people, like Dr. Ullyot's husband, have the idea that if it's exercise, it's got to be too much work, and if it's not work, it can't be exercise. "No pain, no gain"

## Safety Guidelines for Exercise

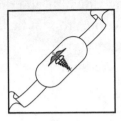

- Know your blood glucose level before, during, and after you exercise.
- Carry a source of carbohydrate with you, such as glucose gel or tablets, a soft drink, or packets of sugar, in case of low blood sugar.
- Try to exercise with a friend or, when you exercise alone, let people know when you are going out, where you will be, and when you will be back.
- Warm up and cool down each time you work out.
- Remember to replace body fluids. Start your workout well hydrated by drinking water before you begin. If you are engaging in aerobic exercise for more than 30 minutes, drink water during the workout.
- Carry visible diabetes identification and money for a phone call. If convenient, consider carrying along a cellular phone.
- Use well-fitting footwear and check your feet every day and after each exercise session for redness, cuts, or open sores. Choose the right shoes for your activity.

seems to be the prevailing attitude. But the truth is, exercise can give you a good workout, with all the benefits to your body—and still be fun. The trick is to pick an activity that you enjoy and do it at a pace that is comfortable for you. You'll be more likely to stick with your exercise plan if you take this approach.

Aim for a workout that is invigorating and slightly challenging but not miserable. If you find that you are uncomfortable the whole time, stop for a few minutes and take a rest, cut back the intensity, or find a new activity. Consider taking up a recreational sport or activity to get in your exercise. Listen to what your body is telling you. If you are in agony, you're not going to stick with that activity, and you are certainly not going to make it a lifetime habit.

The key to a safe and effective workout is to find the pace that is right for you. Then, gear your workouts to get your heart rate into the target range to get the most benefit for your heart and lungs.

## Exercise and Your Blood Glucose Level

Glucose is the fuel that muscles use to keep you moving. You know that the glucose from the food you eat makes its way into the bloodstream. But glucose can also be found in your muscles. Your muscles keep plenty of glucose, stored as glycogen, ready to use for energy.

When you first start to exercise, your body uses the glucose stored in your muscles and liver for fuel. When these stores of glucose run low, your muscles recruit the glucose from your blood. So, during exercise, your blood glucose levels can fall. After you stop exercising, your body replenishes the stores of glucose in the liver and muscle cells. This can further lower blood glucose levels even hours after you have stopped exercising. Because of this, if you exercise in the evenings, you leave yourself vulnerable to hypoglycemia while you sleep. Regular exercise can be a tool for lowering blood glucose levels, but at the same time it puts you at risk for hypoglycemia. This is why monitoring blood glucose levels before and after exercise works to keep you in the game. Exercise-induced hypoglycemia is a concern for people who take insulin or a sulfonylurea or a meglitinide.

Besides directly affecting blood glucose levels, exercise can also affect the action of insulin. It's a fact that the body absorbs insulin differently from one day to the next. Similarly, exercise can affect insulin absorption. By increasing the flow of blood throughout the body, exercise speeds up how fast the insulin you inject gets to work. Injecting into an arm or leg that's then involved in exercise can speed up insulin absorption. So, a given amount of insulin can have different effects from one day to the next, especially if there are differences in your physical activity routine. This makes it doubly important to check your blood glucose levels when you exercise.

For people with type 2 diabetes, especially those who are managing blood glucose levels through diet and exercise alone, big swings in blood glucose levels do not usually occur during exercise. However, if you have type 2 diabetes and are taking insulin, a sulfonylurea, or a meglitinide, your blood glucose levels may drop too low during or after exercise. Like people with type 1 diabetes, you will want to avoid hypoglycemia. If you are beginning an exercise program, it would be smart to monitor your blood glucose levels just to make sure they aren't falling too low.

## Guidelines

Everyone (with or without diabetes) can use the general recommendations for a safe and effective workout, outlined above. This means taking time to warm up and cool down and aiming for an appropriate target heart rate range. People with diabetes, especially type 1 diabetes, also need to take extra care to make sure that blood glucose levels do not swing too

> **TIP**
>
> Check your blood glucose level before you exercise. If your blood glucose level is less than 100 mg/dl, have a snack that has 10 to 15 grams of carbohydrate, such as a piece of fruit or three graham crackers. Then test 15 to 30 minutes later. Don't start exercising until your blood glucose level is over 100 mg/dl.

widely. This is true not only during the activity, but also up to 16 to 24 hours later, as blood glucose is used to replenish glucose stored in muscle tissue.

## Type 1 Diabetes

The way that exercise affects blood glucose levels in people with type 1 diabetes can be a little complicated. Not only do you have to think about blood glucose levels getting too low, you also have to make sure they aren't too high. Having the right amount of insulin on board will help you get the most benefit from your workout or leisure activity. So, take the time to learn how to predict your insulin and food needs by monitoring in all types of situations. This will help you enjoy all manner of aerobic and strengthening exercises open to you.

During mild to moderate exercise that doesn't last too long, your blood glucose levels are likely to fall during and after exercise. This is because the glucose in your blood is being used up faster than your liver can produce more glucose. This is one of the positive benefits of exercise. But if you exercise for longer periods, or if you didn't have much glucose in your blood to begin with, you could experience hypoglycemia. If you exercise on an empty stomach, you'll probably need to snack during or after your workout so that your blood glucose levels don't drop too low.

If you exercise vigorously, or if you do not have enough insulin available, you could experience the opposite effect. A high blood glucose level can go even higher because of exercise. Sometimes during vigorous exercise, the nerves signal the liver to release stored glucose. This can result in a rapid rise in blood glucose levels. These increases can occur even with exercise of moderate intensity if your insulin levels are low. In this situa-

## Avoiding Exercise-Induced Low Blood Glucose

- Exercise 1 to 3 hours after a meal. This is when your blood glucose is highest.
- Try not to exercise when your insulin injection is peaking. If you use rapid-acting or regular insulin, this would mean to avoid exercising within the first 1 to 2 hours after injecting it. Remember that exercise increases blood flow, which speeds up how fast your insulin goes to work.
- If your exercise is going to be of moderate to high intensity or you're going to be working out at a more moderate intensity but for a longer time than usual, think about decreasing the insulin dose that will be working while you exercise. Ask your health care team for guidance.
- Know your own blood glucose response to different types of exercise. Learn this by monitoring often, before, during, and after exercising.
- If you are going to be doing vigorous exercise for an extended period, check your blood glucose 1 hour and again 30 minutes before you begin, to know whether your blood glucose level is stable or dropping.
- You may need to eat during or after exercise if you work out hard or for a long time (an hour or more).
- Know that you may have a low blood glucose reaction up to 24 hours after exercising, depending on how hard and how long you exercised.

tion, ketones can be produced and ketoacidosis can result. That's why it is important to check blood glucose levels both before and after exercising to make sure your glucose levels aren't going too high or too low.

If you are exercising vigorously or for long periods, think about monitoring during the exercise. You may need to eat a snack during the workout. Try snacking on something that is low in fat and has 15 to 30 grams of carbohydrate. If you are really going at it, you may need to repeat this snack based on blood glucose levels. How much food you need depends on what you ate before you began exercising, how hard you are exercising, and what your insulin levels are. When in doubt, always check your blood glucose.

It's never a good idea to exercise within 1 to 2 hours of your last injection of short- or rapid-acting insulin. The insulin will be peaking and your blood glucose levels can fall faster if you're also exercising. Know the action times of your specific insulin(s). Consider what type of insulin you are using and the timing of your injections, exercise, and meals. Try not to exercise when insulin is working its hardest (see Chapter 4).

You'll also want to consider where you inject your insulin. That's because insulin can be absorbed much more rapidly if it is injected close to muscles that are being exercised. The longer you wait between injecting insulin and working out, the less you have to worry about choosing your injection site. Talk to your diabetes care provider or diabetes educator about the kinds of exercise you like to do and the best places to inject your insulin. Also, discuss the timing of your insulin injection, meals, and exercise. Perhaps you can time these events so you won't have to worry about where you inject insulin.

You may need to know which way your blood glucose level is heading, especially if you are about to start an activity in which you can't easily "pull over." If you are about to go for a long run or wind surfing, checking your blood glucose level midstream may not be very convenient. Try checking 1 hour and then 30 minutes before you start. If your monitoring shows that your blood glucose level is coming down, even if you are

TIP

Monitoring your blood glucose levels is a great idea, even if you're not at high risk for hypoglycemia. It can be very motivating to see just how much exercise can reduce your blood glucose level. Try checking before and a little bit after your workout.

still in a safe range, you may want to have a snack to keep it from going any lower. Also, keep in mind when your insulin is peaking.

If you suspect a low blood glucose reaction is coming on, **stop exercising at once.** Take some form of carbohydrate. Don't fool yourself into thinking you can last just 5 minutes longer. Always keep some form of glucose handy just in case you need it while exercising. This can be a soft drink or fruit juice, which will provide sugar and replace water. Or you can use glucose tablets, raisins, or hard candy.

Be on the lookout for hypoglycemia not only while you are exercising, but up to 24 hours later. Keep monitoring your blood glucose levels to detect very low blood glucose.

## Type 2 Diabetes

Regular exercise can be an important part of the management plan for people with type 2 diabetes. Many people with type 2 diabetes find their blood glucose levels are much easier to manage if they exercise regularly. This is because regular exercise increases insulin sensitivity and lowers insulin resistance. And regular physical activity, combined with a balanced, reduced-calorie diet, leads to weight loss—which further lessens insulin resistance.

If you have diabetes complications or other health concerns, you need to be cautious. Be sure to consult with your provider before starting an exercise program. However, be assured that almost everyone can benefit from some form of

## How Do I Keep Motivated?

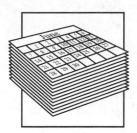

It will take several months for your new, more active lifestyle to become a habit. In the meantime, try these strategies for sticking with it.

- **Schedule your workout and stick to your schedule.** It's as important as any other appointment in your day.
- **Find a workout partner.** On those days when you're tempted to skip your workout, your partner will probably be ready to go. It helps to have a commitment to someone else.
- **Cross-train.** This means having different activities instead of doing the same thing every time. Twice a week, you may lift weights; 3 days a week, you may take an aerobics class; once a week, you may play tennis. This keeps your interest level up and your risk of injury down. By building up your fitness in many areas—strength, flexibility, and aerobic capacity—you'll protect yourself from overuse of any one group of muscles.
- **Set realistic, specific goals.** Don't expect to lose a lot of weight or run a mile without stopping right away. Set both long-term ("I plan to walk 5 days a week for 30 minutes") and short-term ("I plan to walk for 15 minutes 3 days this week") goals.
- **Reward yourself for sticking with it.** Do an easier workout 1 day a week, such as a yoga session. Don't skip the hot tub or steam room if you really enjoy them after your workout. (If you have high blood pressure, ask your provider about hot tub precautions.)
- **Track your progress.** Record noticeable changes like your energy level, the way your clothes fit, your belt size, and the amount of medication you take.

exercise, as long as it doesn't increase your risk of injury. For example, just increasing some daily and familiar activities, such as parking farther from the door, walking short distances instead of driving, and using the stairs instead of the elevator, is an excellent start. Or consider a mild weight-lifting program to increase your strength. You can start strength training using very small weights or no weights at all. Ask your health care team about working out with elastic bands or with isometric exercises.

If you take insulin, you'll need to use precautions to prevent low blood glucose, just like people with type 1 diabetes. See the previous section about type 1 diabetes, and follow those guidelines for reducing insulin or adjusting medications. You'll probably want to try to avoid extra snacks, but talk to your diabetes care provider and educator about what's best for you. If you take sulfonylureas or meglitinides, hypoglycemia is rare but it can occur, so it pays to know what to look for and how to treat it. People who treat their type 2 diabetes by meal planning and exercise almost never have hypoglycemia.

If you are cutting back on calories to lose weight, exercise will speed up your progress. Review your meal and exercise plans with your health care team to be sure you are getting enough vitamins and minerals and you are replacing fluids lost during exercise. If you are on a very-low-calorie diet (fewer than 800 calories per day), your provider should be closely monitoring your exercise and overall health.

If you have difficulty getting around, are obese, or are recovering from heart surgery or stroke, talk to your provider and an exercise physiologist about the best way to begin your exercise program. You'll need to start slowly and build up gradually. Consider joining a wellness or rehabilitation program, or see what kind of program your insurance will cover. The exercise specialists at these types of programs will work with you to create an exercise plan that avoids worsening any health problems you have.

## Exercise and Pregnancy

If you exercise regularly with type 1 or type 2 diabetes, pregnancy is no reason to stop working out, but you may need to lower your workout intensity. If you have gestational diabetes, exercise lowers your blood glucose level and so is considered an effective part of your treatment plan. Staying physically fit during your pregnancy will help you prepare for the work of labor and baby care that lies ahead. Exercise can also moderate your weight gain, increase your strength and stamina, and lower your anxiety level. In some cases, it may help you avoid or delay the start of using insulin.

Exercise during pregnancy does pose some risks. You'll need to consult with your diabetes care provider and your obstetrician about the type of workout you want to do. They will consider your medical history and advise you if it is safe. One thing you definitely should not do is start a new, strenuous exercise program while you're pregnant. This is especially true if you didn't exercise regularly before pregnancy. However, you'll probably be able to begin a new program of low-intensity exercises, such as walking or swimming.

Most women use intensive blood management during pregnancy, to keep blood glucose levels close to normal. If that is your goal, you'll need to be extra watchful for low blood glucose levels caused by exercise. Your glucose level can go very low very quickly. Blood glucose

> **TIP**
>
> Some safe and effective exercises during pregnancy are swimming or aerobics classes held in the pool, walking, and stationary bicycling. Talk to your providers about which exercises are safe for you.

## Keep Your Workout Safe During Pregnancy

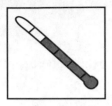

- Monitor your blood glucose levels often, before, during, and after exercise.
- Drink plenty of fluids before, during, and after you exercise.
- Warm up before and cool down after you exercise.
- Keep the strenuous part of your workout to no longer than 15 minutes.
- Keep your heart rate under 140 beats per minute while you exercise (this is about 23 beats in a 10-second pulse count).
- Keep your body temperature under 100°F. Ask your provider about hot tubs or steam rooms.
- Avoid exercises that involve any of the following:
  - lying on your back after your fourth month of pregnancy
  - straining or holding your breath
  - jerky movements or quick changes of direction
- Stop exercising if you feel lightheaded, weak, or very out of breath.
- Ask your obstetrician to show you how to feel your uterus for contractions during exercise. These contractions can be a sign you're overdoing it.

monitoring is your way to keep watch on hypoglycemia. Chances are, you'll already be monitoring your blood glucose levels frequently during your pregnancy. This can help you figure out how exercise affects your blood glucose and when your levels are starting to drop.

# Finding an Exercise That Works for You

There is no single perfect exercise. But there are some types that burn more calories, some that are particularly helpful for developing strength and flexibility, and others that are especially beneficial for your cardiovascular system. Every exercise also has its downside or even risks. For people with heart disease or diabetes, some of the risks of particular types of exercise are important to know. The important thing is to find an activity that is beneficial, and of course fun, but one that won't worsen any of your complications or lead to new problems.

Some activities are not safe for people with certain complications or health issues.

- People with untreated proliferative retinopathy should avoid any activity before their retinopathy is treated. Then get your provider's okay to exercise. Straining or jarring may cause further damage.
- If you have peripheral neuropathy, avoid exercises that traumatize the feet, such as running, jogging, and high-impact aerobics. You may also be at a higher risk for injuring soft tissues and joints because you may not be able to feel when you've overstretched or overdone it.
- If you have autonomic neuropathy, do not exercise until your provider and perhaps an exercise specialist have given you the okay. Your body may not be able to compensate for the exertion of exercise. You may be at high risk for dehydration and low blood pressure. Your aerobic capacity—the ability of your heart, lungs, and blood vessels to support your muscles while they work—and your ability to achieve maximum heart rate may also be limited by neuropathy, so you may have to stick to activities of low in-

## Foot Care: The Agony of the Feet

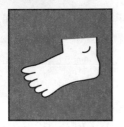 If you're an adult, you'll need to pay attention to foot care. Most children and teens with diabetes don't need to think too much about foot complications.

- Check your feet daily for any red, irritated areas, blisters, corns, calluses, or ingrown toenails. If you detect a problem, call your diabetes provider or podiatrist right away. Don't expect it to get better on its own.
- Well-fitted shoes are worth their weight in gold. They will help keep problems from starting in the first place. Shoes should feel comfortable right away. Don't count on breaking them in.
- If you have neuropathy or decreased sensation in your feet, you can't always trust the way shoes feel as you try them on. You may need to consult your podiatrist or a professional shoe fitter (a pedorthist) to get a correct fit.
- You may want to try special socks designed with extra cushioning for exercise. In truth, any good athletic sock that is made of a blend of cotton and synthetic material will provide warmth and cushioning and will absorb perspiration away from your skin.

tensity, such as walking. You will also need to choose a method other than counting your heart rate to measure workout intensity.

- If you are pregnant, avoid strenuous activities and those that are jarring, especially during the last months.

## Walking

Walking is probably the safest and least expensive form of exercise. It can fit into almost anyone's schedule because it can be integrated into other events and activities. If you have to drive a half mile to the post office, you may as well walk and squeeze in a workout. The only investment you need to make is in a comfortable pair of shoes for walking. In exchange for this—and extra attention to foot care—you get an exercise that conditions the cardiovascular system, the lungs, and the muscles of the arms, legs, abdomen, lower back, and buttocks.

You can benefit your heart and lungs by walking 30 minutes per day, five days per week. You don't have to walk 30 minutes all at once. You get the same benefit by walking 10 minutes three times per day. For example, you might want to park farther from work so that you have a 10-minute walk in the morning and afternoon. You can then add a 10-minute walk at lunchtime, and you have completed your 30 minutes of exercise. If you are trying to lose weight, you will need to gradually increase the length of time to 60 minutes of walking per day.

You might want to purchase a pedometer, an inexpensive tool that counts your steps and may measure the distance and duration of your walk. Approximately 2,000 steps are equal to 1 mile. Start by wearing your pedometer on two or three typical days to find your usual number of steps. Then gradually increase to at least 10,000 steps per day. It can be

**TIP**

Try on shoes in the afternoon, when foot size tends to be a little bigger, while wearing your workout socks. Wear new shoes for short periods at first. Check your feet for red, irritated areas. You may need extra padding in some areas of the shoe to prevent friction.

both motivating and fun to figure out how to add steps into your daily routine.

Walking can be especially invigorating if you move at a brisk pace and travel over hilly terrain. Walking is a lifelong activity, and it is a good way to have a more active lifestyle. It can also help you ease into a more vigorous exercise if you are newly diagnosed with diabetes or are not used to exercising. Maybe you are a little afraid that exercising too vigorously will throw your blood glucose levels out of whack, just when you thought you had things figured out. After walking for a while, you will develop the confidence, stamina, and fitness level to try other activities.

At the beginning, it may take you 30 minutes to walk a mile. An experienced walker can walk a mile in 10 to 12 minutes. A pace of 4 miles per hour or 15 minutes per mile is a good goal to work toward, if you are motivated by keeping track of your time and mileage. For some people, however, paying too close attention to the pace destroys the joy of the activity. Walk at a pace that is both enjoyable and invigorating for you. Some people find that walking with hand weights makes for a more challenging workout, but first check with your provider or exercise physiologist.

## Jogging/Running

Some people would rather jog or run than walk. You get a more intense workout in less time than walking. But jogging is tougher on your joints and feet because each step pounds the foot with three to five times your body's weight. Make sure that you discuss your running or jogging program with your provider before you start to make sure it is safe for you.

To reduce the chances that you'll get injured or drop out of a walking/jogging/running program, take the time to develop

## Counting Cals

Counting the calories you're burning is one way to keep track of your fitness efforts. The numbers of calories burned shown here are for a 150-pound person working out at an average intensity. If you weigh more or work out harder, you'll burn a few more calories. But remember, exercise has more benefits than just burning calories.

| Activity | Notes | Calories burned in 30 minutes* |
|---|---|---|
| Walking at 4 miles/hour | Works the lower body; include some hills | 135 |
| Jogging at 5 miles/hour | Run on soft surface; use well-padded shoes | 240 |
| Swimming, leisurely | The crawl uses the whole body | 200 |
| Bicycling, leisurely | Works the lower body | 200 |
| Ice skating | Nonstop at a moderate pace | 235 |
| Low-impact aerobics | Nonstop at a moderate pace; include arms | 170 |
| Advanced aerobics | Nonstop at high intensity | 240 |
| Tennis, doubles | Keep moving | 200 |
| Tennis, singles | Keep moving | 270 |
| Golf | Carry your clubs and walk the course | 150 |

*Based on metabolic expenditure units given in Ainsworth BE et al.: *Med Sci Sports Exerc* 25:71–80, 1993.

your leg and foot muscles. If you are trying to progress from walking to running, try this: Start walking your normal route or distance. Walk for a few minutes, then try jogging. Jog for as long as you feel comfortable. If you start to feel winded or uncomfortably out of breath, switch to a brisk walk. Don't stop, but keep walking. When you have regained your breath, jog for a little bit. You may find that eventually you will be able to jog the whole distance. Of course, you may want to stick to a combination run-walk or you may want to alternate some days running and some days walking. Do what feels good to you.

Avoid jogging on concrete—it's too hard; try the track at a nearby school or a park instead. Buy a pair of well-padded running shoes, and replace them before they wear out. Choose shoes that fit well and are comfortable from the first time you put them on. If you start to develop any persistent pain, especially in your joints, don't risk further injury. Rest, take a few days off, or try walking instead.

## Strength Training

Strength training with weights is not just for Mr. Universe wannabes. Anyone, old or young, male or female, who wants more strength and endurance can benefit. Well-toned muscles can help in all your daily activities, whether it's carrying groceries, climbing stairs, doing laundry, or changing a flat tire. Strength training can also help prevent osteoporosis and build muscle, even in elderly people. This is important because as people get older, they tend to lose muscle mass and tone. Even people in their 80s and 90s can greatly increase strength through weight training. Another benefit of weight training is that well-toned and larger muscles burn more calories even when you are doing absolutely nothing. So a regular weight lift-

## Safe Strength Training

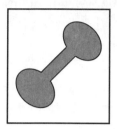

- Talk to your provider before starting any weight-lifting routine. For some people, lifting weights will increase the risk of worsening diabetes complications.
- Always do some sort of aerobic exercise, such as walking, jogging, jumping rope, or jumping jacks, for 5 or 10 minutes to warm up before lifting weights. Cool down after lifting.
- Don't hold your breath while lifting. Instead, breathe in when lowering weights and breathe out when lifting.
- Exercise with a partner or trainer, who can help you if something goes wrong.
- Always allow at least a day's rest between workout sessions, or alternate upper body training one day with lower body training the next.

ing program can help you lose fat and manage blood glucose levels in the long run, both during and in between workouts. But some of these programs can raise blood glucose and blood pressure levels and put pressure on the blood vessels in the eyes. Be sure to talk with your health care provider before you begin.

There are several approaches to weight training. Most people combine weight training with aerobic activity for a complete workout. It can be as simple as lifting a small set of hand weights in your living room. Or you may want to join a gym or health club where you will have access to a whole array of weight machines and exercise equipment. Most weight training programs involve sets of weight-lifting exercises. Each set consists of a series of repetitions. When you first start, do just one set each session. Eventually work your way up to three to six sets each session. As you become stronger, you will also find that you can lift more weight. Then add more weight, a little at a time. Muscles become stronger by lifting heavier loads. Plan your program with your personal goals in mind:

- If you just want to increase your endurance, then choose a weight that you can lift only 15 to 20 times. Rest for a few minutes between each set of repetitions (reps).
- If you want to build both strength and endurance, choose a weight you can lift only 8 to 12 times. Rest for a few minutes between sets of reps.
- If you are geared toward competitive weight lifting, you might want to maximize your strength by lifting only 2 to 6 times. Rest for a few minutes between sets of reps.

## The Best of the Rest

Try yoga to increase your flexibility. Try aerobics classes, especially if you like to dance. Community and senior centers may have equipment available or offer classes that are free or reasonably priced. Try a trial membership at a health club convenient to your home. You could try out their machines to see if there are any you would use at home. You could rekindle your love of tennis, squash, or volleyball. Make an aerobic challenge out of washing the windows or sweeping the deck. When it comes to your fitness, the old saying "use it or lose it" is true!

# Diabetes Complications and Prevention

10

*Perhaps the hardest thing about living with diabetes is thinking about the possibility of complications. The key is the same for all diabetes-related complications: keeping blood glucose levels close to normal can help prevent or delay their occurrence.*

Fred went to the doctor because he was having problems with his vision. He didn't expect a diagnosis of diabetes. And to make it worse, he found out he would also need laser treatments for his eyes. He read that complications arise after living with diabetes for years. It hardly seemed fair that he had diabetic eye disease even before he knew he had diabetes. He wondered what else might be wrong with him.

Elaine was only 16 when she was diagnosed with diabetes. Everyone had told her to take care of herself, and she did the best she could. But back then, they didn't have glucose meters and insulin pumps. Now she was in her 40s and was starting to experience numbness in her legs. It just wasn't fair. She had done all the right things.

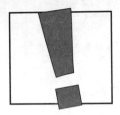

**Warning Signs of Diabetes Complications**

Anytime you "just don't feel right" and can't explain it, you need to tell your provider. Call right away if you notice any of these signs:

- vision problems, such as blurry or spotty vision or flashes
- unexplained, overwhelming tiredness
- discomfort in your legs when walking
- numbness or tingling in your hands or feet
- chest pain that comes on when you start to exert yourself
- cuts or sores that stay infected or take a long time to heal

It's possible that you view your diabetes care from two perspectives: the "close-at-hand" and the "far away." The close-at-hand might be things like daily blood glucose monitoring, making food choices, and reaching next month's fitness goal. Maybe the faraway category contains diabetes complications: something to consider, but not dwell on.

But the truth is, the more you think now about the complications of diabetes and ways to prevent them, the better off you will be. The best way to reduce your risk of getting diabetes complications is to keep your blood glucose levels as close to normal as possible. Doing this not only helps your faraway picture look brighter, your close-at-hand experiences with diabetes will be more meaningful.

## The Glucose Connection

Almost all of the complications of diabetes are caused by having too much glucose in the blood. A major problem—and the

**"But I was just diagnosed! I can't have complications already!"**

Some people have the unpleasant experience of finding out they have diabetes complications soon after diagnosis. Or they find that complications are present at the time of diagnosis. This is more likely if you're diagnosed with type 2 diabetes. The signs of type 2 diabetes may be so subtle that you may have had high blood glucose levels for quite a while without ever realizing it. The damage was occurring even before your diagnosis. Maybe it was a diabetes complication, like problems with your vision, that brought you to the doctor in the first place. Because of your symptoms, your blood glucose levels were tested and you learned you had diabetes.

cause of many health problems associated with diabetes—is that the small blood vessels that carry blood throughout the body get clogged up. Blood can't get to where it needs to be. This causes problems with circulation to the small blood vessels and leads to eye disease (retinopathy) and kidney damage (nephropathy). Too much glucose can also speed up the normal hardening of the arteries (atherosclerosis) that occurs as you age. This decreases blood flow to the heart, which can cause a heart attack, and to the brain, which can cause a stroke. Too much glucose can also damage nerve cells and delay, change, or halt the electrical messages that your nerve cells send throughout your body, especially to the feet.

But the good news is that we know more about why these problems happen to people with diabetes, so we know more about how to prevent them. The Diabetes Control and Complications Trial (DCCT) and the United Kingdom Prospective Diabetes Study (UKPDS) showed that keeping blood glucose levels as close to normal as possible can help prevent or slow the progression of many of the complications of diabetes. The DCCT examined more than 1,400 people with type 1 diabetes for 10 years, and the UKPDS studied people with type 2 diabetes for over 20 years. Those people who kept their blood glucose levels as close to normal as possible ended up with less eye disease, less kidney disease, and less nerve damage.

The volunteers in the DCCT's intensive management group monitored their blood more often—4 to 7 times each day—and injected insulin more often. They stayed in close touch with their health care team. And their hard work paid off. They cut their risk for developing these complications by more than 50 percent. For example, those who kept their A1C levels closer to normal had 76 percent less eye disease, 60 percent less nerve damage, and 35 to 56 percent less kidney damage than the study group who used standard therapy. For more information about the DCCT, the UKPDS, and intensive management, see Chapter 7.

As you are working to lower your glucose levels, it may help to know that any improvement you can make in lowering your blood glucose levels will benefit you. The less time you spend with too much glucose in your blood, the lower your risk for developing diabetes complications.

To manage your glucose, you need to help your body use the glucose you take in as efficiently as possible. If you use insulin, managing blood glucose levels involves matching insulin doses to your food intake and exercise. If you use oral diabetes medications, the technique for managing blood glucose levels is similar, but fine-tuning is harder. And for everyone with diabetes, regular physical activity helps your body get the glucose into your cells where it can produce the energy you need.

Even if you already have one of the complications of diabetes, it's not too late. Most complications can be helped by lowering your blood glucose levels, even if they have already developed. You may be able to decrease your symptoms by managing your blood glucose and taking other steps to healthier living. So, if you have already decided to live a more healthy lifestyle—exercising regularly and choosing more nutritious foods, for example—you're on your way to preventing complications.

## Other Things You Can Do

### Quit Smoking

The role of smoking in causing lung disease is well known. But smoking is even more risky for people with diabetes. Over time, smoking damages your heart and circulatory system by narrowing your blood vessels. When blood flow to cells is restricted, the cells in your body can die. This damage can lead to heart disease, impotence, and amputation. Coupled with the already high risk for people with diabetes, the effect can be devastating. If you smoke now, talk to the members of your health care team about strategies that can help you quit.

### Eat Healthy Foods

You may already be using a meal plan low in saturated fat and cholesterol with lots of whole grains, fruits, and vegetables and a moderate amount of protein. Maybe you have cut down on salt to lower your blood pressure. If you have decided to lose weight, you also need to watch the total number of calories you eat. By making wise food choices, you can reap benefits far beyond keeping your blood glucose on target. You can also reduce your risk of cardiovascular disease. And healthy eating habits are contagious. Your family will benefit, too.

### Lower Your Blood Pressure

High blood pressure, or hypertension, puts a strain on your body, especially your heart, blood vessels, and kidneys. In addition, high blood pressure can accelerate the progression of eye and kidney complications. You can lower your blood pressure by losing weight and exercising. For some people, limiting salt intake helps lower blood pressure. You may also take medications to keep your blood pressure at or below the recommended level of 130/80.

### Exercise Regularly

Exercise helps people with diabetes in several ways. It can delay or help stop cardiovascular disease. It can help clear glucose out of your blood, so that cells can use it for energy. This lowers blood glucose levels and in some individuals may lower the amount of insulin needed. And it can give you a positive way to cope with stress. For people who are overweight, exercise helps in weight reduction, and losing weight lowers your insulin resistance. Exercise just helps your body work better. See Chapter 9 on working with your health care team to design an exercise program that is safe for you.

## Dealing with Complications

Despite your best efforts, you may some day develop complications from diabetes. Factors you can't control—your age, race, and genetic makeup—can affect your risk of developing complications.

**FACT OR MYTH?**

**"I give up. It's just not worth the trouble. No matter what I do, I'll get diabetes complications."**

Unless you've been dealt an incredibly poor genetic hand, this is a diabetes myth. Blood glucose levels are at the root of this disease, so it makes sense that keeping blood glucose levels as close to normal as possible will stop or slow down diabetes complications from occurring. People studying diabetes and seeing patients with diabetes have suspected this connection for decades. But it took the DCCT and the UKPDS to prove it.

You are not predestined to get diabetes complications. It's true that one study found that, after 20 years of diabetes, 95 percent of the people in the study had some evidence of retinopathy. But early retinopathy can be successfully treated without impairing vision. Like diabetes, heart disease and high blood pressure run in families. If you have genes that make you more susceptible to, for instance, poor circulation, your body might react more to the effects of high blood glucose. Do high blood pressure, obesity, or cardiovascular problems occur in your family? These are health conditions that are worsened by high blood glucose levels. If health problems that are aggravated by the effects of diabetes are in your family gene pool, you have even more reason to work hard to lower your blood glucose levels.

If you have been taking steps to prevent complications, you may feel cheated if you develop a diabetes-related health problem. You may have many of the same feelings you had when you were first diagnosed with diabetes—anger, fear, guilt, or denial. You may feel overwhelmed that on top of dealing with diabetes and the ordinary stresses of everyday life, you now have new health problems to contend with. You may feel tired of having worked so hard to prevent complications, only to have them develop anyhow.

But there are treatments for diabetes complications, and they are getting better all the time. The earlier the signs of complications are found, the more effective these treatments can be. So be sure you are getting up-to-date information on treatments and prevention (see p. 86 for a complete diabetes care schedule). Read all you can and ask your diabetes care provider and other members of your health care team—don't rely on hearsay from friends and relatives who may not be up on the latest research.

The remainder of this chapter is in sections that explain some of the most common complications of diabetes, with emphasis on ways to detect, prevent, and treat them:

- cardiovascular disease
- retinopathy (eye disease)
- nephropathy (kidney disease)
- neuropathy (nerve disease)
- infections

If you are interested in information about lipid abnormalities, look in the section on cardiovascular disease. If you want information about amputation, see the section on infections. If you need information about impotence or sexual problems, see Chapter 11.

## Cardiovascular Disease

There are several kinds of cardiovascular disease, and they are all due to problems in how the heart pumps blood or how

## Your Risk, in General: Cardiovascular Disease

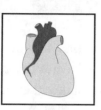

People with diabetes are

- 2 to 4 times more likely to get heart disease;
- 5 times more likely to have a stroke than people without diabetes;
- at risk for cardiovascular disease, which

causes more than half of the deaths in older people with diabetes.

blood circulates throughout the body. Blood flows through the blood vessels in your body to deliver all the oxygen, glucose, nutrients, and other substances needed to run your body and keep your cells alive. When blood can't get to cells and tissues, they can become damaged or die.

Most of the cardiovascular complications related to diabetes have to do with a blockage or slowdown in blood flowing throughout the body. Diabetes can change the chemical makeup of some of the substances found in the blood, and this can cause the openings in blood vessels to narrow or to clog up completely. This is called atherosclerosis, or hardening of the arteries, and diabetes seems to speed it up.

Blood vessels can become clogged in several ways. If there are too many lipids (fats) in the blood, such as cholesterol and triglycerides, they can collect in the walls of the blood vessels. Diabetes changes the number and makeup of proteins that deliver lipids to cells. But if you lower your blood glucose levels, these so-called lipoproteins will return to normal and do their job of delivering and removing lipids to cells in your blood vessels. Blood lipids can also accumulate if you eat too much fat and cholesterol. And if there is also too much glucose in the blood, these lipids are more likely to clog blood vessels. That's why it is important to pay attention to fats in your diet if you have diabetes. By keeping your glucose levels on target and limiting your saturated fat intake, you can prevent clogging of your blood vessels. Diabetes can also affect the platelets in your blood, which play a role in blood clotting. Diabetes can cause blood platelets to churn out too much of a substance that causes blood to clot, and this can also cause blood vessels to narrow.

When blood vessels narrow or clog because of cardiovascular disease, the blood supply to the heart, brain, and other tissues and organs can be restricted. If blood to the heart is slowed for a time, it can cause chest pain known as angina. Angina is not itself a disease, but it can give a warning that something is slowing the flow of blood to the heart. A complete stoppage of blood is a heart attack. When the blood flow to the brain is cut off, this can cause a stroke. Blockages in the arteries of the legs can cause leg pain known as intermittent claudication.

## Hypertension

Hypertension, or high blood pressure, can also contribute to cardiovascular disease. Hypertension itself usually has no symptoms. If you have it, you probably won't even realize it unless you have your blood pressure checked. Hypertension is especially common among people with type 2 diabetes. Over 70 percent of people with diabetes also have high blood pressure or use medicines to treat hypertension.

High blood pressure not only increases your risk for heart disease but also increases your risk for other diabetes complications. The recommended blood pressure for most people with diabetes is <130/80 mmHg. Along with exercise, weight loss, and watching salt intake, many people with diabetes also take one or more medications to lower their blood pressure. The most commonly used are angiotensin-converting enzyme (ACE) inhibitors and angiotensin receptor blockers (ARBs). These lower blood pressure and help protect your kidneys. Diuretics, beta blockers, and calcium channel blockers may also be used. It will take time to figure out the best medicine plan for you. Be sure to keep in close contact with your health care team during this time and let them know if you are experiencing any side effects from these medications.

If you have hypertension, your heart is forced to work harder than usual. This extra stress can damage the lining of your arteries. If this goes untreated for a long period, a type of fatty tissue called atheroma can form. This can cause your arteries to narrow or become completely blocked. Even by itself, hypertension can damage small blood vessels and capillaries, especially in the eyes and kidneys. If you have hypertension on top of diabetes, there is an even greater chance that your arteries may become clogged. The risk of further damaging tissues and further aggravating cardiovascular disease increases dramatically if you have both hypertension and diabetes.

## Prevention

There are six things you can do to prevent cardiovascular disease:

- stop smoking
- lower your cholesterol levels
- lower high blood pressure
- lower high blood glucose levels
- exercise
- ask your provider if taking aspirin will benefit you

All of these actions will help keep your large blood vessels open for blood to flow to all your vital organs, and you will lower your risk of developing cardiovascular disease dramatically.

## Blood Lipid Abnormalities

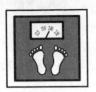 Abnormal lipid profiles are quite common in diabetes, especially type 2 diabetes. Lipid abnormalities, hypertension, obesity, and type 2 diabetes seem to go hand in hand. That has led researchers to ask whether lipid abnormalities are the result of obesity, and ultimately, type 2 diabetes. If you and other family members have severely high levels of cholesterol and other blood fats, you may have a lipid disorder that is not related to diabetes.

There are several kinds of lipids in your blood. HDL cholesterol is sometimes called good or "helpful" cholesterol. This lipid helps remove deposits from the insides of your blood vessels and keeps them from getting blocked. The target levels for HDL cholesterol in your blood are above 40 mg/dl for men and above 50 mg/dl for women. You can raise your HDL cholesterol level by getting more exercise, avoiding saturated fats, choosing more omega-3 and omega-6 fats, and lowering your triglyceride levels.

LDL, or bad, cholesterol can narrow or block your blood vessels, which can lead to a heart attack or a stroke. The target level for LDL cholesterol in your blood is below 100 mg/dl. High levels of LDL cholesterol are usually treated with medications called statins.

Triglycerides are another kind of lipid in the blood. It is recommended that you keep your triglyceride level below 150 mg/dl. Triglyceride levels are closely linked to blood glucose levels and can usually be lowered by making these changes:

- lowering your blood glucose levels
- losing weight
- increasing physical activity

## Blood Lipid Abnormalities (*Continued*)

- eating a healthy, low-fat, high-fiber diet
- taking medications called fibrates

A visit with a dietitian can help you make healthy food choices. Here are some things to consider if you are prescribed drugs to lower blood lipids and cholesterol:

- Watch carefully for changes in your blood glucose levels; even if you have type 2 diabetes, you may want to monitor your blood glucose level several times each day.
- Start new drugs one at a time, if possible; some medications can interfere with the breakdown, absorption, and removal of other medicines.
- Know that many kinds of medications are used to treat high lipid levels and that side effects may occur; report anything unusual to your provider.

### Treatment

If you develop cardiovascular disease, the preventive measures listed above can still help you. Even if you are being treated for cardiovascular disease, taking preventive steps can slow or stop the progression of the disease. A low-cholesterol, low-fat diet that is rich in fiber can further lower your levels of cholesterol (the blood vessel–clogging culprits).

But sometimes, prevention alone isn't enough, especially if you have had cardiovascular disease for a while. You may need medication to reduce blood clotting, to lower cholesterol levels, or to reduce high blood pressure. If your blood vessels are already blocked or significantly narrowed, you may need surgery to remove the blockage. Angina can also be treated by both preventive and surgical steps. The goal is to increase the amount of oxygen going to the heart.

Several different surgical procedures are now commonly used to remove the blockages of blood vessels. **Balloon angioplasty,** while not performed as often as it used to be in people with diabetes, is a procedure that uses a balloon at the tip of a long tube. A cardiologist inserts the tube into the blocked artery and then inflates the balloon. This opens up the blocked vessel. A metal stent, or ring, may be left in place to help the blood vessel stay open. **Atherectomy** is another kind of minor surgery used to open blood vessels. With this technique, the cardiologist bores a hole through a blocked blood vessel. Laser surgery can also be used to melt away blockages with an intense beam of light. All of these surgeries can remove smaller blockages and require little recovery time.

A more severe blockage calls for more serious surgery. Cardiac surgeons can create a detour around the blocked artery through arterial bypass surgery. Maybe you already know someone who has had a single, double, triple, or even quadruple bypass surgery of the heart. Surgeons can construct one, two, three, four, or even more detours, if there are multiple blockages. To do this, surgeons remove a part of a larger artery from the chest wall or from a vein in the patient's leg and attach it above and below the blocked blood vessel. Now, instead of running up against a wall, blood can flow around the blockage and through the new blood vessel.

Intermittent claudication, or leg pain, is not a nerve problem but a sign of a circulatory problem. It can be relieved by exercise, quitting smoking, drug therapy, and surgery similar to that for blocked heart arteries. Strokes are usually treated by a combination approach. Treatment to lower blood glucose and lipid levels and blood pressure, therapy to help the person recover mental and physical abilities, and medications that reduce blood clotting are all effective common approaches. Sometimes surgery is needed.

People with cardiovascular disease are advised to be physically active and to eat foods that protect the heart and blood vessels. Because of diabetes, you'll also need to manage your blood glucose levels and perhaps lose weight as part of your recovery.

## Retinopathy

One common complication of diabetes is retinopathy, a disease of the retina, the light-sensing region of the inner eye. The retina acts like a miniature "movie screen" in the back of your eye, on which the images you see are projected. Retinopathy is caused by damage to the blood vessels that supply blood to the retina.

You probably won't even notice any changes in your vision when diabetic retinopathy first begins. The only way to detect the changes in blood vessels found in the early stages of disease is to have a dilated eye exam by an ophthalmologist or optometrist. And early detection is the key to keeping this disease from interfering with your vision. Detected early enough, retinopathy can be slowed or stopped altogether.

Retinopathy is more common among people with type 1 diabetes, but people who have had type 2 diabetes can also develop it. There are two major forms of retinopathy. In one type, called nonproliferative (or background) retinopathy, blood vessels can close off or weaken. When this happens, they leak blood, fluid, and fat into the eye. Although this can lead to blurry vision, it does not cause blindness, unless there is leakage in the macula, the area of the retina near the optic nerve that is responsible for most of our vision.

Nonproliferative retinopathy can progress to a more serious, although less common, form of eye disease called prolifer-

## Your Risk, in General: Retinopathy

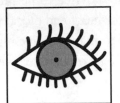 Diabetic retinopathy is estimated to be the most frequent cause of new blindness among adults aged 20–74 years. After 20 years of diabetes

- nearly all people with type 1 diabetes show signs of retinopathy, and
- more than half of all people with type 2 diabetes develop some signs of retinopathy.

ative retinopathy. This occurs when new blood vessels sprout, or proliferate, in the retina. This may seem like a good thing, but the new vessels don't grow in the way they should. Instead, they grow out of control. They are fragile and rupture easily during exercise or even while sleeping, especially if you have high blood pressure. When this happens, blood can leak into the fluid-filled portion of the eye in front of the retina. This can block the light coming into the eye and impair vision. In addition, scar tissue can form on the retina. The scar tissue often shrinks, and when that happens, it can tear the layers of the retina apart. This damages your eyesight. Glaucoma, or high pressure within the eye, and cataracts occur more often in people with diabetes. If found early, glaucoma can be treated.

Retinopathy can also cause swelling of the macula of the eye. Because the macula is that central portion of the retina that allows you to see fine detail, when it swells, vision can be impaired and blindness can result. This condition is known as macular edema.

## Prevention

There are several reliable ways to lower your risk of impaired vision from retinopathy. First, get a yearly eye exam from an eye doctor (ophthalmologist or optometrist). Adults with type 1 diabetes need a dilated eye exam within five years after the onset of diabetes. Adults with type 2 diabetes need an eye exam shortly after diagnosis. Your eyes should be dilated for the exam. The early detection of any eye problems is critical to keeping your vision.

Second, keep your blood glucose levels as near to normal as possible. The DCCT found the most striking results of intensive management in preventing retinopathy. The UKPDS showed that people with type 2 diabetes who lowered their blood glucose and blood pressure also lowered their risk of retinopathy. So the third step is to lower your blood pressure. The fourth is to stop smoking.

The bottom line, whether you have type 1 or type 2 diabetes, is that you can significantly reduce your chances of developing retinopathy or of having your retinopathy worsen. See your eye care specialist if one of the following occurs:

- your vision becomes blurry
- you have trouble reading
- you see double
- one or both of your eyes hurt
- you feel pressure in your eye
- you see spots or floaters
- you lose peripheral vision

## Treatment

The best way to treat proliferative retinopathy, oddly enough, is with light—an intense beam of light called a laser—using a procedure called photocoagulation. An ophthalmologist aims the laser beam at the retina. This creates hundreds of tiny burns in the retina. These burns will destroy abnormal blood vessels, patch leaky ones, and slow the formation of new fragile blood vessels. If you have the more serious form of retinopathy, proliferative retinopathy, or macular edema, photocoagulation can usually prevent blindness.

Photocoagulation may not be for everyone, however. It may not work if the retina has bled a lot or has detached. In these cases, a surgery called a vitrectomy can remove the excess blood and scar tissue, stop the bleeding, replace some of the vitreous humor—the clear jelly-like substance that fills the eye—with salt solution, and repair the detached retina.

If you need either of these procedures, choose an ophthalmologist who specializes in retinal disease and who has a lot of experience in treating patients with diabetes. Don't put off visiting your eye specialist. **The earlier you get treated, the greater your chances of preventing blindness or further eye damage.**

## Nephropathy

Your kidneys are your body's filter units. They work 24 hours a day to rid your body of the toxins that your body makes or takes in. Toxins from the blood enter the kidneys by crossing the walls of small blood vessels along its border. In people with nephropathy, these tiny blood vessels, called capillaries, are unable to filter out the impurities in your blood. They begin to leak, allowing some of the waste products that should be removed to stay in your blood, and some of the proteins and nutrients that should remain in your blood to be lost in the urine. Symptoms of kidney disease usually occur after much kidney damage has already been done and may be subtle: fluid

## Your Risk, in General: Nephropathy

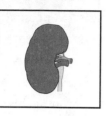

- Approximately 43 percent of new cases of end-stage renal disease (kidney failure) are due to diabetes.
- Of all people with diabetes, around 30 percent have nephropathy.
- Native Americans, Hispanic Americans, and African Americans are at a greater risk than Caucasians with type 2 diabetes.

buildup, sleeplessness and tiredness, vomiting, or weakness. Fortunately, damage can be detected early through a urine test for small amounts of protein.

When you first develop diabetes, you may have an excess of protein in your urine. This is usually a temporary condition. Unchecked hypertension and a period of hyperglycemia before diagnosis could contribute to this condition. But the more obvious symptoms of kidney disease take a long time to appear. The kidneys have so much extra filtering ability that noticeable problems will not appear until 80 percent of the kidneys are damaged.

Not everyone with diabetes develops nephropathy. Severe kidney damage is more common in people with type 1 diabetes than in those with type 2. However, kidney damage can also result from high blood pressure, and many people with type 2 diabetes also have hypertension. Years of high blood pressure can damage the delicate filters in the kidneys, leading to less efficient removal of waste products from the blood. The good news is that there are steps you can take to reduce your risk of nephropathy.

## Prevention

The most important thing you can do to prevent kidney damage is to keep your blood glucose levels close to normal. The DCCT showed that people in the intensive management group reduced their risk of kidney disease by 35 to 56 percent. Another important step you can take is to keep your blood pressure in the target range. If your blood pressure is high, the delicate capillaries in your kidneys can become damaged. Two things that you can do to lower high blood pressure are to keep a healthy body weight and to eat less salt. If kidney damage is advanced or if you cannot reduce your blood pressure with these steps, you may need one or more medicines to lower blood pressure. ACE inhibitors and ARBs are blood pressure medications that also preserve kidney function.

## Treatment

The earliest sign of kidney disease is finding small amounts of protein in the urine (microalbuminuria). Your urine needs to be checked once a year starting 5 years after the diagnosis of type 1 diabetes, or starting at the diagnosis of type 2 diabetes. This can be done at your provider's office, or you can do the test at home and mail it in. Make sure your urine is tested for *microalbuminuria*, not just *proteinuria*. If you have this early sign of nephropathy, the first step is to bring your blood glucose levels into the target range. In the DCCT, people with microalbuminuria who were in the intensive management group cut their risk of progressing to a more serious stage of kidney disease in half. To reap this benefit, these study participants kept an A1C of 8.1% or lower. You may also be advised to begin a diet low in salt. Blood pressure medications called ACE inhibitors or

ARBs are usually prescribed, even if your blood pressure is in the recommended range. ACE inhibitors and ARBs decrease the rate of progression of kidney disease.

If your kidney disease becomes more advanced, more will need to be done. A low-protein diet may be recommended. If the kidneys fail, they are no longer able to do their job of filtering out toxins from your body. This condition is known as **end-stage renal disease.** At this point, the only two treatment options are dialysis and kidney transplantation. Both remedies are ways of replacing the kidneys.

Dialysis uses a machine to artificially do the job that the kidneys are no longer able to do. There are different types of dialysis, but they all accomplish the same thing—removing toxins from the blood. One type of dialysis, called hemodialysis, removes the blood from an artery (usually in the arm), filters it through a machine, and returns it to a vein. If you need hemodialysis, you will most likely go to a dialysis treatment center three times a week for 2 to 4 hours. Or you may be able to have a trained caregiver come to your home to provide hemodialysis.

The other type of dialysis is called peritoneal dialysis. Here, instead of using a machine to filter the blood, the abdominal cavity, or peritoneum, serves as the filtering site. A solution called a dialysate is poured through a small tube into the abdomen, where it is allowed to sit and collect waste products. Waste products from the blood are exchanged in the peritoneum. After a few hours, the dialysate, which now contains the wastes, is drained out of the abdomen. This process can be performed manually by letting gravity carry the dialysate into the cavity and drain it out again. Or, a machine can carry out the exchange, usually overnight.

Transplantation is usually more effective than dialysis. A new kidney functions as well as your old ones did before disease. However, it depends on the availability of a kidney and requires taking drugs that suppress the immune system to prevent rejection of the new kidney. A genetically near-identical donor is desirable, but not essential. A relative may be willing to donate a healthy kidney, or a kidney may become available from someone who has just died. People often go on dialysis while waiting for a transplant. Some people choose to have a pancreas transplant at the same time. Pancreas transplants are always from organ donors who have died.

Transplantation has its risks as well. It is major, expensive surgery and requires good cardiovascular health. The drugs you must take to prevent immune rejection of the new kidney may put you at a greater risk of developing infections. And the new kidney will face the same pressures as the old ones did.

## Neuropathy

Your body's nervous system controls virtually everything you do and every move you make. From moving your muscles and digesting your food to breathing, blinking, and thinking, the nerves in your body serve as your body's electrical circuits. They are the wires that send and receive signals from your brain that tell other cells to do what they need to do.

Diabetes usually doesn't impair the brain and spinal cord (central nervous system). But the nerves in the rest of the nervous system can be damaged. They may be unable to send messages, send them at the wrong times, or send them too slowly. And because the nerves send signals to so many places in your body, nerve damage can cause a range of effects. Maybe you have pain in your feet or hands. Or perhaps you are having trouble with digestion or bladder or bowel control. You may experience sexual dysfunction or loss of sensation or feeling or find that your muscles are weak. All of these symptoms could

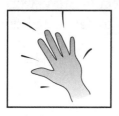

**Your Risk, in General: Neuropathy**

- About 60 to 70 percent of people with diabetes have mild to severe forms of neuropathy.
- Autonomic neuropathy occurs in 20 to 40 percent of people with long-standing diabetes.

be caused by diabetic neuropathy. Often, they come and go or are severe for only a short period. These symptoms can also be caused by other health problems. Be sure to tell your provider about any symptoms you are experiencing. Lowering your blood glucose levels may help improve these symptoms. Neuropathy is more likely to affect people who have had diabetes for a long time or who have had high glucose levels for some time.

No one really knows for sure why high blood glucose causes nerve damage. It may be that proteins coated with glucose cause direct damage. Or high levels of glucose may upset the chemical balance inside nerves. Or the blood supply to nerves may be cut off or constricted, and nerves may not receive the oxygen they need. Single nerves can also get squeezed by the tissues surrounding them. However, neuropathy can have causes other than diabetes.

## Prevention

The DCCT showed that people with type 1 diabetes who intensively managed their diabetes reduced their risk of neuropathy by 60 percent. Nerves need a constant blood supply to function properly. Keeping blood vessels healthy will protect the nerves they supply. It's also important to stop smoking and exercise regularly to help keep the nervous system in prime working condition. Alcohol is also a direct toxin to nerves and can be another cause for neuropathy.

## Types of Neuropathy and Treatment

There are many types of nerve damage. Our nervous systems are so complex, it's often hard to decide exactly what type of neuropathy is present. Complicating this is the fact that high blood glucose levels can damage nerves in two ways: directly and by slowing down or stopping their flow of blood. Sometimes it's hard to know whether a problem is caused by nerve damage or by circulation problems.

*Distal Symmetric Polyneuropathy.* This type of neuropathy, also called peripheral neuropathy, can strike the nerves in many parts of your body. Sensation can be either decreased or increased with neuropathy. The treatment is determined by the symptoms. If sensation is decreased, your feet can feel numb, or you can lose the ability to determine temperature or the position of your feet. If you have lost sensation, you need to pay special attention to care for your feet and protect them from injury. You can step on something and not feel it or burn your feet with your bath water. If you don't realize it and treat it, you can get an infection.

Dealing with the pain of neuropathy can be difficult. Many people find that their pain gets better when their glucose levels are lower. Some even notice that their pain will be worse when their blood glucose levels go up temporarily. Walking may also help to decrease calf pain.

Several types of medications can be used for pain. Nonsteroidal anti-inflammatory drugs (NSAIDs) are generally the first medications that are tried. Others include low doses of antidepressants, antiseizure medications, and drugs designed specifically for neuropathy pain. Medicines that contain narcotics are generally not used unless the pain is very severe. Lidocaine patches can be used to numb the area, and a high-potency cream (capsaicin) can be rubbed on the area.

If these therapies aren't effective, ask for a referral to a pain clinic. There are also less conventional methods to treat the pain. Biofeedback training, hypnosis, relaxation exercises, acupressure, acupuncture, and use of a TENS (transcutaneous electrical nerve stimulation) unit have all been effective for some people.

*Focal Neuropathy.* This is a condition due to damage to a single nerve or group of nerves. It may develop when the blood supply to a nerve is shut off because of a blockage in the blood vessel that supplies the nerve. Or it could result from a nerve being pinched. Focal neuropathy can injure nerves that sense touch and pain as well as nerves that move muscles. Fortunately, it is not usually a permanent condition. It usually goes away within 2 weeks to 18 months.

**Carpal tunnel syndrome**, a type of focal neuropathy, occurs about three times more often in people with diabetes than in the general population and more often in women than in men. It occurs when the median nerve of the forearm is squeezed in its passageway, or tunnel, by the carpal bones of the wrists. It can cause tingling, burning, and numbness and can make you drop things you are holding without even realizing it. Suspect carpal tunnel syndrome if you have tingling in your hands or fingers that goes away when your arms are relaxed down at your sides. Carpal tunnel syndrome is often treated with splints, medication, or surgery to remove the pressure on the nerve.

*Autonomic Neuropathy.* Some of your nerves control parts of your body that you don't move voluntarily. These are called autonomic nerves, and when they become damaged, autonomic neuropathy can result. Autonomic neuropathy can take many different forms:

- **Gastroparesis:** Your stomach and intestines slow down or become less efficient at emptying, leading to feeling full after a few bites of food, erratic glucose levels, nausea and vomiting, constipation, or diarrhea.
- Nerves to the bladder can become damaged, causing diminished sensation of bladder fullness and an inability to completely empty the bladder. Because urine can then stay in the bladder for long periods, you are at high risk for developing urinary tract infections.
- **Erectile dysfunction:** Men may find that they cannot have an erection even though they may still have sexual desire.
- Women may experience vaginal dryness and a decreased sexual response.
- Autonomic neuropathy can also affect blood pressure. You may find yourself feeling lightheaded or dizzy when you stand because of a drop in blood pressure. This is called orthostatic hypotension. Or when you exercise, your blood pressure may go way up.
- Nerves to the skin may cause too much or too little sweating or very dry skin.
- Nerves to the heart may fail to speed up or slow down your heart rate in response to exercise. That is one of the reasons it is important to get a checkup before starting any exercise program. If your heart rate doesn't respond as it should to exertion, you won't be able to use a standard method, such as counting your pulse, to find your target heart rate during and after a workout.

*Treatment.* Different types of autonomic neuropathy call for different treatments. Feeling full or bloated may be helped by eating small frequent meals instead of three large ones. Medications, such as metoclopramide, can help food to move through your stomach. There are other medications and dietary adjustments that you can use to treat constipation or diarrhea.

Incontinence, or urine leakage, can be treated by training in bladder control and timed urination using a planned bladder-emptying program. Rather than waiting until your bladder feels full, you can try urinating every 2 hours. Men sometimes find it easier to urinate sitting down. Applying pressure over the bladder may also be helpful. If these steps don't work, oral medication may be needed. Or you may need to use a catheter or have surgery. Fecal incontinence (passing stool involuntarily) is treated in a similar way, with medicine for diarrhea and biofeedback training.

If you are experiencing a sudden drop in blood pressure when you stand up, there are several treatment options. If you drink alcohol or take medications, such as diuretics, ask your provider about stopping them. Other options include medications for low blood pressure, raising the salt content of your diet, or raising the head of your bed. However, low blood pressure in itself is not unhealthy. It only becomes a problem if it makes you dizzy or disoriented. Try to stand up more slowly and avoid staying still for long periods to prevent fainting. When you get up in the morning, sit on the edge of the bed before you stand up.

Sometimes neuropathy can trigger a cascade of diabetes-related complications. For example, many people who have had diabetes for a long time develop a condition known as Charcot's foot. This disorder usually affects weight-bearing joints, such as the ankles. It may start with a loss of feeling and thinning of bones in the feet. This can lead to a painless fracture. Because the injury doesn't cause pain, it can go unnoticed and untreated. You may continue walking on the fracture, making matters worse. Muscle shrinking (atrophy) and joint damage can occur and add to the damage, which can become severe enough to deform the foot. The key to treating Charcot's foot is early non–weight-bearing. This involves keeping weight off the joint and wearing special footwear. If you notice any swelling in a joint, especially in your ankle or foot, see your provider right away.

## Infections

High blood glucose levels put you at greater risk for infection. The white blood cells attack the invading bacteria, viruses, and fungi that can cause infections. An excess of glucose makes the white cells less effective. This can keep them from reaching and killing their targets—the invading germs that cause infection. To make matters worse, some of the invading pathogens feed on the extra glucose in the blood, making infection even more likely. People with diabetes tend to have more infections: in the mouth, ears, gums, lungs, skin, feet, and genital areas and in the incision areas after major surgery.

Other complications of diabetes can add insult to injury. When neuropathy affects the bladder, the bladder is more likely to become infected. Neuropathy can make you unaware that you need to urinate, which increases the risk for bladder infection. If neuropathy affects your arms, legs, or feet, you may be less likely to notice a cut or burn, because you will not feel pain. Left untreated, even minor skin abrasions can sometimes lead to infection.

There are several reasons why your legs and feet are prone to infection:

## Your Risk, in General: Infections

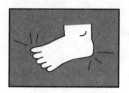 • Although the rate of kidney infections is about the same in people with or without diabetes, people with diabetes are twice as likely to need to be hospitalized to treat the infection.

• Almost one-third of people with diabetes have severe gum disease.

• Recurrence of tuberculosis was found to be 5 times more common among Native Americans with diabetes compared to those without diabetes.

■ neuropathy numbs legs and feet, making you unaware of injury and infection

■ injury opens the door to infection

■ diseased blood vessels slow blood flow to the legs and feet, impairing the healing process

■ high blood glucose disables the body's immune cells, the white blood cells

It doesn't matter where in the body an infection happens to start—the gums, vagina, skin, or feet. Infections need to be treated. They can quickly get worse and cause serious problems.

*Oral Health.* People with diabetes are at high risk for gum disease and periodontitis, so you need to be extra vigilant about brushing and flossing daily. Have your teeth cleaned at least every 6 months. Bacteria love to feast on the areas between

## What's a Foot Ulcer?

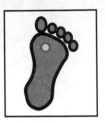

The word **ulcer** probably brings stomach problems to mind. But foot ulcers are more common in people with diabetes than stomach ulcers.

An injured or infected area of the bottom of the foot can develop an ulcer. Layers of skin are destroyed by the infection, which causes an open area or hole. Foot ulcers are serious business. If you discover that you have a foot ulcer, you need to see your provider that day or go to an emergency room.

If untreated, the ulcers may go as deep as the bone and infect the bone, too. You'd be surprised at how quickly this happens. When infection is very deep, a part of the foot, or even the entire foot and leg, may need to be removed to save the person's life. So don't underestimate the importance of daily foot care, especially if you have any loss of feeling in your feet.

your gums and teeth. If bacteria set in, they can destroy the bone in your tooth socket. This can cause sores on your gums. If gums are inflamed, or infected, they will pull away from the teeth and jaw bone, and the situation can get even worse. Bacteria will multiply in the newly created gap. The teeth may even become loose and fall out. If periodontitis is severe, your dentist may need to scrape the plaque from your teeth and remove tissue from around the root of the tooth.

*Infectious Diseases.* Common infectious diseases such as influenza or pneumonia are often more serious for people with diabetes and are more likely to result in hospitalization. Flu vaccines are recommended every year for adults and children (over the age of six months) with diabetes. All adults need a one-time pneumococcal vaccine.

**Vaginal Infections.** Many women with diabetes also find that they are susceptible to vaginal yeast infections. This is due to the yeast *Candida albicans,* which flourishes in a moist environment nourished by high levels of glucose.

*Candida* or other vaginal infections can happen to women regardless or their age, sexual activity, or hygiene. They occur more often after menopause because estrogen levels are lower. Estrogen helps to protect the vaginal lining. Infections are also more likely to occur just before your period, during pregnancy, or after you take antibiotics for another infection.

Signs of a vaginal infection include the following:

- vaginal itching and burning
- thick, white discharge
- redness and tenderness
- foul-smelling green or gray discharge
- painful intercourse

You can buy antifungal products to treat yeast infections. These products come as creams or suppositories that are placed directly into the vagina, usually at night. The type and strength of the product determine how long you will need to use the medicine. Some work in one day, while others need to be used for seven days. They work by destroying the bacteria that cause the infection. Your pharmacist can help you choose one that will work for you.

It is important that you follow the directions exactly for how to use the product. Be sure to use it for the entire time, even if your infection seems better. Even though it may seem to be gone sooner, the infection is more likely to return if the treatment is not completed. If your infection is not better at the end of the time for the product you are using, or it comes back right away, make an appointment to see your primary care provider or gynecologist. They can prescribe stronger medications. Your infection may be caused by different bacteria that do not respond to the over-the-counter therapies. Using a condom during sexual intercourse while you have the infection may help to prevent it from reoccurring.

Keeping your blood glucose close to your target range can help to prevent infections in the future. Avoiding irritating products such as bubble bath and douches may help prevent infections for some women.

Vaginal infections are annoying and can be painful, but they usually respond quickly to treatment. Although it may be tempting to ignore the infection or wait for it to go away, it can become more serious if not treated.

**Foot Problems.** Your feet deserve special attention. No matter how much you weigh, pound for pound, your feet carry a heavy load. Because they are vulnerable to injury, you need to check them every day for signs of injury and infection. This is doubly important if you have neuropathy, because you may not feel pain due to an injury or abnormality, such as shoes that don't fit correctly. Check your feet every day for blisters, sores, ulcers, calluses, corns, or other visible problems. Check inside your shoes each time you put them on. Make sure that the lining is smooth and that there are no objects inside. See your provider or a foot specialist if you have any concerns. There is a lot you can do to protect your feet and legs. See Chapter 3, page 77, for pointers on foot care.

Your diabetes care provider needs to examine your feet at each visit. Taking your shoes and socks off when you go into the exam room will be a good reminder for him or her. Once each year, your feet should be examined more thoroughly. Sensation will be tested with a monofilament and a tuning fork, and your provider will check your reflexes and pulses.

Keeping the blood flowing to your feet is an important aspect of foot care. To do this, take steps to lower high blood pressure and cholesterol levels. If you smoke, ask your health care team for help in quitting.

If a foot or leg infection is not treated, a part of the foot or leg may need to be removed to save the rest of it from being infected. Amputation is traumatic and is always the last resort. The surgeon will remove as little of the limb as possible to make walking possible. After the limb heals, you will most likely be fitted with a prosthesis. Today, prosthetic limbs are lighter and more comfortable than the clunkier models of the past.

# Diabetes and Sex | 11

*At several different times in your life, you are bound to have concerns about how diabetes affects your sexual health. Even though it may be tough to voice what's bothering you, talk to your health care team.*

Most people would rather have a tooth extracted than discuss their sex life with a doctor or nurse. But, the truth is that diabetes can affect your sexual performance, your choices of birth control, and how you respond to the aging of your reproductive system. It is worthwhile to open the lines of communication with your health care team. Rest assured, they will not be shocked by your questions, and there are ways of coping with any problem you might face.

For men with diabetes, the major concern is impotence— worry about erectile dysfunction (ED) or anxiety about how to treat it if it happens. Men and women both may share concerns about birth control and safe sex. For women with diabetes, sexual problems may include poor vaginal lubrication and pain during intercourse or diminished sexual desire and problems achieving orgasm. In addition, women need to deal with the effects of sex hormones on blood glucose levels, throughout the menstrual cycle and as they experience menopause. Women with diabetes have extra challenges as they prepare for pregnancy and carry a growing baby. Don't face these important issues alone just because they concern your sexual life. Sex is a part of each of our lives as humans and belongs in a healthy life.

## Glucose Levels and the Estrogen Cycle

### Menstruation

Andrea had been living with type 1 diabetes since she was a teenager and had been doing reasonably well. Last year, she decided to try to more closely monitor her blood glucose levels. Through hard work, she mastered balancing her insulin doses with her food and exercise but noticed that things became more difficult about a week before her period. Her blood glucose levels were much higher than usual, even though she was careful to do everything she always did to manage them. Her provider asked if she might be eating more than she thought during these times, but she knew that wasn't true. What was happening?

At first, you think you're just imagining it. You're going along and everything seems fine. You're in good spirits, eating well, getting regular workouts, and your blood glucose levels are on target most of the time. Then, for some unexplained reason, everything seems out of whack. Maybe your blood glucose levels are too high. Or maybe they're too low. Then you check the calendar. Oh, yeah—it's that time of the month.

If you have trouble keeping your blood glucose levels on target just before your period starts, you are not alone. A survey of 200 women with type 1 diabetes showed that in the week before their periods, 27 percent had problems with higher-than-normal blood glucose levels and 12 percent had lower-than-normal blood glucose levels. Another study revealed that among women under the age of 45 who were hospitalized for diabetic ketoacidosis, half were within several days of starting their periods. And a survey of more than 400 women revealed that nearly 70 percent experienced problems with blood glucose levels premenstrually. The problem was more common among women who considered themselves to suffer from the moodiness associated with premenstrual syndrome (PMS). Just what proportion of women have problems with their blood glucose levels before menstruation is uncertain. Many studies are based on surveys conducted after the fact and do not take exercise and eating patterns into account.

## Sex Hormones and Insulin Resistance

From the onset of menstrual cycles until menopause, every month a woman's reproductive system revolves around the task of ovulation—releasing an egg ripe for fertilization. The follicular phase of the menstrual cycle begins the day your period starts and lasts for about 12 to 14 days until you ovulate, or release the egg. During the early part of this stage of the cycle, the female sex hormones estrogen and progesterone are at their lowest levels. Another hormone, follicle-stimulating hormone, is produced, which turns on estrogen production. This causes the ovary to release an egg midway through the cycle. After egg release, the luteal phase takes over. A second pituitary hormone, luteinizing hormone, triggers the ovary to produce estrogen and progesterone. These hormones cause the lining of the uterus to thicken, in preparation for a possible pregnancy. If fertilization does not occur, the ovary stops making estrogen

and progesterone. The sudden loss of estrogen and progesterone cause the shedding of the uterine lining, and menstruation occurs.

Some women find that the high levels of estrogen and progesterone about a week or so before menstruation affect their
blood glucose levels. Researchers aren't exactly sure why, but
they have some clues. Insulin works by binding to receptor proteins that sit on the surface of cells. After insulin binds, it sets
off a "relay race" within the cell that in the end allows glucose
to enter the cell. When levels of progesterone and other progestin hormones are high, insulin action within cells is affected.
This leads to temporary extra insulin resistance—the cells no
longer respond to insulin the way they should. The result is that
blood glucose levels may be higher than usual and then drop
once menstruation begins.

However, higher than normal estrogen levels may actually
increase sensitivity to insulin by improving insulin action.
When this occurs, the increased insulin action can lead to blood
glucose levels that may be lower than usual before menstruation.

Not all women experience changes in blood glucose levels
before menstruation. Some studies have shown no differences
in blood glucose levels throughout the menstrual cycle. Some
women experience bloating, water retention, weight gain, irritability, depression, and food cravings, especially for carbohydrates and fats. If you have a tendency to crave these foods,
they could also be contributing to high blood glucose levels
before your period.

**Steps for Staying on Target.** If you suspect that your blood glucose levels are affected by your menstrual cycle, there is a way
to find out for sure. If you are already recording your blood glucose levels on a daily basis, look over the past few months.

Mark the date that your period started for each month. Do you see any pattern? Are your blood glucose levels higher or lower than normal during the week before your period? If you are not recording your blood glucose levels, now may be a good time to start.

If you find your blood glucose levels harder to manage on a monthly basis, there are some steps you can take to get things back on track. Changes in blood glucose levels could be due to normal changes, PMS, or both. Some women find that they need to adjust their insulin dose before their period and again once they start. Think about charting your symptoms along with your glucose levels. It will also help your detective work to note how you are feeling throughout the month, not just before your period, to see whether you can detect any sort of pattern.

If you have unexpected blood glucose readings—either too high or too low—or wide swings in your glucose levels around the time you get your period, there are some strategies you can try.

Try one strategy at a time, so you know which one is the most effective. If your blood glucose levels tend to rise about the time you expect your period, consider these options:

- If you use insulin, gradually increase your dose. Work with your health care team to add small increments, so that insulin levels are higher the last few days of your cycle, when blood glucose levels normally rise. One to 2 additional units of insulin may be all it takes. It will take a little trial and error to figure out the right dose for you. As soon as menstruation begins, estrogen and progesterone levels drop. When this happens, return to your usual dose of insulin to lower your risk of hypoglycemia.
- Eat at regular intervals, when possible. This will keep your blood glucose levels from swinging too much. Large blood

glucose swings could contribute to some of the emotional and physical symptoms of PMS, which may in turn make variations in blood glucose levels worse.

- Try to avoid eating extra carbohydrates. Keep a handy supply of crunchy veggies—for example, celery, radishes, or cucumbers—and dip them in fat-free salsa.
- Cut back on alcohol, chocolate, and caffeine. They can affect both your blood glucose levels and your mood.
- Be especially careful about your salt intake, which causes bloating. Use pepper, fresh or powdered garlic, cayenne pepper, or scallions to add some zing to food.
- Try to exercise regularly. Many women find that regular exercise diminishes mood swings, prevents excessive weight gain, and makes it easier to manage blood glucose levels.

If you have a tendency toward low blood glucose before your periods, consider the following options:

- If you use insulin, work with your health care team to gradually decrease the amount of insulin you take a few days before your period starts. A decrease of 1 or 2 units of insulin may do the trick.
- Reducing diabetes medications may help, especially if you are concerned about having to take extra food. Ask your provider about the safest way to go about this.
- Try spreading your carbohydrate intake over the course of the day. Multiple small meals can help to even out your glucose levels.
- Eat a small amount of carbohydrate foods before you exercise.

If your periods are irregular and your blood glucose swings are unpredictable, try to chart your ovulation to see whether

## Predicting Ovulation

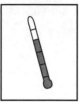

Finding out when you ovulate can help you figure out when you can become pregnant. It can also help you predict when your period will occur.

- Ovulation prediction kit: Available over-the-counter in most pharmacies, these tests can tell you when you ovulate based on a simple urine test. This is probably most helpful for planning a pregnancy.
- Basal body temperature: Take your temperature for 2 minutes each morning before you get out of bed. A chart of these temperatures from month to month will show a pattern. Your body temperature is relatively constant. But, just before ovulation, there is usually a dip of 0.5 to 1.0 degrees. At ovulation, body temperature can rise 0.5 to 1.5 degrees. When you notice the rise in temperature, you know that you are ovulating. Mark this date on your calendar. After ovulation, your body temperature will remain elevated until a day or two before your period, when it decreases. Among women with irregular periods, the interval between menstruation and ovulation can vary, but the interval between ovulation and the next period is usually constant—about 14 days. Using this method, you can predict when your next period will occur, even if you are irregular.
- Vaginal secretions: Although this varies a lot between women, immediately after menstruation, you probably secrete very little fluid and your vagina is relatively dry. As you approach ovulation, you may begin to secrete some vaginal fluid. It will probably be wet, but not too sticky. When ovulation occurs, the secretions become very sticky, about the consistency of egg whites. With training, some women can use their vaginal secretions to tell when they are ovulating.

you can tell when your period will occur so you can adjust your treatment plan. If you are taking insulin, you may want to try intensive diabetes management, perhaps with an insulin pump. This may give you the flexibility you need to deal with changes in blood glucose levels on a daily basis.

## Menopause

Rita has type 2 diabetes. She had learned to deal with it but was now going through menopause. Her gynecologist suggested hormone replacement therapy, but she just wasn't sure. What were the risks? She had heard that these hormones could cause cancer. And how would it affect her diabetes and the A1C level she had worked so hard to achieve?

Menopause is a process, not an event. It proceeds slowly, often lasting 8 to 10 years. It begins when your body slows down its production of estrogen and progesterone, the hormones that set the stage for pregnancy. Ovulation and menstruation become irregular. Some months you may ovulate and have a period, other months you may not. It can begin before you turn 40, but many women continue to menstruate well into their 50s or 60s. The average age for U.S. women having their last period is 51. Your mother's age at menopause is highly predictive of yours.

Menopause can throw your diabetes management plan out of balance. That's because you may have learned to adjust your plan around your normal hormonal fluctuations. And the hormones that keep your menstrual cycle going—estrogen and progesterone—can also affect blood glucose levels. In some women, high levels of progesterone and other progestin hormones may decrease the body's sensitivity to insulin. High levels of estrogen tend to improve insulin sensitivity. As you start the transition of menopause, you'll want to pay close attention to the effects it will have on your blood glucose levels.

Some women find that they gain weight during menopause. This can increase the need for insulin or oral medication. Many women find that they need to eat less and exercise more to maintain their weight. But this time of life can be very positive for many women. They are free from some of their responsibilities and can spend more time taking care of themselves.

***Facing New Risks.*** Without so much progesterone circulating through your body, you may have greater insulin sensitivity. That's good news. But losing estrogen can increase your insulin resistance. And the lack of these hormones can also cause other changes, some of which can affect diabetes complications.

Having diabetes increases your risk for heart attack and stroke two to four times above the risk for people without diabetes. Women without diabetes are protected against cardiovascular disease until menopause. But this is not the case for women with diabetes. Diabetes overrides the protective effect of estrogen. If you have diabetes, your risk for heart attack and heart disease is six times that of a woman without diabetes.

Total cholesterol levels tend to rise and levels of "good," or HDL, cholesterol tend to drop after menopause. For some women, hormone replacement therapy may increase triglycerides, a common problem in type 2 diabetes. High blood glucose levels can make this situation even worse. Keeping your blood glucose, blood pressure, and cholesterol levels on target can help.

Estrogen also helps to maintain strong bones. As estrogen levels fall, your bones can lose some of the minerals that hold them together. This can lead to osteoporosis, a condition in which bones are brittle and easily broken. Eating calcium-rich foods, taking calcium supplements, and participating in regular weight-bearing exercise, such as walking, can help. Hormone replacement therapy can increase bone density and lower your risk of osteoporosis. Other medications to combat osteoporosis are available.

Many women with diabetes find they are more prone to vaginitis and yeast infections once they enter menopause. Yeast and bacteria can irritate the vaginal lining if they grow out of control. They thrive in warm, moist places with a good supply of food (glucose). Even before menopause, you are more likely to develop yeast infections when your blood glucose levels are high. After menopause, the risk increases. That's because estrogen normally nourishes and supports the vaginal lining. Without it, yeast and bacteria have an easier time growing. These infections are not related to sexual activity or personal hygiene.

***Hormone Replacement Therapy.*** You may have a hard time trying to decide whether to take hormone replacement therapy. It is a complicated issue. On one hand, estrogen can decrease the risk of osteoporosis and vaginitis and alleviate hot flashes. On the other hand, it can increase the risk of breast cancer and uterine cancer. When estrogen and progesterone are administered together and in the correct doses, the risk of cancer of the uterus or endometrium is reduced. Research on this very important issue is ongoing; not all questions are answered. Earlier studies suggested that hormone replacement therapy protected against heart disease. But more recent controlled studies indicate that hormone replacement therapy may actually increase your risk for heart disease and stroke.

The current recommendation is to take the smallest dose of hormone replacements for the least amount of time possible to control symptoms. There are different types of hormonal therapies available. Most combine estrogen and progesterone. Some treatments also include small amounts of testosterone, which helps improve bone mass and may improve sex drive.

For some women, estrogen and progesterone replacement can cause frequent or irregular bleeding, even after menopause is complete. Sometimes, bleeding occurs at the start of treatment and disappears as therapy continues. Along with the protection these hormones can give you, there are also potential effects on blood glucose levels, although these are usually minor. There is evidence that estrogen replacement increases insulin sensitivity. Adding a progestin hormone may counteract this. Blood glucose monitoring will help you figure out the effects.

Whether you decide to use hormone replacement therapy is up to you. Many factors can influence your decision. If you have a personal history of breast or endometrial cancer or blood clotting problems, hormone replacement therapy may not be for you. If you have a family history of breast cancer or have had uterine fibroids or fibrocystic breasts, you should know that hormone replacement therapy increases your risk for also developing these problems. On the other hand, if you have a personal or family history of osteoporosis or suffer from hot flashes, hormone replacement therapy may be in order.

As a woman with diabetes, you need to play an active role in your overall health care throughout menopause and beyond. You have more at stake during this time in your life than do women without diabetes. As with other issues related to your sexual health, it's important that you discuss concerns with your provider and other health care team members.

## Hormone Replacement Therapy and Diabetes

After menopause, if you use hormone replacement therapy, add these tests to your diabetes plan. Any tests that give abnormal results should be repeated more frequently.

- Have your A1C tested two to four times a year. This test tells you about your blood glucose levels over the long term.
- Have your cholesterol and triglyceride levels checked as recommended by your provider. The progesterone in hormone replacement therapy can sometimes cause cholesterol levels to rise.
- Have yearly eye exams and kidney function tests.
- Have a yearly mammogram to detect breast cancer.
- Have a yearly Pap smear and gynecologic examination to detect cancer of the cervix, uterus, endometrium, and ovaries.

## Birth Control

Practicing birth control and safe sex are important for anyone, but they are especially important for women with diabetes. The outlook for women with diabetes and their babies has improved dramatically in recent years. Part of the reason is that more women are planning pregnancies and getting the guidance and care they need before conception and during pregnancy.

A baby's organs are formed in the first six weeks after conception. Most women are not even sure that they are pregnant during this critical time. High blood glucose levels can interfere with this development, and the baby has a greater chance of a birth defect. Also, when blood glucose levels are high, the risk of spontaneous miscarriage may double in early pregnancy. You increase your chances for a healthy child when you plan your pregnancy and have an A1C level that is as near to normal as possible before you conceive. In fact, when blood glucose levels are close to normal, the risk for birth defects is about the same as for women without diabetes. Choosing and using an effective form of birth control allows you to plan your pregnancies.

## For Women

Women with diabetes have the same birth control options as other women. The pill, intrauterine device (IUD), barrier methods, and spermicides are all ways to reduce the risk of unplanned pregnancy. The rhythm method, in which women predict ovulation and avoid intercourse during fertile times, is generally not a sufficiently reliable method of birth control for women with diabetes. A tubal ligation may be an option if you are sure you never want to become pregnant, because it is nearly impossible to reverse.

Many birth control methods work by altering hormone concentrations. The methods of birth control that rely on hormones, such as birth control pills and the IUD that releases progesterone, can affect your blood glucose levels. Birth control methods that don't rely on hormones are not likely to change your blood glucose levels. Which method you choose will depend on your own personal and family health history and your individual preferences. If you have any special concerns, be sure to bring them up with your health care team.

***Hormonal Methods.*** Oral contraceptives ("the pill") are the most popular and effective birth control method available. Hormonal methods of birth control prevent pregnancy by preventing ovulation. Hormonal methods are available as pills, patches, vaginal rings, and by injection. Hormonal contracep-

### Pill Precautions

 If you use the pill or other hormonal contraceptives

- check your blood glucose levels frequently, especially during the first couple of months.

Some women need to slightly increase their insulin dose. By keeping complete records, you and your health care team can decide whether you need to make changes in food, activity, or diabetes medication.

- have your A1C, blood pressure, cholesterol, and triglyceride levels checked 3 months after you go on the pill, and then as often as recommended.

tives are about 95 to 99 percent effective. But whether the pill is right for you depends on many factors.

There are two types of birth control pills on the market today: pills that contain estrogen and progesterone and pills that contain only progesterone (called mini pills). A newer form of oral contraceptive is based on a 90-day cycle rather than 28 days. This means you only have four periods a year. Hormones can also be given in a patch, through a small circular device (ring) inserted into your vagina, or by injection. The patch contains both estrogen and progesterone. You leave it on for 21 days and then remove it for seven days. The vaginal ring also contains estrogen and progesterone. You insert it deep into your vagina and leave it there for 21 days. The injection is called Depo-Provera and contains only progesterone. It is given at your provider's office every three months. Before committing to any long-lasting method, you may want to try a progesterone-only pill, which you can stop at any time, to see how you respond.

In general, hormonal methods of birth control are safe for women with diabetes. If you are over 35 and smoke, or you have a history of heart disease, stroke, high blood pressure, peripheral blood vessel disease, or blood clots, these methods may be risky for you.

If you've found that your insulin sensitivity varies at certain times of the month, being on the pill, patch, ring, or injections may help smooth out your blood glucose levels. By providing a steady dose of hormones, blood glucose swings can be kept to a minimum.

Some women find that oral contraceptives increase insulin resistance. If your blood glucose levels are affected, your insulin or your dose of oral diabetes medication can be adjusted. Taking the lowest possible dose or the mini pill can also help.

*IUD.* The IUD is a small T-shaped object that is placed into the uterus by a provider. IUDs prevent sperm from reaching the egg or from implanting in the uterus. One type contains copper and others contain progesterone. IUDs can remain in place for one, five, or ten years, depending on the type. IUDs are generally recommended for women who have had one or more children. When properly inserted and retained, IUDs are about 95 to 98 percent effective in preventing pregnancy.

*Barrier Methods.* Barrier methods of birth control include the diaphragm, sponge, cervical cap, and condoms. Barrier methods prevent the sperm from reaching the egg. The diaphragm is a shallow rubber cup that fits tightly over the cervix, the entrance to the uterus. The diaphragm is coated with spermicidal jelly before you insert it. The diaphragm is put into place just before intercourse and needs to be kept in place for at least 6 hours after intercourse and then removed. It is 80 to 94 percent effective for preventing pregnancy. The effectiveness depends on the user's ability to place the device correctly, use of spermicidal jelly, and leaving it in place for the full time. Your gynecologist will fit your diaphragm and teach you how to place it properly and check to be sure it is covering the cervix.

The sponge contains spermicidal jelly and is placed into the vagina over the cervix. It can be inserted up to 24 hours prior to intercourse and needs to be left in place for 6 hours afterward. Sponges are 80–91% effective.

The cervical cap is a small, thimble-shaped barrier device that fits tightly over the cervix to prevent sperm from entering the uterus. It is used with spermicidal jelly.

The female condom is another barrier method of contraception. It is a larger type of condom that you insert into your vagina up to eight hours before intercourse. You remove it afterward, taking the sperm with it. It can also help protect against sexually transmitted diseases. It is 74 to 79 percent effective.

***Spermicides.*** These work by killing sperm and can be purchased without a prescription. There are several types: foam, gel, cream, suppository, or tablet. They can be used alone or to increase the effectiveness of barrier methods. They are 72 to 90 percent effective.

***Sterilization.*** If you are sure you never want children or don't want any more children, you may want to consider surgical or nonsurgical sterilization. With the surgical method, the fallopian tubes are tied off to prevent eggs from reaching the uterus. With the nonsurgical method, tiny spring-like coils are placed into the fallopian tubes. Material embedded into the coils irritates the lining of the tube, causing scar tissue to grow. After about three months, there is enough scar tissue to block the tubes. Done correctly, these methods are almost 100 percent effective in preventing pregnancy. In very rare cases, a fertilized egg may reach the uterus, resulting in pregnancy, or may grow outside the uterus, resulting in an ectopic pregnancy. You'll need to be certain about your decision to be sterilized, because it is nearly impossible to reverse.

### For Men

Although the choices are more limited, men also have options for birth control. The most popular is the condom, a thin sheath that fits over the penis before intercourse. It prevents the sperm from entering the woman's vagina. When used correctly and along with a spermicide, the condom is about 85 to 90 percent effective in preventing pregnancy. The condom should be put on before intercourse and can be removed soon afterward. Condoms also help prevent the spread of several sexually transmitted diseases, including gonorrhea, chlamydia, and AIDS.

Men who are certain they do not want to father any or any more children can opt for a vasectomy. This is a simple procedure that prevents the release of sperm into the seminal fluid. When the man ejaculates, the semen contains no sperm, but men still experience the full pleasure of intercourse. However, it is very difficult and expensive to reverse a vasectomy, and you'll need to be certain about your decision. Some men opt to store some of their sperm before vasectomy for possible in vitro fertilization or artificial insemination, should they decide they want children at some later time.

## Sexual Health

Diabetes can affect sexual functioning and fulfillment for both men and women. The good news is that sexual health is getting

---

### Avoiding Lows after Sex

If you use insulin, you need to be watchful for low blood glucose during or after sex.

- Check your blood glucose first: This may slow you down a bit, but it's better than having to deal with a low blood glucose later.
- Eat just before or right after active sex, just as you would if you were exercising.
- Consider having a snack before going to sleep for the night.
- If you use an insulin pump, you may want to disconnect it during lovemaking to avoid going low. The length of time you can safely keep the pump off without an injection depends on how active you are. Ask your health care team for advice about this.

---

more attention, and there is more help available. If you are having any problems related to sexual issues and you want help, talk to your health care team. If you don't feel comfortable talking with your provider, perhaps you need to find a health care professional with whom you do feel comfortable discussing personal matters.

Your provider will evaluate your concerns and help you sort out the causes. There are many factors that can result in sexual difficulties, including medications, hormonal changes, problems caused by diabetes, and your emotional health. If your sexual problem appears to be due to a physical cause, you may be referred to a gynecologist or urologist. If stress or anxiety is contributing to your problem, a visit with a mental health professional may be in order. Depression, which is more common among people with diabetes, can also contribute to problems with sexual fulfillment and performance.

## Women

Many women with diabetes at one time or another experience some sexual difficulties. In fact, one study showed that 30 to 40 percent of women with diabetes reported that they have problems with sexual functioning, refrain from sexual relations, and are generally not satisfied with sex. But for women, long-term blood glucose levels and diabetes complications don't appear to have a direct effect on sexual functioning. For most women with diabetes, the problem is caused by lack of arousal. There is a very strong link between mind and body. If a woman does not feel in the mood for sex, then her body does not respond the way it needs to in order for her to enjoy it. If she is not emotionally ready or interested in sex, then she will be less likely to enjoy it physically.

This is probably true for all women, but there are certain reasons that it is especially true for women with diabetes. Women's sexual health can be affected by many issues:

- vaginal infections that affect how you feel physically and how sexy you feel
- bladder infections that can cause intercourse to be painful
- hormonal changes due to your menstrual cycle or menopause
- vaginal dryness
- lack of sexual desire
- fear of pregnancy
- depression and medications used to treat depression

*Infections.* Vaginal infections (yeast infections, vaginitis) are more common among women with diabetes. Blood glucose gives the bacteria an excellent medium to grow. These infections do not have anything to do with how clean you are, your age, or sexual activity. While vaginal infections do not directly affect your sexual health, they can affect how sexy and desirable you feel. You can buy over-the-counter antifungal products to treat these infections. If the infection does not clear up within a week, contact your health care provider for stronger medicine.

Women with diabetes are also at risk for bladder or urinary tract infections (UTIs) for the same reason. Signs of a bladder infection include feeling like you need to go to the bathroom more often, painful urination, painful intercourse, and blood in the urine. If you think that you have a bladder infection, call your health care provider right away. These infections usually respond quickly to antibiotics. Some women find that cranberry juice helps to treat or prevent these infections. Cranberry juice contains sugar—1/3 cup has about 15 grams of carbohydrate, equal to 1 carbohydrate serving. If you drink cranberry juice, even as a treatment for these infections, you will need to count it as part of your carbohydrate intake. Cranberry pills you can buy over the counter may be an alternative that will not affect your blood glucose levels.

*Hormonal Changes.* Many women find that during their menstrual cycle, and especially around the time of their period, their blood glucose levels are erratic, and they have less energy for everything, including sex. During menopause, hormone levels change, and some women find that their blood glucose levels go up and down. Mood changes and hot flashes are also common during this time. Although menopause does not affect sexual desire, some women find that they have vaginal dryness that can cause sexual relations to be painful or uncomfortable. You can buy lubricating gels (e.g., water-soluble jelly) that can help. You can also ask your provider about estrogen creams.

*Lack of Sexual Desire.* Some women find that they are just too tired. They are coping with busy lives, caring for children and grandchildren, working, and trying to find some time for themselves. Diabetes adds additional stress and work to their lives. High blood glucose levels add to feeling tired and run down. Because of nerve changes related to diabetes or simply due to getting older, some women find that they need more stimulation to fully enjoy sex.

Depression is more common among people with diabetes. Depression usually causes people to feel less interested in sex. In addition, some of the medications used to treat depression can affect sexual desire.

For women using insulin, worries about low blood glucose reactions during sex can get in the way. Women with either type 1 or type 2 diabetes may feel less desirable or that their bodies are less attractive as they get older and perhaps heavier. Having complications from diabetes can also cause you to feel less desire both emotionally and physically.

There are things that you can do:

- If you have dryness, infections, or are worried about getting pregnant, talk with your diabetes care provider or your gynecologist.
- If you are worried about your blood glucose levels, do a quick check before you have sex. Knowing that you are not likely to have a reaction can help you relax and enjoy yourself. You may also want to keep something to treat a low glucose by your bedside so that if you do go low, you won't have to get up.
- If you feel sad and blue or if your sadness is affecting your desire for sex, talk with your provider. There are medicines that will work for depression that do not affect your desire for sex.
- Help set the stage to get into the mood. Take time for yourself and your partner. Let your partner know what will help you to feel more romantic and in the mood.

## Men

Paul had been diagnosed with type 2 diabetes a few years ago. He had been keeping his blood glucose levels in check, but had recently been traveling quite a bit. He wasn't exercising very often and was eating out most of the time, and he also noticed that he had put on a few pounds. But the worst part was the effect on his sex life. For the past several months, it had become increasingly difficult to sustain an erection. And he had been unable to achieve an erection the last dozen or so times he attempted sexual intercourse. Now he had just given up trying.

Among men, the diagnosis of diabetes brings with it the concern about impotence or erectile dysfunction (ED). But, are problems with erections really more common in men with diabetes than men without diabetes? Because so many men suffer in silence, it's difficult to count how many men with and without diabetes actually have a problem. Here's what we do know:

- ED is age related. It is primarily a problem among men over 40, with and without diabetes.
- Of all men with diabetes over the age of 50, it is estimated that 50 to 60 percent have some degree of ED.

ED has a range of severity. The numbers about ED count all types, from occasional to complete impotence. Complete impotence occurs much less often. So just what is impotence? Being impotent means that most or all of the time, the penis fails to become or stay hard enough for sexual intercourse. If, on occasion, you fail to maintain or achieve an erection, you're not impotent. You are also not impotent if you experience a decrease in sexual desire, have premature ejaculation, or if you fail to ejaculate or reach orgasm. If you are impotent, you can't achieve or maintain an erection. However, many of these other problems can also occur with impotence.

ED can be caused by physical or psychological factors or both. The most common causes in men with diabetes are blood-vessel and nerve-related damage. If you have experienced neuropathy or cardiovascular complications of diabetes, you are at risk for ED. The way to reduce your risk is to keep your blood glucose levels as close to normal as possible. In addition, it will help to quit smoking, decrease your alcohol intake, and keep blood pressure near normal. Psychological factors, depression in particular, are also common culprits in men with diabetes.

Figuring out why ED occurs can be difficult. Sexual desire begins in the brain, and signals are sent through the nervous system to the blood vessels to trigger an erection. The male sex hormone testosterone is also involved in sexual desire and achieving erection.

Hearing so much about ED can create fear that contributes to the problem. And if you know that you are at increased risk because you have diabetes, you may even expect it to happen. For instance, you may be unable to have an erection if you feel pressured to perform. Sometimes, not being able to maintain an erection can create fear and anxiety that can eventually lead to ED. Worry and stress can decrease your brain's response to testosterone. However, because your nerves and blood vessels are in working order, you might have erections during the night. Most healthy men have several erections each night while they sleep. There are simple tests you can do to find out whether you are having erections in your sleep. This means that the problem is not physical and may reassure you that you'll be able to recover your ability to have erections.

ED caused by physical problems usually comes on slowly and gets worse with time. Early symptoms include a less rigid penis during sexual stimulation and when you wake up. Over time, men with ED may not be able to sustain firm erections long enough to enjoy sexual intercourse.

Some of the side effects of diabetes can directly cause ED. Blood vessel damage is a common cause of erection problems in men with diabetes. When blood flow to the penis is reduced, the penis no longer can become erect. A frequently used test for this is an ultrasound study of the penis. Sound waves are used to measure blood flow through the arteries and veins. Another test involves injecting a drug or mixture of drugs into the penis to cause an erection. The drug is injected in such a way that it bypasses the penile nerves. If the injection causes you to have an erection, damaged blood vessels are not the cause. If you don't have an erection, it means there may be some damage to your blood vessels.

Nerve disease is also a culprit. When the nerves that signal the penis are damaged, erection can be impaired. You may be referred to a urologist to find out if the nerves in your penis are affected.

Because ED can also, in rare cases, be caused by low amounts of testosterone, your testosterone level may also be measured. If it is too low, your problem may be caused by a hormonal problem not related to diabetes.

Also be aware that certain medications can cause temporary ED. Tell your provider about all the medications you are using—even over-the-counter remedies. Drugs frequently used to treat high blood pressure, anxiety, depression, and peptic ulcers can all be factors. If you have signs of trouble and suspect that it may be related to a new medication you are using, tell your provider. There may be other medicines you can use. But don't stop taking the medicine. Smoking and alcohol consumption can also contribute to erection problems.

*Treating ED.* There are several treatments available. In choosing a treatment, find one that is most compatible with the needs and desires of both you and your partner.

There are several drugs available for treatment, and many men with diabetes have found them to be effective. Sildenafil (Viagra) and vardenafil (Levitra) can help to stimulate and maintain an erection 30 to 60 minutes after taking a pill. Tadalafil (Cialis) is similar but lasts for up to 36 hours. Ask your provider about these drugs if ED is a problem for you.

Another option is to inject a form of the drug alprostadil directly into the penis. This induces an erection that lasts about 30 minutes to 1 hour. Side effects include bruising and prolonged erection. Some men also develop scarring in the penis, which occasionally results in a permanent curvature during erection. There is a suppository form known as muse that can be inserted in the tip of the penis 5 to 10 minutes before sex.

Another option uses a vacuum pump to create an erection. A cylinder is placed around the penis. A small vacuum pump pulls air out of the container, creating a vacuum. This causes blood to flow into the penis, triggering an erection. To maintain the erection, the container is removed and replaced with a rubber band. This provides an erection for about 30 minutes. The rubber band can cause bruising if kept on for more than 30 minutes. Entrapment bands or external support devices are also available.

You can also have a pump device called a penile prosthesis surgically implanted into the penis to produce erections. Your best bet is to visit a urologist with experience in this type of implant. Be sure to ask about the risks, which can include infection and the need for further surgery in case the device doesn't work correctly.

Testosterone injections or patches can be prescribed if a low hormone level is the problem. The injections are usually given every 3 to 4 weeks. Men are at risk for prostate cancer and should not take testosterone unless they have abnormally low levels and have been evaluated for prostate cancer.

It may also help for you and your partner to work with a therapist who knows how to deal with sexual issues.

All the treatments for impotence have risks or drawbacks. You may decide to seek no treatment. Some men and their partners choose to express their sexuality in ways that do not involve intercourse. If you do want to consider treatment, you need to tell your provider even if you are not asked. Your provider can only help you if you let him or her know about your concerns.

# Pregnancy

In the past, it was common for women with diabetes who became pregnant to experience serious problems, such as miscarriage, stillbirth, or a baby with birth defects. Today, it is very common for women with diabetes—either type 1 or type 2—to have safe and healthy pregnancies. Although women with diabetes and their unborn children face additional risks because of diabetes, these can be kept to a minimum through careful blood glucose management, before and during pregnancy, and intensive obstetrical care. For this reason, all women with diabetes need to plan ahead before becoming pregnant.

## Before You Become Pregnant

When you decide to start a family, the first step is to meet with your health care team to consider the specific challenges you face. You may be concerned that your baby could develop diabetes. You may be worried for your own health. It's important to get a good idea of how much extra work and expense may be involved before you become pregnant. Your glucose levels

FACT OR MYTH?

**"My sister with diabetes had a baby, and it nearly killed her. It's just not a safe thing to do."**

Women with diabetes can and do have healthy babies all the time. It doesn't cost them their lives or health, either. The survival rate for pregnancy is no different between women with and without diabetes, as long as the woman with diabetes takes care to practice tight blood glucose management and treats any diabetes complications before becoming pregnant. And chances are excellent that her baby will be just as healthy as a baby born to a mother without diabetes.

But there are risks. High glucose levels early in pregnancy may cause miscarriage or improperly formed organs in the baby. High glucose levels later in the pregnancy put the mother at risk for hypertension and preterm labor as well as possible worsening of any diabetes complications. High blood glucose levels later in pregnancy can cause the baby to grow too large and cause problems with delivery.

Pregnancy puts stress on any woman's body. This is why it is so important that you and your health care team keep a close watch on your health before and throughout your pregnancy. But here's the good news: When women with type 1 diabetes who have been pregnant are compared to women with type 1 diabetes who have never been pregnant, about the same number of women in each group show signs of diabetes complications. Being pregnant doesn't seem to raise your risk for complications over your lifetime.

*(Continued)*

With newer insulins, self-monitoring of blood glucose levels, and improved techniques for early detection and treatment of complications, women with diabetes have entered an era of expanded possibilities. Don't let old-fashioned thinking stop you from working toward having a healthy baby.

may also be an issue: The mother's blood glucose is directly related to the risks to the growing baby. You also need a complete evaluation of your overall health and to check for any complications from diabetes. Because your diabetes management may change, meeting with a dietitian or diabetes educator will help.

***Genetics.*** Whether you are a potential mother or father with diabetes, you may have concerns about your child someday developing diabetes. The best time to assess the genetic risk of your child developing diabetes is before pregnancy.

Type 1 diabetes is caused by an autoimmune attack on the pancreas that destroys the insulin-producing cells. A child born to a parent who has type 1 diabetes is at slightly greater risk of developing type 1 diabetes than children of parents without diabetes. The risk is slightly higher when the father has type 1 diabetes. Researchers have identified genes that could play a role in type 1 diabetes. But it is not yet clear what percentage of children who inherit a "diabetes" gene go on to develop diabetes or what environmental factors are also involved.

If a baby is born to a mother who is age 25 or older and has type 1 diabetes, that baby has a 1 percent risk of developing diabetes. If the mother is younger than age 25 at the time the child is born, the risk increases to about 4 percent. If the father has type 1 diabetes, the risk for the child of developing diabetes is about 6 percent. Each of these risks is doubled if the parent with type 1 diabetes developed it before the age of 11. If both parents have type 1 diabetes, the risk is not known but is probably somewhat higher. A child born to parents who do not have diabetes has a 0.3 percent risk of developing the disease.

Development of type 2 diabetes seems to depend on both genetic and lifestyle factors. Type 2 diabetes tends to run in families. Research on families with type 2 diabetes shows that you can inherit genes that increase your tendency to develop type 2 diabetes. Studies of twins have shown that genetics play a very strong role in whether a person develops diabetes, especially type 2 diabetes. Obesity also tends to run in families, and families tend to have similar eating and exercise habits.

If you have a family history of type 2 diabetes, it may be difficult to figure out whether your diabetes is due to lifestyle factors or genetic susceptibility. Most likely it is due to both. But just because you may have a tendency toward developing type 2 diabetes does not mean that insulin resistance cannot be prevented or reversed. In a large national study called the Diabetes Prevention Program (DPP), participants who lost a modest amount of weight (5–10% of total weight) and participated in a moderate amount of exercise (150 minutes of walking per week) were able to delay or prevent type 2 diabetes even in the face of genetic susceptibility.

If you are concerned or have questions about the likelihood of having a child with either type 1 or type 2 diabetes, ask your provider to refer you to a medical geneticist or genetic counselor. They are trained to assess the contributions of genetic and environmental factors in causing many diseases, including diabetes. They will know the results of the latest diabetes and genetics studies and studies to prevent diabetes in high-risk individuals.

*Mother's Health.* Before becoming pregnant, you need a thorough physical exam. Any problems that could jeopardize your health or that of your baby will be assessed. These problems include high blood pressure, heart disease, and kidney, nerve, and eye damage. If you have any of these complications, they need to be treated before you try to conceive. Even kidney transplant recipients who are otherwise healthy have had babies. Your A1C level will be measured, as well as your thyroid function, if you have type 1 diabetes. In addition, your exam will include a review of all the medications, herbs, and supplements you are taking to make sure they are compatible with a safe pregnancy.

In rare cases, diabetes-related problems may be so serious that it's safer to avoid pregnancy. If you have untreated high blood pressure, cardiovascular disease, kidney failure, or crippling gastrointestinal neuropathy, think carefully about this decision. Pregnancy can make these conditions worse, or they can lead to related problems, such as stroke or heart attack.

If you have any signs of heart disease, such as chest pain on exertion, an electrocardiogram may be done. Signs of nerve damage will also be checked. If the nerves that control heart rate or blood pressure have been damaged, this can affect how you will respond to the physical stress of pregnancy. Neuropathy can also affect how well your body nourishes you and your growing baby, so tell your provider if you have had persistent problems with nausea, vomiting, or diarrhea.

Your prepregnancy exam will also include an evaluation of your kidneys. In women with high blood glucose levels and untreated kidney disease, kidney function can worsen during pregnancy. Fortunately, pregnancy does not appear to have long-lasting effects on kidney function. If you have kidney problems, you need to be prepared for a potentially more difficult pregnancy. This can include problems with edema (swelling) and high blood pressure. If you have been treated with ACE inhibitors or ARBs for kidney disease or high blood pressure, your medication will probably be changed. Taking these drugs during pregnancy can cause kidney problems for the baby.

You will also be referred to an ophthalmologist who will examine your eyes, especially the retina—the part of your eye that senses visual images. Your pupils will be dilated so that the back of the retina can be checked for damage caused by diabetes. Untreated diabetic retinopathy may get worse during pregnancy and should be treated and stable before you become pregnant. You will continue to get your eyes examined throughout the pregnancy.

> ## TIP
>
> The ideal health care team for your pregnancy includes your diabetes care provider, an obstetrician experienced and interested in treating pregnancy complicated by diabetes, a pediatrician interested in the care of infants of mothers with diabetes, a registered dietitian, and a diabetes nurse educator experienced in teaching women how to intensively manage their diabetes.

*Glucose Management.* Although birth defects occur in 1 to 2 percent of all babies born to women without diabetes, they occur more often among babies born to women with diabetes. These problems include abnormalities of the central nervous system, heart, and kidneys. The risks cannot be completely eliminated for anyone. But you can lower your risk to the same level as mothers without diabetes by keeping your blood glucose levels as close to normal as possible before and during the first trimester of your pregnancy.

Why is well-controlled blood glucose important **before** conception? You want your blood glucose levels to be as favorable to your developing baby as possible. All the baby's major organs are formed during the first 6 to 8 weeks of pregnancy, which may be before you know you're pregnant. In several studies, women who had an A1C of 1 percent above normal (i.e., less than 7 percent) before conception lowered their baby's risk of birth defects to 1 to 2 percent, the same as women without diabetes. Babies of mothers who began intensive diabetes management after conceiving were more likely to have birth defects. In addition, it takes time to find a diabetes management plan that will work for you. This takes some trial and error as well as patience. It may take too long if you wait until you are pregnant.

Before you become pregnant, you probably will intensify your daily diabetes care. If you have type 1 diabetes, you will begin or fine-tune your plan by using several insulin injections each day or switching to insulin pump therapy. If you have type 2 diabetes, using oral diabetes medicines during pregnancy is not recommended because they may harm the baby. You will probably need to begin insulin therapy. Many women with type 2 diabetes who in the past have managed without medication find that they need to use insulin during pregnancy.

Your A1C level will be measured frequently. It is recommended that your A1C level be less than 1 percent above a normal A1C level (less than 7 percent) before you stop using birth control. It might also be helpful for you to record your basal body temperatures (see the box on predicting ovulation on page 343) so that you know when you can and do conceive. This will be useful to know for decision making later in pregnancy.

*Expenses.* Having a baby is a major financial investment for any parent. Your pregnancy will include the added expenses involved in tight blood glucose management. But, it used to be worse: Before self-monitoring of blood glucose, a woman could easily spend half of her pregnancy in the hospital. Now the major expenses are fetal monitoring and blood glucose monitoring instead of hospitalizations.

Before you conceive, check with your insurance company about what is covered. Your insurance plan may cover more during your pregnancy with the appropriate documentation. Some of the items that need to be covered are listed below.

- You will need to see both your obstetrician and your diabetes health care provider frequently—perhaps every week or every 2 weeks for most of your pregnancy. You will learn to make adjustments in insulin dose based on blood glucose values. This takes time and practice and lots of support from your health care team.
- Your health care should include nutrition counseling with a registered dietitian and diabetes education. You will likely learn how to count carbohydrates and adjust insulin doses.
- You'll need to check blood glucose values often to make sure you are within your target ranges. Many pregnant women do seven or more tests each day. Test strips are the big expense in monitoring.
- You may need to do ketone monitoring each day. This will protect you against surprise ketoacidosis as well as starvation ketosis, which can occur after a low blood glucose value, when carbohydrate intake is very limited, or when calorie intake is lower than needed. This means buying ketone strips.
- If you treat your type 2 diabetes with oral diabetes medications, you'll probably need to switch to insulin before you become pregnant. This means paying for insulin pens or syringes and insulin, plus training from an educator on how to give insulin and to adjust your dose.

## Once You Are Pregnant

*Blood Glucose Management.* The first step is to choose blood glucose targets for your pregnancy. The targets given in the box on page 370 are an example. Talk to your health care team about

## Sample Target Blood Glucose Ranges During Pregnancy

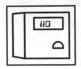 You'll need to set blood glucose target ranges. Talk with your team about choosing target ranges to meet your needs. For instance, your first trimester goals may be a little higher.

- before meals: 60 to 90 mg/dl
- one hour after meals: <120 mg/dl

how to personalize blood glucose target ranges to your health and your lifestyle.

In the first trimester, targets are designed to help you minimize the risk of birth defects or miscarriage. In the second and third trimesters, the targets will help to prevent your baby from growing too large. If you have trouble staying in the range, or if you have frequent or severe hypoglycemia, talk to your health care team about revising your treatment plan or your targets.

Women with type 2 diabetes usually need to use insulin during pregnancy. So may many women with gestational diabetes. Women who use insulin will find that they need to increase their insulin dose over the course of the pregnancy to reach these targets. You may also need to make adjustments in the kind of insulin you take and how often you inject. Usually, the amount of insulin you take increases with each trimester. This is because the hormones of pregnancy, which increase in effect over time, create more and more insulin resistance. Some women need to increase their insulin dose by as much as two or three times, especially in the last trimester. This does not mean that your diabetes is getting worse. You and your provider need to decide together when and how to make any changes in your insulin schedule or dose.

*Food and Exercise.* Your eating habits may need to change during pregnancy to help you stay on target. And you also will want to make sure that you are eating foods that provide adequate nutrition for you and your baby. You will probably have a visit with your dietitian even before you become pregnant. In general, choose nutritious foods that are part of any healthy eating plan (see Chapter 8). Women with gestational diabetes may be able to manage their blood glucose levels more effectively by limiting their carbohydrate intake to 35 to 40 percent of calories.

Your dietitian will help you tailor your meal plan to your recommended weight gain. A weight gain of 22 to 32 pounds over the 9-month period is normal. Women who are underweight to begin with may be advised to gain more. And women who are very overweight may be advised to limit their weight gain. Checking your urine for ketones each morning will help you know if you are getting the carbohydrates and insulin you need.

## Help with Nausea

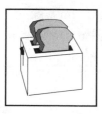

- Eat dry crackers or toast before rising.
- Eat small meals every 2 1/2 to 3 hours.
- Avoid caffeine.
- Avoid fatty and salty foods.
- Drink fluids between meals, not with meals.
- Take prenatal vitamins after dinner or at bedtime.
- Always carry food with you.
- Talk with your health care team. They may have helpful suggestions. Also tell them about any herbs or supplements you may be using. These may make nausea worse.

Eating five or six small meals a day may help your efforts to stabilize your blood glucose. This eating pattern may also help with "morning sickness," which is often worse when the stomach is empty. Morning sickness is not limited to mornings, and nausea can occur day or night, often accompanied by vomiting. If you have morning sickness, there are some dietary steps you can take to feel better. It can help to keep some starch, such as Melba toast, rice or popcorn cakes, or saltines or other low-fat crackers, close at hand to eat if you become nauseated. Some women find it helps to prevent morning nausea when they eat a small snack at bedtime or before they get up in the morning.

It is important to maintain physical activity during pregnancy, as long as your overall health permits it. Being fit prepares you for the physical stress of labor and delivery and the busy days that follow. It is usually safe to continue with any exercise you were doing regularly before pregnancy. But pregnancy is not the time to take up any new, strenuous activities. See the section on exercising during pregnancy in Chapter 9.

***Glucose Monitoring.*** You will probably need to check your blood glucose levels several times each day. If you take insulin, you may monitor before and after meals and at bedtime. If you have type 2 or gestational diabetes and are managing it through meal planning and regular exercise, you will need to check more frequently than you are used to.

You may want to check your blood glucose at these times:

- once before each meal
- 1 to 2 hours after each meal
- at bedtime
- during the middle of the night, around 2 a.m.

If you take insulin and keep your blood glucose levels near normal, you are more likely to have episodes of low blood glucose. During pregnancy, a blood glucose of 70 mg/dl is considered to be a low blood glucose. In addition, your early warning symptoms of hypoglycemia may change. Some women develop hypoglycemia unawareness during pregnancy (see Chapter 5). You may have less shaking and sweating and more rapid development of drowsiness or confusion. Monitoring frequently helps you know whether you are close to being low. There is no evidence that hypoglycemia is dangerous for the baby. But, a hypoglycemic episode can be dangerous for the mother-to-be. In addition to testing before and after exercise, always check your blood glucose before you drive. Be prepared for severe low blood glucose by carrying a glucagon kit and training several people you see daily how to use it (see Chapter 5).

***Obstetrical Care.*** Because of the risks to you and your baby, you'll need more frequent visits to your obstetrician, perhaps every two weeks for the first part of your pregnancy and weekly during the last month. The reason for these visits is to make sure that your baby is developing as expected and that you stay in good health. You will be screened for neural tube defects early in pregnancy (around weeks 15 to 18) by measuring the concentration of alpha-fetoprotein in your blood. You'll need an ultrasound test early in your pregnancy (to show when your baby was conceived) and several more throughout your pregnancy to follow the baby's growth. A fetal echocardiogram may be done around the middle of your pregnancy. Other monitoring includes counting your baby's movements for an hour each day and fetal movement and heart rate monitoring during the last 6 to 12 weeks of pregnancy. These tests help ensure your baby's well-being and will assist your health care team in deciding when to deliver your baby.

## Birth

In the past, babies born to women with diabetes tended to be large. This problem, called macrosomia, was the baby's response to having extra amounts of glucose from the mother's blood. To reduce the risk of delivery problems or stillbirth, these babies were usually delivered by inducing labor or a cesarean section (C-section) before or during the 37th week of a 40-week pregnancy. Now, because more women are able to manage their diabetes more intensively and better tests are available to monitor the baby's health, most women can deliver close to their due date.

Macrosomia is less common, but sometimes the baby is too large or the woman's pelvis is too small for a safe vaginal delivery. Trying to deliver a too-large baby vaginally can result in shoulder damage or respiratory distress for the baby. In this case, a C-section is performed.

Your blood pressure will be checked frequently throughout your pregnancy. High blood pressure can be a sign of preeclampsia, a serious condition that occurs more often in women with diabetes. Preeclampsia may also lead to early delivery, often by C-section.

Labor is work, and usually you will not be able to eat. You will probably get an intravenous catheter (IV) so that fluids or calories can be given as needed. Your blood glucose levels will be monitored frequently during labor. You can be given insulin either as injections or through the IV. Many women don't need insulin during active labor.

Your baby will be closely watched after birth. He or she is at risk for hypoglycemia and will have frequent blood glucose monitoring during the first 24 hours after birth. Hypoglycemia occurs because the baby has been putting out enough insulin to deal with high glucose levels in the uterus. This does not mean your baby has diabetes. Jaundice is also common and may require therapy with lights. If your baby was delivered early or is very large for his or her age, your baby will also be evaluated for respiratory problems. It is not unusual for these babies to be in an intensive care nursery for a short time so that they can be watched very closely.

## After Delivery

If you have type 1 diabetes, you may require less insulin for the first few days after delivery. If you have type 2 diabetes, you may not need insulin at all during this time. Your insulin needs will gradually go back to your prepregnancy level in about 2 to 6 weeks.

The postpartum period may be one of unpredictable blood glucose swings. Your hormones and body chemistry are in flux. You are recovering from a major physical challenge. And you are probably exhausted from caring for your baby. If you find that keeping your blood glucose on target poses a greater challenge, try not to get too discouraged. If you find that you feel overwhelmed by trying to care for a new baby and diabetes or you are feeling depressed, contact your health care team. They can help you find sources of support or make a referral for evaluation or counseling. It's not a sign of weakness to need help at this time. Your baby needs a healthy mother!

If you had gestational diabetes, your blood glucose levels will most likely return to normal after delivery. Nevertheless, you need to be tested for diabetes 6 weeks after your baby is born. A few women continue to have diabetes after they deliver. If this is the case, you will be referred to a diabetes care provider. If your postpartum glucose test is normal, you are still at greater risk for developing diabetes than women who never had gestational diabetes. If your postpartum test reveals a

## "Because I had gestational diabetes, I might get diabetes when I'm older."

This is true. Gestational diabetes is a temporary form of insulin resistance that usually reveals itself about halfway through the pregnancy. This is when the hormones of pregnancy normally create extra insulin resistance. Most women are able to overcome this extra resistance to insulin. However, for women with gestational diabetes, either their pancreas is not able to make the additional insulin that is needed or their body's cells become less efficient at taking up glucose from the blood.

Women who have had gestational diabetes are at greater risk for getting diabetes again. They have a 2 in 3 chance of developing gestational diabetes during future pregnancies. Also, their risk of developing type 2 diabetes 5 to 15 years after they had gestational diabetes rises to between 40 and 60 percent, compared with about a 15 percent risk in the general population. Obesity increases the risk of getting type 2 diabetes after having gestational diabetes to a 3 in 4 chance. Women who have had gestational diabetes can reduce their risk of developing diabetes closer to a 1 in 4 chance by keeping a healthy body weight (see Chapter 1).

higher than normal blood glucose level, but not diabetes, your risk of developing diabetes in the next 5 years is high. About 60% of women with gestational diabetes eventually develop type 2 diabetes. The good news is that you can delay or prevent type 2 diabetes in the future with modest weight loss and moderate activity. Losing the weight you gained with your pregnancy may be enough to lower your risk. You also need to have your blood glucose level checked once a year to detect any changes. Ask to have your glucose levels tested earlier in the course of any future pregnancies. Remind all providers that you had gestational diabetes. Some drugs, such as steroids, can raise your blood glucose levels just as pregnancy did.

Don't forget that you can become pregnant again soon after you give birth. Even if you have not had a period, you can still ovulate. And breastfeeding does not necessarily prevent you from becoming pregnant. So, before you resume having intercourse, be sure you are using effective birth control.

Although virtually every aspect of your life may seem turned on its head after the birth of a new baby, the four basic management tools remain the same: insulin or oral diabetes medication (oral diabetes medications cannot be used while you are breastfeeding), blood glucose monitoring, meal planning, and exercise. Exercise may be the last thing you are thinking about after the baby is born. But as soon as you feel well enough and you have your doctor's okay, taking your baby for a daily walk can help you feel better and more relaxed.

**Highs and Lows.** Hormonal changes, emotional shifts, irregular sleep patterns, and fatigue may hide or change your symptoms of high or low blood glucose. You may find it hard to tell the difference between "after-baby" blues, such as unexplained crying or moodiness, and low or high blood glucose. Fatigue, feeling spacey, weakness, or forgetfulness can be caused by both high and low blood glucose and by lack of sleep. If you're not sure, play it safe and check your blood glucose.

With a new baby depending on you, it's critical to guard against hypoglycemia. Test often; if you feel hypoglycemia coming on, treat it right away, whether or not you can test. Keep items such as glucose tablets, hard candy, or regular soda handy in several rooms. Make sure that those around you know how to spot your signs of low blood glucose; teach them what you want them to do if you don't seem like yourself. Keep a glucagon kit on hand.

If you have had hypoglycemia unawareness in the past, be vigilant not to let your blood glucose get too low when you are alone with your baby. Get help with middle-of-the-night feedings, or make it a habit to eat a snack then. Take care to test before you get into the car to drive. Don't nap or sleep on an empty stomach. Remember that your best protection is still frequent blood glucose monitoring and regular snacks and meals.

Having a new baby can affect your diabetes care habits, especially if you have other children to care for. You may find that your baby's unpredictable schedule and your own erratic sleep patterns make it difficult for you to eat or snack when you need to. Using multiple injections may make your life easier and give you more flexibility. Although it is tempting to put your infant's needs before your own, taking care of yourself is important for both you and your baby.

## Breastfeeding

The ideal food for your baby is your own breast milk. You will need about 300 additional calories per day while breastfeeding, so you may want to schedule another visit with your dietitian. Your hunger level may change, and you may need some help trying to balance your meals and your baby's meals with your insulin doses.

The extra energy your body uses to make breast milk can cause your blood glucose levels to become erratic. Throughout the time you breastfeed, continue checking your blood glucose level often. And make sure you have a source of fast-acting sugar, such as glucose tablets or orange juice, handy while breastfeeding. When your baby is ready to nurse during the day, eat your own snack or meal, plus a glass of water or low-fat milk, as you feed your infant. It helps to have the snack or meal portion ready so you don't have to prepare your food while the baby is waiting to be fed. This provides your body with fluids and helps prevent a low blood glucose. During nighttime feedings, have a snack yourself. Otherwise, you might have a low blood glucose reaction, especially if you have been up several times in the night.

# Coping with | 12
## Diabetes

*Many people with diabetes feel blamed or criticized for their efforts at diabetes care. When someone you care about has diabetes, simply listening to how he or she feels about living with diabetes can be the most loving and helpful act.*

Jeanne was sailing along, enjoying life. She had just turned 30, started a new job, and bought a horse, all in the last 2 months. She lived for the thrill of cantering her horse across the hills and through the woods almost every day. But then one day after a long ride, she felt dizzy and collapsed in the barn. She was rushed to the hospital, and that's when she found out she had diabetes. She always thought diabetes affected older, sedentary people, but she was young and active. It just wasn't fair. She felt angry and was determined to show everyone that she could live just fine without worrying about diabetes.

Hilda, a 60-year-old widow, had just retired from nursing. A few months later, her youngest daughter got married. She thought she would enjoy the peace and quiet, but instead she just didn't feel quite right. During her yearly medical exam, she found out she had diabetes. As a former nurse, she knew all about diabetes, but never thought it would happen to her. Even though she knew how to manage, she couldn't help feeling alone, helpless, and down in the dumps. She just couldn't motivate herself to do what she knew she needed to do.

When you found out you had diabetes, you were probably given a lot of new information about how to manage the disease. You may have made changes in your lifestyle, eating habits, and daily activities. You may have started taking oral medications or insulin and checking your blood glucose on a regular basis.

Having all this thrown at you at once can be overwhelming. In the midst of trying to sort out all the new information, you probably also experienced many different feelings. Maybe you tried to shrug diabetes off. Maybe you felt imperfect or that your body had failed you. Or perhaps you felt angry and wanted to find something or someone to blame. Maybe you felt sad, blue, or out of sorts. Diabetes can cause feelings of depression and isolation, anger, frustration, fear, and guilt. You may have experienced all of these different emotions initially and at different times as you live with diabetes. Even as you are trying to absorb the diagnosis and a lot of new information, it is equally important to pay attention to your feelings.

## Dealing with Your Feelings

The emotions you experience as you deal with diabetes are generally negative ones. But these negative feelings may actually be useful. For example, denial can be part of nature's way of letting the news of diabetes sink in gradually. Even anger can be an ally in dealing with diabetes if you are able to channel your anger into energy that helps keep you motivated.

The key to dealing with your emotions is to understand your feelings and not try to suppress or deny them. Learning to understand how you are feeling and how your feelings influence your actions is the first step in dealing with your emotions.

## Denial

If your first reaction to the news that you have diabetes was to try not to think about it, to wish it would go away, to tell your-

---

### Food for Thought

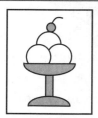

If you're having trouble knowing where to start making changes to manage your diabetes, try out this series of questions. They will help you identify what's important to you and help you to make a positive step.

- What part of living with diabetes is the most difficult or unsatisfactory for you?
- How do you feel about this situation?
- How would this situation have to change for you to feel better about it?
- Are you willing to act to improve this situation for yourself?
- What steps could you take to bring yourself closer to where you want to be?
- Can you pick out one thing that you can do to improve things for yourself?

self you would deal with it later, or to convince yourself that the diabetes care providers don't know what they are talking about, then you may be experiencing denial. Denial is not necessarily a bad thing. It can help you adjust to living with diabetes. By putting your emotions on hold, you can better deal with the shock of absorbing all the new information. By pretending you don't have diabetes or that diabetes is not that big of a deal, you can avoid feeling overly stressed out, angry, or depressed as you learn about diabetes and begin to care for yourself. Eventually, however, denial is no longer helpful or protective. In fact, it can be just the opposite. People who continue to deny the seriousness of diabetes are less likely to take positive steps to manage their blood glucose levels and ultimately to prevent the complications of diabetes.

If you feel overwhelmed, talk to your spouse or close friends or your diabetes care provider or educator. It may help to take one step at a time. Don't try to change everything all at once. Pick one area that is meaningful for you and start there. Remember that every step in the right direction is a big step. You may want to consider joining a support group, joining a chat room or newsgroup on the Internet, or seeking counseling. It can be reassuring to know that you have many of the same concerns as others, and they may be able to offer you ideas about ways to cope with diabetes.

## Anger

When you find out you have diabetes or over the course of living with diabetes, you are likely to experience feelings of anger and frustration. You may feel that life is treating you unfairly. You may feel frustrated when all of your hard work doesn't seem to be paying off. Or you may find that feelings of anger coexist with feelings of denial, depression, or anxiety. You may find yourself feeling angry whenever you think of having diabetes or when confronted with some of the problems it brings. Or you may find that you flare up more quickly in situations that have nothing to do with diabetes. It's as if you are using all of your strength and coping skills to deal with diabetes. There's not much left to deal with life's other stresses and strains.

All of these feelings are a common reaction to dealing with a difficult condition. It is normal to feel angry over something you feel you can't control. Trying to manage blood glucose levels is often frustrating.

Start to keep track of your angry episodes and the events that trigger your anger. Keep notes or a journal if possible. After a few days or even weeks, sit down and review your observations. Try to figure out if there is any sort of pattern. See if there are any particular situations or people that make you angry. Does your anger typically occur after sitting in a traffic jam? Or does it occur when people start to ask you about your diabetes?

A good way to deal with anger and other bad feelings is to recognize the feelings, realize they are common, and find ways to channel your energy.

Sometimes just identifying the triggers may be enough. You may also need to avoid those situations that cause you to become angry. If you find yourself getting hot under the collar every time your spouse asks you about your blood glucose, don't wait until things build up to an angry outburst. In a calm moment, explain that it bothers you. Let your spouse know how he or she can be helpful.

You may discover that you have angry feelings because you haven't completely come to terms with your diabetes. If this is the case, think about joining a support group, talking with other people, or seeking the help of a professional counselor.

You can let anger eat away at you and make you miserable, or you can think of it as unharnessed energy. Use that energy to do something positive. Your anger may be telling you that you are due for a change in your life. Educate yourself about diabetes. Learn ways to handle anger without taking it out on others or yourself. For example, go for a walk, count to ten, or walk away from the situation. Many people find that seeing a professional counselor can be helpful initially and as they live with diabetes.

## Handling Stress

People with diabetes, as well as doctors and researchers, have long suspected that stress can affect blood glucose levels. Although there is no clear evidence that stress alone can cause any disease, it is possible that it can bring on or worsen symptoms in someone already headed for disease.

Stress is a double-edged sword for people with diabetes, as with many chronic diseases. Stress may contribute to the symptoms of the disease, and living with diabetes can trigger stress. How to handle diabetes and its associated stress is different for everyone. But you may find the strategies you use to handle other stresses can help with diabetes-related stress.

Stress is influenced by both the individual and the environment. Each of us defines what situations we see as stressful and how we respond to the stress. Both positive and negative situations can be stressful. Change almost always is. How stressful we perceive it to be depends on how good or harmful we find it to be and what else is going on in our lives. Something can feel stressful one day and not the next. Stress can have an effect on your blood glucose levels. Your body prepares for stress by sending out hormones. High or fluctuating blood glucose and ketone levels may result. If stress is short-lived and repetitive, levels of blood glucose and ketones may "bounce" considerably. Some people actually experience a low blood glucose level with an acute stressor.

It's usually helpful to first recognize how you act when you are stressed out. Do you anger easily and take your feelings out on others? Do you cry easily or become depressed or withdrawn? Perhaps you feel emptiness or apathy. Maybe you reject help from those close to you or want extra attention from them. Maybe you come down too hard on yourself.

One way to deal with a stressor is to eliminate it. If we can't eliminate the stress, we need to find a way to deal with it. This is called coping. Everyone needs a variety of coping skills to use in different situations. Each person deals with stress in his or her own way. We usually behave in ways that are familiar to us. Some of these strategies work and some leave us feeling tense, tired, angry, or sick. Some, such as smoking, drinking too much, and drug abuse, cause other problems. Other techniques and ways of dealing with stress can help us to feel more in control, relaxed, and less tense after a stressful event. To determine if a strategy is effective, ask yourself, "Did it work? Did I feel better both temporarily and later? Is this an effective strategy to use in the future?" There are three important factors in coping: having enough information, feeling in control, and having the support of others.

Some of the following stress management strategies might work for you:

- Find someone to talk to and who will listen when something is bothering you.
- Join a support group.
- Form a discussion or networking group on any topic or activity that interests you.
- Take up a new hobby or sport, learn a musical instrument, or join a dance class.
- Exercise—join a health club, sign up for an aerobics class, or just take a walk every day.
- Engage in volunteer work.
- Sign up for a class that interests you.

## Progressive Muscle Relaxation

- Close your eyes and breathe slowly and deeply.
- Start with the muscles in your face, working your way down to your feet and toes.
- Inhale. Raise your eyebrows. Tense them. Hold for a count of 3. Relax your eyebrows. Exhale.
- Inhale. Open your mouth and eyes wide. Then close your mouth and eyes tightly. Squeeze. Hold for a count of 3. Relax your eyes and mouth. Exhale.
- Inhale. Bite down on your teeth. Hold for a count of 3. Relax your jaw. Exhale.
- Inhale. Pull your shoulders up. Hold for a count of 3. Relax your shoulders. Exhale.
- Inhale. Tense all the muscles in your arms. Hold for a count of 3. Relax your arms. Exhale.
- Inhale. Tense all the muscles in your chest and abdomen. Hold for a count of 3. Relax your chest and abdomen. Exhale.
- Inhale. Tense all the muscles in your legs. Hold for a count of 3. Relax your legs. Exhale.
- Inhale. Tense all the muscles in your feet. Curl your toes. Hold for a count of 3. Relax your feet. Exhale.
- Inhale. Exhale any tension that may be lingering in your body. Breathe in energy. Take several more deep, slow breaths. Enjoy feeling relaxed.
- Gradually open your eyes.

- Think of something you can do that relaxes you and do it— read a book, take a bubble bath, get a massage, or watch a movie.
- Spend time with friends or alone, whichever will replenish you more.

- Pray or meditate.
- Do a relaxation exercise.
- Take a vacation or even a night away.
- Get a babysitter to give you some extra time alone or with your spouse.

Recognize that everyone has choices in life and you make your own choices. Pace yourself. Make it a point to identify and anticipate stresses, and create ways to deal with them ahead of time. You may not be able to control traffic jams, an angry boss, or a crying baby, but you do have some control over the way you react to these situations.

## Depression

Everyone gets the blues now and then. It's easy to feel blue when there is too much stress in your life, when sad things happen to you or your family, or simply from the everyday strain of living with diabetes. Learning new ways to cope with stress, figuring out what is important for you, solving the problems that you can, practicing your religion, and getting support are some ways to get past the blues. Taking care of your diabetes can also help. People with type 2 diabetes who have blood sugars closer to normal report feeling more zest for living and an improved quality of life.

People with diabetes often say that they feel sad, scared, and angry all at the same time. Clinical depression is more common among people with diabetes, occurs more frequently, and lasts longer, compared with the general population. It can occur any time—when you are first diagnosed or after you have been dealing with diabetes for years. Depression can coexist with other feelings, such as denial, anxiety, or even anger. When you are depressed, it is often harder to pay attention to your diabetes.

People respond to depression in different ways. Some find that they aren't hungry at all, while others eat to feel better. Some people sleep all of the time, while others find that they toss and turn. It is also common to withdraw from family and friends or to stop doing things that you enjoy. If you experience any of the following, you may be depressed:

- You no longer find pleasure in activities you once enjoyed.
- You have trouble falling asleep at night or wake up once you have fallen asleep.
- You feel tired during the day.
- You no longer enjoy eating the foods you once liked.
- You find yourself eating more or less than you used to.
- You either gain or lose weight.
- You have a hard time concentrating.
- You have a difficult time sitting still.
- You cannot seem to make even the most trivial decision.
- You experience feelings of guilt or a lack of self-worth.
- You feel that everyone else would be better off without you.
- You entertain thoughts of suicide or think of ways to hurt yourself.

If you have any of the above symptoms or if you have been feeling sad or hopeless for more than a few weeks, talk to your health care provider. There may be a physical reason for your feelings of depression—a change in medication or high blood glucose levels, for example.

If there are no physical causes, ask to be referred to a mental health professional. Seeing a mental health professional does not mean there is something wrong with you as a person. It simply means that you may have a medical problem that affects your emotions.

You may see a psychiatrist, psychologist, psychiatric nurse, licensed social worker, or other mental health counselor. Your counselor may recommend psychotherapy, medications, or both. Many people find successful relief from depression from a combination of the two. Many emotional problems are caused by chemical imbalances in the brain, and antidepressants can help you get back on track.

It is important to recognize the symptoms of serious depression and seek help right away. Unfortunately, when you feel depressed, you probably feel even less able to seek help. But it is the best thing you can do to get your life and health back on track.

## Ending Alcohol Abuse

If you have diabetes and your blood glucose levels are on target, it is generally safe to drink alcohol occasionally. But if you drink too much or have trouble controlling how much alcohol you drink, you may have an alcohol abuse problem.

Alcohol abuse is even more dangerous for people with diabetes. Many of the complications of diabetes—including nerve damage, eye problems, high blood pressure, kidney disease, and heart disease—can worsen with excessive alcohol use. Alcohol abuse is especially hard on the liver, where your body stores glucose. If your liver is damaged by alcohol, your blood glucose levels may become erratic, and you are more likely to have hypoglycemia. Long-term alcohol abuse can interfere with how you take care of your diabetes.

Ending alcohol abuse can be very difficult, but it is crucial for many reasons, including your diabetes care. If you have a problem with alcohol, or think you might have, there is help available to you. Talk to your provider, or call your local chapter of Alcoholics Anonymous (AA). Your health care team can help you find the treatment you need to begin the path to recovery.

## Managing Anxiety

Everyone feels nervous or anxious from time to time, especially in a stressful situation. This is normal and, often, even helpful. Anxiety is a survival mechanism that can help you get through a difficult situation. If you are face-to-face with a man-eating bear or have to give a lecture before 1,000 people, for example, feeling a little anxious can help you get through the ordeal. But if you find that you feel nervous or anxious in situations that are not stressful to most people or if your anxiety is so intense and long-lasting that it interferes with day-to-day living, you may have a more serious problem called an anxiety disorder. The issue is not that your worries are unfounded, but that your worries are more intense, frequent, or last longer than others experience in a similar situation. Feelings of anxiety can coexist with feelings of depression.

If you experience any of the following, you may have an anxiety disorder:

- You feel restless, feel irritable, and have difficulty concentrating much of the time.
- You tend to feel very worried or concerned about almost everything.
- You feel tired or easily fatigued.
- You have problems sleeping.
- You avoid people or places.
- You feel panicked or scared for no reason.
- You are not able to stop thinking about something.
- You feel like you have to do something over and over again, such as washing your hands or checking door locks.

■ Your muscles feel tense or you experience frequent headaches.

If your worries or concerns are beginning to interfere with daily living or prevent you from enjoying the things you once enjoyed, it is time to seek help. First, try talking with your provider. Your anxiety could have a physical cause.

If there is no physical cause, you may be referred to a mental health counselor. Through medication, counseling, or a combination of both, your mental health counselor may help you find a way to handle or decrease your feelings of anxiety.

## Boosting Your Self-Esteem

It is much easier to meet life's challenges with a healthy dose of self-esteem. You do better in your work, studies, and personal relationships, and you are more likely to go after what you want out of life when you feel good about yourself. But, unfortunately, diabetes can gnaw away at your sense of self-worth.

Some people with diabetes blame themselves for having the illness or its complications. Or they think less of themselves because they feel different. This can happen whether you are a child, a teenager, or an adult. Some people even wonder if they are being punished when they get diabetes.

Many of our feelings of self-worth stem from the messages we were given as children (both positive and negative) and the messages we give ourselves as adults. One way to boost your feelings of self-worth is to give yourself affirming and positive messages. Recognize your good qualities and give yourself a break, even if no one else does.

When you are feeling good about yourself, write down a list of all your strengths and positive qualities. Include things you are especially good at doing. When someone pays you a compliment, add it to the list. Then on days when you are feeling down, take out the list and remind yourself of what a great person you are. If you have trouble coming up with things to put on the list, ask those around you who like and love you. Often your friends and family are quicker to recognize your strengths than you might be.

## Taking Charge

One of the ways you can take charge of your diabetes is to learn to be assertive. Most conflicts do not arise out of differences of opinion but out of gaps in communication. If you are unable to assert yourself, you might find it difficult to talk about your diet or how much time you need to take care of your diabetes. Or you may be reluctant to have your needs interfere with those of the people around you. Assertive communication means that both your needs and the needs of the other person are equally important and respected. Assertive statements often begin with "I". For example, "I find it helpful when you don't keep chips in the house." This statement is more effective than a blaming or aggressive statement ("You always try to undermine everything I do") or reacting passively and being inwardly resentful.

Try out these skills that can help in the workplace, in social situations, and at home with your family:

- **Learn to say no.** A simple "no, thank you" communicates to yourself and to others that "I respect myself enough to act in in my own best self-interest, and I respect you enough to know that you will understand."
- **Maintain courtesy.** Courtesy is the cornerstone of effective and assertive communication. It relays the assumption that you will treat your needs and those of others equally and that neither will suffer at the other's expense.

- **Be direct.** Direct communication while maintaining courtesy is as important as saying "no" at the appropriate time.
- **Meet your own needs.** Hypoglycemia is an example of an urgent situation in which you must be assertive. Don't put off treatment because you are afraid of offending someone with whom you are interacting.
- **Be firm.** It is important to be firm with both yourself and others. Make a plan about how you will handle certain situations. If pressured, explain your decision directly to others.
- **Maintain self-respect.** If you respect yourself, it will be easier to be assertive.

## Making Choices

Diabetes is largely a self-managed illness. Unlike more acute illnesses, you give almost all of your own care. Even if they wanted to, the members of your health care team cannot manage your diabetes for you on a daily basis. Your provider, nurse, and dietitian do not live with you and cannot insist that you follow their advice. As much as your family and friends can be of help and offer support, they cannot manage your diabetes for you either. It is up to you. You are free to decide how much or how little you do to care for your diabetes. Because you benefit from the results of your choices, you have the absolute right to make these decisions.

Many things in our lives are not of our own choosing. Diabetes is not something most people would choose to have. But while you cannot change having diabetes, you do have choices to make about how you live with it and your attitude toward it. No matter how constrained you may feel, there are always choices you can make.

Freedom brings responsibility as well. In fact, freedom and responsibility are two sides of the same coin. Because the choices you make affect your outcomes, you have a great deal of responsibility for your own health and quality of life. It can be overwhelming. There are things that you can do to help you accept this much responsibility.

First, learn all that you can about diabetes. The more you know, the more you are able to weigh the positives and negatives of the choices you have to make. Ask your provider for a referral to a diabetes education program in your area. Second, work with your diabetes care provider to develop a plan to manage your diabetes that matches your goals and abilities. Be honest about what you can and cannot do. Remember, you are the one who has diabetes and lives with it each day. You are the expert on yourself and your life. Third, be honest with yourself. It may be tempting to shift the decisions to your health care team or blame the people around you for your outcomes. But when we do not accept responsibility, we become victims of our situation.

If you are struggling with this level of responsibility, there are some questions that you can ask yourself to try to understand more about why you feel this way.

- What stands in the way of accepting responsibility for my diabetes?
- What are the negatives of feeling forced to behave in certain ways?
- What are the positives of feeling controlled by diabetes?
- What are the negatives of accepting responsibility for diabetes care?
- What are the benefits of accepting responsibility for diabetes care?
- What one thing can you do this week to take charge of diabetes care?

Power comes from accepting responsibility for our choices and our lives. Taking responsibility for managing your diabetes gives you power and control over your diabetes and your life.

## Your Emotions and Diabetes

***Is depression more common among people with diabetes?*** Most studies find that depression is more common, that it recurs more frequently, and that it lasts longer among people with diabetes than in the general population. Whether you believe this applies to you probably depends on whether you think "depression" is having the occasional "blues" or if you use the more clinical definition of chronic feelings of hopelessness. Everybody, diabetes or no diabetes, goes through periods of feeling down, along with low energy and not caring to be involved in things going on around them. Depression is serious when these feelings go on for long periods or are interfering with your quality of life or your ability to care for your diabetes.

Erratic blood glucose levels can also cause some of these feelings. Having high blood glucose for a long stretch brings on fatigue and sleepiness. It can sap your energy and keep you from getting involved with activities. It can be hard to tell if you are feeling depressed or feeling bad because your blood glucose is high. So in addition to the fact that having to deal with diabetes day in and day out can give you the blues, high blood glucose levels can add to the blues. It can become a vicious cycle. The only way to stop it is to seek help.

***Can diabetes affect my sense of self-worth?*** Having a chronic disease like diabetes can make it harder to feel good about yourself. You may feel "damaged," just because of diabetes. Being different can make the teenage years even more painful than usual.

How you feel about yourself can affect how you care for your diabetes. Do you believe you deserve to spend the time, effort, and money it takes to care for your diabetes? How do you show yourself respect? If you do it by making choices, others will respect your needs, too. If you need to check your blood glucose right now, do it. Don't be worried about asking others to wait for you while you check.

***Can stress affect blood glucose control?*** Yes. Stress affects your body's hormone balance. Your body produces powerful hormones in response to a difficult or "fight or flight" situation. These hormones get your body ready for quick action by breaking down stored forms of glucose into blood glucose. This sends your blood glucose levels up. If you have type 1 diabetes, you probably don't have enough insulin on board to cover the higher glucose levels. If you have type 2 diabetes, your levels are likely to remain too high because of insulin resistance. Your body also releases stress hormones in response to situations such as illness or surgery.

***Can stress cause diabetes?*** Stress doesn't directly cause diabetes. However, for people already headed in that direction, it can push them along a little faster. Perhaps you've heard stories of people whose diabetes began after a stressful experience, such as a severe illness or a car accident.

In type 1 diabetes, the immune system mistakenly destroys the insulin-producing cells of the pancreas. This is a process that usually takes many months, perhaps even years, before enough cells are lost so that diabetes starts. A person on the way to getting type 1 diabetes makes less and less insulin. A stressful experience increases the need for insulin. So, the insulin demands brought on by a stressful experience could overwhelm the body's ability to produce insulin.

In type 2 diabetes, the body loses its ability to respond to insulin. As this happens, the pancreas makes less and less insulin. Adding stress-produced hormones, which create more resistance to insulin, could bring on the first symptoms of diabetes.

**Why do my feelings change so quickly? Is it because of my diabetes?** Trying to meet the never-ending demands of life with diabetes can make anyone feel frustrated, or up one minute and down the next. It's easy to feel cheated when you've met your end of the bargain by doing all that you can but your blood glucose levels don't reflect your efforts. Wide swings in blood glucose levels can also cause your emotions to change.

If you suspect that this is happening, consider doing some investigative testing. If your mood swings are related to blood glucose fluctuations, talk to your health care team about other ways to manage your diabetes.

Tell the people close to you who want to support you about how you feel. And if you need more help to deal with mood swings, ask for a referral to a psychologist or other mental health counselor. You don't have to be alone with diabetes. There is help and support available if you ask for it.

# Diabetes and Family Life 13

*Diabetes affects all family members. It can be tough to balance the needs of everyone, but with practice, families can learn to cope and support each other.*

Ever since he had been diagnosed with type 2 diabetes 2 years ago, Richard had a hard time staying on track. Most of the time he ate about the right amount of carbohydrates, but he still needed to lose about 25 pounds. He knew he was eating too many fatty foods, and he couldn't resist potato chips, which always seemed to be in the house. To Richard, that seemed to be a big part of the problem. His family never really understood that he needed help to manage his diabetes. If anything, they seemed to be undermining all his efforts.

Stacey had always managed her type 1 diabetes almost effortlessly. She loved to exercise and had always been very diligent about counting carbs, monitoring frequently, and taking her insulin. But the demands of family life were getting to her. It was okay when the kids were little, but now her three kids were in school and life was full of their activities. Driving them between ballet class, soccer and softball practice, and piano lessons was taking its toll. Her husband was often late getting home from work, so it all fell to her. Now she was having a hard time keeping everything on track. One week, she'd had a close call—a low blood glucose level while driving her kids to soccer. They were running late, and she didn't have enough time to monitor. She felt like there was just no time to take care of herself and her diabetes.

## Balancing Family Demands and Diabetes

Life is tough enough. Whether you are married, have children or grandchildren, live with your parents, or have just struck out on your own, it's difficult enough to balance all the stresses of modern life. Work, school, financial matters, child rearing, retirement, or divorce are all hard enough to deal with without the additional burden of diabetes. It may be easier to eat what you want and to exercise when you want if you live alone, but friends and family still enter into the picture. You need their support and understanding and they need yours. If you live with others, you need to take their needs into account as well as your own. People who are most successful at managing their diabetes have the cooperation and support of their family and friends. It helps when you don't feel alone in meeting the challenge of learning to live with diabetes.

### How Diabetes May Affect Your Family

Maybe at first it seems as though you should be able to handle things on your own. After all, your family can't hold your hand

and watch you do everything. It is still up to you to manage your diabetes, right? Yes. But having diabetes is bound to affect your family. Life can be demanding. Finding out you have diabetes may upset the delicate balance of your juggling act. You can't tend to your 2-year-old when you're in the middle of giving yourself an insulin shot. Your partner may begin to resent having you check your blood glucose and take insulin just as you're getting dinner on the table. And sex can lose some spontaneity if you have to eat a snack just when the mood is striking.

One way to enlist your family's support is to look at your schedule and routines. Probably the best way to approach this is to enlist their support right away. Hold a family meeting and explain how important it is to coordinate insulin doses, exercise routines, and meals. Ask for suggestions as to how your needs can fit into the family routine. Perhaps other family members can do a little more, or it may mean enlisting some outside help.

You may already feel stretched to the limit. Planning meals, checking your blood glucose, and exercise all take time. It's often helpful to write down your usual activities or sit down with your day calendar and try to figure out how to best fit it all in. Don't be afraid to acknowledge that you can't do it all and that something is going to have to give.

Scheduling might not be the only change. Maybe you decide to eat or cook differently. Again, open communication will help. Explain that you are not going on a diet and are not going to force your family into spartan eating conditions. The recommendations for people with diabetes are basically guidelines for healthy eating. The key is getting your family's input. No one likes to be forced into doing something they don't like to do. If you are trying to lose weight, you may need to eat smaller portions or to avoid some high calorie foods that your family enjoys. If this gnaws at your willpower, ask your family not to eat it in front of you, to have it less often, or to not always keep it in the house.

Let your family know that you might have mood changes. Recognize that your family members will also have feelings about your illness. Learn to talk about your feelings, and try to establish open channels of communication. Sometimes you'll be cranky because of the diabetes, and sometimes you will feel cranky because of life's demands. They may express their concern for you by asking frequently about your diabetes or trying to pretend it doesn't exist. They may also express their concern by reminding you to take care of your diabetes. It may feel like nagging or that they are becoming the "diabetes police." If this is a problem, let them know how they can express their concern in a way that feels supportive to you. Learn to work with your family members to talk about how you and they are feeling and what to do about it. Maybe you just need a snack or maybe you need to go for a walk. Or maybe your spouse or children need a break. Recognize when there is a problem, and talk about solutions.

Finally, your family should know what to do in an emergency. Make sure they understand the signs of hypoglycemia. Often people with diabetes having a low blood glucose episode will deny there is a problem or refuse treatment even though they may be in danger. Make sure your family members can recognize the signs of hypoglycemia and know how to deal with it.

## What Your Family Can Do

Sometimes problems arise among family members when they don't really understand the disease. If your teenager is grumpy because he has to wait for you to take an insulin shot before you drive him to the mall, it may be because he doesn't understand how important it is. And if your spouse is waving potato chips under your nose when you are trying to cut back, she may not understand the importance of your goal to eat healthily. Many people think that treating diabetes is as simple as taking insulin a few times a day. Keep in mind that you have the right to ask for the support you need.

As a first step, each family member needs to understand what diabetes is, how it is managed, and how to handle emergencies. There is lots of help available. Books, magazines, pamphlets, libraries, support groups, on-line message boards and chat rooms, and medical professionals can all be of assistance. Take a family member with you to some of your health care appointments. By keeping a running list of questions or issues with which they may be concerned, your family can get answers to their questions firsthand. Many diabetes education programs encourage family members to attend. The more information they have, the more they can help you and learn to integrate your diabetes management plan into the daily family routines.

Your family can also help with your eating plan. For many people, this is the most difficult adjustment to make after being diagnosed with diabetes. You may want to change some of the foods you eat and when you eat them. It will help you tremendously if the members of your family are willing to accommodate your new plan. Your family may object to eating different food and may resent eating on schedule. But eating well for diabetes is not really a special diet, it just means eating sensibly. Whether you have diabetes or not, eating large amounts of sugar, fats, and salt isn't good for your health.

Exercise is also an important part of diabetes management, and your family can participate. Exercise benefits everyone, not just those with diabetes. Ask your family to join in, walking or jogging alongside of you. If not, tell them how they can encourage your efforts. Consider some activities that you can do together. Plan family activities that involve some form of exercise—walking the dog, a nature walk, or a bicycle trip to the corner store. The more you can get your family involved in exercise, the easier it will be for everyone. An evening family stroll or bicycle ride might add to the quality of life for all family members. In addition, helping your children keep fit and at a healthy weight lowers their risk for developing diabetes.

Depending on your family, you can expect different responses to your diabetes and different levels of enthusiasm for helping you work toward your diet and exercise goals. Some may partake wholeheartedly, looking at this as a team effort. Other families or family members may resent making changes when they aren't even sick. You need to find the approach that works best for you. In some situations, you may be better off if you go it alone.

## Finding Other Sources of Support

Support is important, so if your family isn't able to be supportive or you live alone, you may need to look elsewhere for an extra boost.

*American Diabetes Association.* One place to start is the American Diabetes Association (ADA). Check the Resources section at the end of this book for the ADA office nearest you.

ADA can tell you about support and educational groups that you can attend. By participating in these groups, you can meet other people with diabetes and health care professionals. Whether you are seeking more information or want to talk to people who share your experiences, a support group may be just the thing. You may be able to find a diabetes care partner, and you can support each other.

In addition to education and support groups, ADA can mail you a packet of information on request. They can also answer any questions you may have about the disease or some of the practical issues in managing diabetes: health care, health insurance, and referrals. They also have books, magazines, and publications available that may help.

***Health Clubs.*** You might also consider joining a health club. Although this is a source you may not have thought of, developing a diabetes management program really means developing healthy living habits. And people who actively participate in the local health club or fitness center may share similar goals, whether they have diabetes or not. The club may even offer a personal trainer who can be a tremendous help to you. You might also meet other people with diabetes.

***Counseling.*** Sometimes, despite the help of support groups, and even with a supportive family, you might need extra help. Coping with diabetes and all of the feelings that go along with it is not an easy process. There are bound to be times when you will need extra support. Your friends and family may not have all the skills you need. Or new issues may arise during the course of your life or the course of your disease.

Whatever your situation, you may want to consider some form of individual or group counseling for those times when you need extra help. It might help you to sort out any difficulties you may be having to work with a professional who can be an objective source of support. A professional therapist can help you examine your problems. Depending on your individual needs, you may want individual, marriage, or family therapy.

You might seem a little put off by the idea of seeing a therapist. Maybe it conjures up negative images, or maybe you think seeing a therapist indicates that there is something wrong with your mental state. Nothing could be further from the truth. Counseling is a healthy way of helping people deal with some of life's difficult problems.

Counseling involves an ongoing conversation between you and your therapist. Your therapist will help you explore your thoughts and feelings and examine how you interact with others and the decisions you make. Your therapist may encourage you to tell your story, starting from the beginning. This may help you find a new perspective on the problems in your life and discover the patterns in your actions. He or she may also offer suggestions that may help you see the situation from another viewpoint and may help you find new ways of coping.

One of the most important aspects is to find a therapist you trust. You need to feel comfortable with your therapist and feel that he or she is helpful. It often means finding the right personality match. Someone who works well with one person may not necessarily be compatible with someone else. So don't be too discouraged if the first therapist you see doesn't fit your needs. You may need to talk to several before you find one that feels right.

Living with diabetes means adjusting to the complex interplay between family relations, personality, emotions, lifestyle habits, and diabetes management. Therapy will help you learn to take the initiative and necessary action to take charge of your diabetes as well as the conflicting emotions that go along with it.

*Group Therapy.* While some people benefit from one-on-one encounters with a therapist, others gain more from weekly group therapy sessions. And many people find the combination of approaches to be a double benefit. These groups can foster mutual support, encourage camaraderie, and help combat the depression and isolation that often goes along with a diagnosis of diabetes. Sometimes talking things out with other people helps you to find fresh solutions.

There are many types of settings and formats for group therapy. Some meet in hospitals, clinics, community agencies, and even in therapists' private offices. Group therapy should include a trained therapist, a careful selection of group members, and a social structure that includes rules for behavior. All therapy groups share the principle that talking about feelings, ideas, and experiences in a safe, respectful atmosphere increases self-esteem, deepens self-understanding, and helps a person get along better with others.

The group setting gives each member a chance to see how others react to his or her feelings about diabetes and observe how he or she incorporates diabetes into family, work, and play. Group therapy has special advantages for people with diabetes. It can help you

- learn that you are not alone;
- discuss feelings, worries, and concerns that you may never have dreamed of discussing anywhere else;
- discover new approaches to old problems;
- explore who you are and who you are not;
- reduce stress, which in turn may lead to better health.

## Don't Forget Your Partner

If you have diabetes, you know that it can take an emotional toll. But you're not the only one who may feel the stress. Your family members, especially your partner, is likely to share in the burden. If you shut out your partner completely, he or she may feel isolated and helpless. He or she may feel a need to "rescue" you and resent being left by the wayside. But if you shift too much of the burden to your partner, he or she may resent having to spend too much effort trying to help you and feel that you should be doing more to help yourself. Many spouses dislike being put in the position of parent or nursemaid.

Your mate may worry when the decisions you make about caring for yourself seem wrong. He or she may fear the consequences of what will happen, either in an emergency situation or down the road, if you neglect your health. Maybe you feel that your spouse is nagging too much. Maybe your spouse feels that you are deliberately undermining his or her efforts to support you. However you are feeling, it is important for both of you to realize that nobody is perfect. And often many of these feelings are due to love, concern, stress, or fear. It is important to acknowledge that these feelings—and probably many other conflicting emotions—do exist. Try to share them honestly when neither of you is feeling pressured or stressed out. By sharing your feelings and communicating openly, you and your partner may be drawn closer together rather than driven apart.

You might need help learning to communicate. Admitting to this is a sign of strength, not a weakness. Confide in your friends. Speak with your spiritual counselor. Consider seeking the help of professional counselors who are trained in coping strategies for people with chronic disease. Your health care professional or local ADA office may be able to help you find the skilled professional you need to talk to.

And finally, don't forget to lighten up. Humor can help you get through stressful times. Laughter helps lighten the load, relaxing us in the process.

## Diabetes and Children

Jenna and Drew were just like any other brother and sister. Sometimes they fought, but most of the time they got along fine. Then Jenna, at the age of 10, was diagnosed with type 1 diabetes. Now all the attention was on her, it seemed to 8-year-old Drew. Everything from family meals to outings seemed to revolve around Jenna. Their parents, Gail and David, couldn't understand why Jenna and Drew weren't getting along anymore. Drew was getting whiny and demanding. Why couldn't he cooperate at a time when they needed it most?

## Suggestions for Family Members

Caring about someone who has diabetes offers special challenges. Here's how you can help:

- Get an education in diabetes care.
- Be supportive, but don't take on the role of caretaker.
- Learn to listen without offering advice or criticism.
- Be flexible and open to new ways of eating and spending free time.
- Plan for emergencies.

Any kind of change can upset the family dynamic. How you treat your children and how they interact with each other can be influenced by many factors. And having a child diagnosed with diabetes is a big change that is likely to affect the entire family in ways you never thought possible. At a time when you, your child, and other children are probably fearful about what the future holds, you will likely be confronted with feelings of anger, resentment, and jealousy. At a time when you are trying to gather information and help your child manage his or her diabetes, it is difficult to keep all the family relationships running smoothly at the same time.

If you have a child with diabetes, your top priority will be to help your child manage the disease while trying to live as normal a life as possible. You will also want to help the rest of the family make a smooth transition into accepting the changes that are inevitable.

### Dealing with Your Child's Diabetes

The first step in helping your child manage his or her diabetes is to learn all you can. Other chapters in this book and Internet resources are a good starting point (see the Resources section at the end of this book for ideas). You will also want to talk to your child's care provider and diabetes educator. Try to schedule an appointment that is long enough so that all your questions and concerns can be addressed. In general, you will need to know how to check your child's blood glucose, how to give insulin, how to use a meal plan, and how to figure out an insulin dose and give injections. You will also want to know the extent to which your child can begin to take responsibility for her own care. If your child is only 2 years old, it is unrealistic to expect her to give herself insulin or test for blood glucose, but if your child is 10, she may very well be capable of checking her blood. Children mature at different rates. Some may be ready to give their own injections at age 7, but others may not be able to do it until age 11 or older. In doing your research and helping your child develop a treatment plan, don't forget that every child is different. What works for one child may not work for your child. You already know a lot about your child and what will work best for your family.

After you meet with your child's diabetes care provider, you will also want to meet with a diabetes educator. A diabetes educator can help you learn to coordinate your child's overall diabetes management plan. This includes balancing your child's meals with his insulin schedule and physical activities. You will also want to meet with a dietitian and work out an eating plan. Make sure to take into consideration your child's likes and dislikes, how your family usually eats, any cultural or religious influences, how to include treats, and how to handle special events. You will help your child and your family if you all eat the same foods. Don't prepare one dish for the rest of the family and a special meal for your child with diabetes. Make sure to involve your child in the meal planning, and ask him what foods he would like to include in his eating plan.

Also talk to your child's teachers and school officials or day care providers about any special needs your child has. (For more on diabetes at school, see page 440.) Once you and your child figure out the daily routine and work out ways to deal with special events and circumstances, you will both feel better about living with diabetes.

## Dealing with Your Own Feelings

When you first find out your child has diabetes, you may be overwhelmed with feelings of shock, disbelief, sadness, anger, or even guilt. It can seem so unfair. You may experience self-doubt as you wonder whether you can give your child the care she needs. With all the stresses in your life and all the demands on your time and energy, it may seem that you just won't be able to handle it all.

It can be overwhelming, especially at first. As you learn more about diabetes, you will also learn how to help your child live like any other kid. It may take a little work as you figure out how to balance your child's meals with insulin injections and physical activities. You may find that your child takes it all in stride and that the hardest part may be coming to terms with your own feelings.

Don't forget that your child is looking to you for guidance. Your attitude will have a direct impact on how your child sees himself and how he comes to terms with his new lifestyle. If you take your child's diabetes in stride, it will be easier for your child to accept it. If you react with anxiety, apprehension, and fear, so will he. Deal with diabetes in a matter-of-fact way. Don't downplay your child's fears or concerns, but address them in a straightforward fashion.

When you are anxious and concerned about your child, it is tempting to do everything for your child. But even very young children need to have some say in their diabetes care plan. Let your child assume some of the responsibility with taking care of her diabetes, such as helping to plan meals or snacks. Gradually increase the amount of responsibility your child has. But at the same time, make sure your child is able to take on this responsibility. You aren't really doing your child a favor if you let her diabetes care slide. Treat shots and blood glucose tests as givens, with no exceptions. As soon as your child sees that these are nonnegotiable, she will be more likely to cooperate. The best way to establish diabetes care habits is for them to become a way of life.

## Dealing with the Rest of the Family

If you have more than one child, the time you spend taking care of diabetes is bound to cause some tension in the family. Siblings may feel jealous of the child with diabetes because of all the attention that he is getting. On the other hand, siblings may give your child with diabetes too much attention, and your child may feel like his siblings are on his case. He may feel that everyone is breathing down his neck.

The best way to deal with diabetes in the family is to treat it openly. Explain what is happening to the other children and other family members, and ask them to be patient as you work things out. Even young children can understand simple information. Try to schedule special times with your other children who may feel left out, or ask if they want a job in the overall care of your child with diabetes. A sibling could help record blood glucose readings, for example. In general, you will want to treat your child's diabetes matter-of-factly. Once your child and her siblings come to accept diabetes as a part of your family routine, feelings of anger, jealousy, and fear usually begin to subside. However, if you continue to experience family turmoil, you might want to consider family counseling. Talk to your child's provider and diabetes educator for help in finding a family counselor.

## Your Child's Changing Role

Just how much you can expect your child to handle with respect to his diabetes care will change as he matures and will depend on his personality. If your child is an infant or toddler when diagnosed, you will be completely responsible for your child's care. But you can and should still keep him involved. You will have to see that your child gets his shots at the right time and you will have to check his blood glucose and evaluate the results, but you can give your child a voice. Let him pick the injection spot or the finger to poke. This is a good way for your child to get used to having a say in his care. It will help him to develop a sense of responsibility so that you can gradually help him assume more and more of his own diabetes care as he grows older.

If your child is in preschool, you are still responsible for making sure she is eating based on the plan you have worked out together, doing blood glucose checks whenever necessary, and taking the right type and dose of insulin at the right time. But there is nothing wrong with letting your child begin to take over some of these tasks, with supervision. Insulin pens may make it easier for your child to help with his shot. As your child matures, he can take on more and more of the tasks. You may want to consider an insulin pump. This can give her much greater flexibility and independence but is also a big responsibility. As your child matures during this period, it is essential that she learn to take responsibility for her own care and decisions, because she will often be with friends or at school and out of your watchful vision.

Adolescence is bound to provide the greatest challenges to both you and your child with diabetes. There will be times when your teen resents you and blames you for all the ups and downs of diabetes. This is a normal part of becoming independent and would happen whether or not he had diabetes. He may try to rebel by neglecting his diabetes care. Your child may try to deny her diabetes in an effort to fit in and appear just like everyone else. It can be hard to take insulin, count carbohydrates, and check glucose readings at school or when she is out with friends. It may help to remind her that the best way to fit in and keep diabetes from interfering with her life is to keep blood glucose levels on target. A bout of severe hypoglycemia or DKA will surely make your child feel different. Make sure he understands the consequences of his decisions, both now and in the future. You might suggest that your child visit a diabetes educator on his own. This gives your child a chance to ask questions and establish a relationship that can be helpful in the future as well. When your child is treated more like an adult, she may act more like an adult. It is critical that she understand that it is up to her to take charge of her care.

It is not uncommon for your children and teenagers to feel depressed. Eating disorders, especially among girls, are common. One type of eating disorder among teens with diabetes involves skipping insulin. This allows a person to eat and not gain weight. If you start to suspect that your child is depressed or developing any sort of coping problem, eating disorder, or behavioral problem, seek the help of a professional counselor immediately (see page 264 for more on eating disorders).

## Handling Emergencies

Whether your child is a toddler or a teen, it is important that you, your child, and those close to him be aware of the signs that could signal an emergency. Severe hypoglycemia (low blood glucose) or hyperglycemia (high blood glucose) are both emergency situations. Hypoglycemia can lead to unconsciousness and coma. Hyperglycemia can lead to DKA, a life-threatening situation. To prevent either situation, learn to recognize the warning signs, check your child's blood glucose right away, and treat promptly. Talk to your child's provider in advance about what to do if your child's blood glucose levels fall too low or rise too high.

*Hypoglycemia.* Recommended blood glucose levels are different for children and adults, because of children's high risk and vulnerability to hypoglycemia, relatively low risk of complications before puberty, and developmental and psychological issues. The blood glucose levels at which hypoglycemia is treated are also often higher than the standard recommendations for adults. Any time your child's blood glucose level falls below the value you have established, he or she may have hypoglycemia. Signs of hypoglycemia include nervousness, shakiness, sweating, irritability, impatience, chills, clamminess, rapid heartbeat, anxiety, light-headedness, and hunger. When hypoglycemia begins to affect the brain, your child may also appear sleepy, angry, uncoordinated, or sad. She may also experience nausea, blurred vision, tingling or numbness in the lips or tongue, nightmares, crying out during sleep, headaches, or strange behavior. In severe stages, confusion, delirium, personality changes, and unconsciousness can occur.

If your child is experiencing any of the symptoms of hypoglycemia, have him check his blood glucose right away. If you don't have time to check, treat anyhow.

To treat hypoglycemia, give your child a fast-acting carbohydrate. This could be 2 to 5 glucose tablets, 2 tablespoons of raisins, half a can of regular (not diet) soda, 3 to 4 ounces of juice, or 5 to 10 jelly beans, LifeSavers, or gumdrops. In general, you want to give your child 15 to 30 grams of carbohydrate. Wait 10 to 15 minutes and test again. If her blood glucose is still low, give another dose of carbohydrate.

| Plasma Blood Glucose and A1C Goals for Type 1 Diabetes by Age Group | | | |
|---|---|---|---|
| | Plasma blood glucose goal range (mg/dl) | | |
| Values by age (years) | Before meals | Bedtime/ overnight | A1C (%) |
| Toddlers and preschoolers (<6) | 100–180 | 110–200 | ≤8.5 (but ≥7.5) |
| School age (6–12) | 90–180 | 100–180 | ≤8 |
| Adolescents and young adults (13–19) | 90–130 | 90–150 | <7.5* |

*A lower goal (<7%) is reasonable if it can be achieved without excessive hypoglycemia.

If your child is unable to eat or shows any signs of severe hypoglycemia (confusion, delirium, or unconsciousness), she needs help right away. Call for emergency help. The quickest way to raise blood glucose levels is to give an injection of glucagon. Ask your child's health care provider or diabetes educator to show you how to give a glucagon injection and under what circumstances to give it. Glucagon requires a prescription. Make sure your child wears an ID at all times identifying her as having diabetes.

*Hyperglycemia and DKA.* High blood glucose levels due to insufficient insulin can lead to DKA. This is a life-threatening condition that requires immediate action. Symptoms of DKA include extreme thirst, dry parched mouth, fruity-smelling breath, and sleepiness or confusion. Your child may also have warm, dry skin with no sweating, or vomiting or stomach pain. Check her blood glucose and her urine for ketones. If your child has moderate to high levels of ketones, call your diabetes care provider right away. Talk to your provider or diabetes educator in advance to develop an action plan for when to call or go to the emergency room. In general, you should call immediately if

- ketones are present in the urine,
- vomiting occurs more than once, or
- your child has trouble breathing.

# Diabetes in the Real World | 14

*Before you developed diabetes, did you know much about it? Most people don't. One of the opportunities that comes with having diabetes is educating others in the workplace, the schools, and our society about what you need to live well with diabetes.*

Okay, so you've finally figured out a diabetes management plan. You've met with your diabetes educator and learned all you can. You met with your dietitian and figured out an eating plan that works for you. You've even talked with an exercise physiologist to come up with an exercise program that you can handle. This would all be very manageable if it weren't for one thing: the real world.

Sure, you could monitor your blood glucose 4 to 7 times a day, exercise once a day, eat specific meals on schedule, and give yourself insulin 2 to 4 times a day. But most of us don't live a life with much leisure. We work, go to school, take care of family, travel, pursue outside interests, or tend to other responsibilities.

With everything else going on in your life, taking care of your diabetes may seem next to impossible. Whether you hold down a job or go to school, working your diabetes care into the rest of your day presents special challenges. And as if that weren't enough, even if you do manage to balance the demands of work, school, and diabetes, you may face discrimination.

Fortunately, you can learn to integrate your diabetes care into everything else you do. The better you plan and communicate with others around you, the better you will be able to take care of your diabetes—and still do all the things you want and need to do in the real world.

## Diabetes in the Workplace

Jason had spent his whole career in the job he loved: nursing. When he moved to a new city, he immediately found a position in the intensive care unit of the city's biggest hospital. He enjoyed working the night shift from 11 p.m. to 7 a.m. even though it meant keeping odd hours. But a few months after starting his new job, he was diagnosed with type 2 diabetes. He worried about whether he would be able to care for his diabetes while working such an erratic schedule.

Anne had just graduated from college. She had been living with diabetes since her early teens and had learned how to manage it reasonably well while attending classes, studying, working out at the gym, and even partying with her friends. And now she had landed an exciting sales job. It would mean lots of traveling all over the country with occasional overseas visits, business luncheons, and cocktail parties. But how could she ever manage her diabetes with all that traveling and while keeping such crazy hours?

For Jason and Anne, new jobs and new schedules certainly mean big changes. Without a doubt, they will both have to learn to make frequent adjustments in their diabetes care. As teachers, police officers, cooks, doctors, nurses, electricians, engineers, firefighters, athletes, factory workers, farmers, and corporate executives, there's really no end to the types of work people with diabetes can do. It hasn't always been this way. Today, thanks to the Americans with Disabilities Act, which guarantees your rights in private employment and local government, and the federal Rehabilitation Act, which ensures your rights in federal government employment, there are more and more opportunities for people with diabetes. Diabetes affects each person differently, and each person should be evaluated based on what he or she can do. As long as you are qualified, you can go after almost any job you desire.

## Work Schedules

You may have an easier time managing your diabetes if you have a regular work schedule. But if your job entails working the late shift or traveling all over the globe, diabetes doesn't have to keep you from pursuing it. Most people can make the necessary adjustments with help from their health care team. If your employer or prospective employer questions your ability to manage a job with irregular work hours, explain to them how you are able to manage your diabetes. Emphasize that you are in charge of your diabetes and the discipline you exercise in taking care of your diabetes is the discipline and determination you will bring to the workplace.

*Night Shift.* When you work the night shift you may feel out of sync with the rest of the world. While everyone else is eating breakfast, you're ready for your bedtime snack. And adjusting to conventional hours on your days off can also be a challenge. Nevertheless, with careful planning and monitoring, you can learn to make adjustments so that your new routine works for you.

Let's say you're working the 11 p.m. to 7 a.m. shift. If you get home at 8 a.m. and plan to sleep through the day, you may need to adjust your insulin dose to prevent hypoglycemia while you sleep. It may be easier to use a more intensive approach to your diabetes. For example, you could take an injection of long-acting insulin at the same time every day and rapid- or short-acting insulin before your meals. An insulin pump may also work well. Your health care team can help you make changes.

On the other hand, maybe you prefer to stay up until noon and sleep through the afternoon and early evening. In that case, your normal morning insulin dose may work just fine. But you may have to make adjustments in your evening dose. If your job calls for some nights on and some nights off, then you will need to check your blood glucose levels more often and fine-tune your insulin dose.

If you have type 2 diabetes and are not taking insulin, you may still have to accommodate your work schedule. And if you are taking oral agents, eating at a particular time may make a difference. It may be as simple as making sure you eat a snack before sleeping or changing the times you eat and exercise. Whenever you are getting used to a new routine, more frequent blood glucose monitoring will help you decide how to best adjust your daily routine to keep your blood glucose levels in balance.

**Erratic Hours.** You may not work the night shift, but you have the sort of job that makes you keep odd hours. Perhaps a meeting with clients has you eating later than usual. Or your job may demand lots of traveling. Even in the most conventional job setting, there are probably going to be occasions when you're eating or exercising at a different time. Whether it happens all the time or once in a blue moon, you'll need to learn how to make adjustments to accommodate changes in routine.

For example, if you're going to eat a late lunch, try eating your afternoon snack or part of your carbohydrates at your normal lunchtime, and you'll be able to hold off for a while until you eat your full meal. You may also need to delay giving your insulin until your meal time. It will take a little trial and error, but you will soon figure out how to make adjustments. If you do tend to keep a crazy schedule, talk to your health care team about an insulin plan that allows for maximum flexibility. Afterwards, check and record your blood glucose levels and evaluate how well your plan worked.

Exercise can also be affected by changes in schedule. If you are used to a lunchtime jog, but a noontime lunch meeting keeps you from your normal routine, your blood glucose will probably be higher that afternoon. You can compensate by eating less, or, if you're taking insulin, injecting a little more insulin than usual. If you take your run later in the day, you may find it necessary to eat a larger snack than usual. Whenever changes in routine require adjustments, be extra diligent about monitoring to keep your blood glucose on target and to learn how to make future adjustments. And be sure to always keep a snack on hand in case your glucose level goes low.

## Driving and Operating Heavy Equipment

If you operate heavy equipment, if you are involved in public safety jobs like law enforcement or firefighting, or even if you drive an automobile, it is important to always be aware of your blood glucose levels. This is especially important for people who take insulin or oral medications that can cause a low blood glucose reaction. A low blood glucose reaction in these situations can result in serious injury to yourself and others and can have serious employment consequences. Federal law requires an employer to evaluate each person with diabetes as an individual, looking at the job in question and how diabetes affects that person. There are a few exceptions.

The federal government does not allow people who take insulin to enter the armed forces or to pilot commercial airplanes. However, some people who take insulin have been able to remain in the armed forces when diagnosed with diabetes, and some people who take insulin can pilot small, noncommercial planes. The federal government used to ban people who take insulin from driving large trucks or buses on interstate routes but has now set up an exemption program for individual evaluation of each potential driver.

When you drive or operate heavy equipment keep the following guidelines in mind:

- Check your blood glucose level before you leave your house or start work. If it's low (70 mg/dl or less), treat it. Recheck 15 minutes after your first check to be sure your blood glucose level is rising. Otherwise, it is not safe to drive or operate equipment. If your glucose is not on the rise, treat again and wait until your blood glucose level has come back up.
- Always take along a fast-acting source of carbohydrate— glucose gel or tablets, hard candy, juice boxes, or raisins. Also keep them in your glove compartment so you will always have something available. If you feel even minor symptoms of low blood glucose while driving or operating heavy equipment, stop and check your blood glucose. Driving with a low blood glucose level is dangerous. It is better to be a few minutes late or to take a little longer getting the job done than to risk an accident.
- If you can't check your blood glucose and you feel hypoglycemic, stop what you are doing and treat the symptoms.

Don't start driving or working again until the symptoms pass. It's a mistake to think you can hold out until you get to wherever you are going or finish up the job.

- Wear or carry diabetes identification.

## Discrimination

A few years ago, David worked in a research lab at a university. He was told by his supervisor not to administer insulin at his desk or he would face termination. David obliged, but resented that he couldn't take care of his diabetes the way he wanted. Eventually, he found another job, but had to take a pay cut and give up some retirement benefits. He always wished he had stood up to his supervisor and stayed with the job he loved.

Paula, who had been managing her type 2 diabetes for several years, was told that she would have to switch from working the day shift to a rotating shift schedule or face termination. This would wreak havoc with her diabetes care, but she didn't want to lose her job.

Jon was enjoying his dream career. He graduated from a military academy and was now serving as a second lieutenant in the U.S. Air Force. But after he started feeling dizzy on duty, a physical exam revealed he had type 1 diabetes. His commanding officer put him on medical hold while his case was being reviewed. He feared he would be discharged.

Today there are laws to protect against discrimination in the workplace. But unfortunately, discrimination against people with diabetes still exists. Sometimes people with diabetes are told outright they won't be hired because of their diabetes. But other times discrimination can be more subtle. Did you get passed over for a promotion because of your work performance or because your boss was afraid your diabetes might interfere with the added responsibilities? Did you fail to get that job offer because you weren't qualified, or because you told the employer you have diabetes? Sometimes it's hard to know. The best thing you can do to guard against discrimination in the workplace is to do the best job you can and understand your rights.

In 1990, the Americans with Disabilities Act (42 U.S.C. 12101 et seq.) was signed into law. This law protects qualified individuals with disabilities from being discriminated against. It covers all private sector employees who work for companies that employ 15 or more people and people who work for state or local governments. The Rehabilitation Act of 1973 provides similar protection for people who work for the executive branch of the federal government or who work for companies or contractors that receive federal funding. The Congressional Accountability Act provides the same coverage for employees of the legislative branch of the federal government. Under these laws, employers cannot discriminate against you if you have a disability, are qualified for the job, and can carry out the work with or without reasonable accommodation by the employer. All states have their own anti-discrimination laws and agencies responsible for enforcing those laws. Some state anti-discrimination laws provide more comprehensive protection than do federal laws. In principal, employers are not allowed to discriminate, but in practice some discrimination still occurs. Some employers are slow to change workplace policies, such as bans on hiring anyone who takes insulin, unless they are challenged in court.

The federal Rehabilitation Act, the Americans with Disabilities Act, and the Congressional Accountability Act require employers to give people with disabilities an equal opportunity.

Perhaps you have been working hard to keep your blood glucose on target and to prove to yourself and to others that you are healthy. So it may be difficult to think of diabetes as a "disability." But this legal term is necessary to defend your rights.

As a result of three Supreme Court decisions in 1999 (referred to as the Sutton trilogy), a person with diabetes must show that she or he still meets the definition of "disability" after taking mitigating measures such as insulin or oral medication. Diabetes doesn't go away simply because someone takes medication, so it is important to explain to the courts the multifaceted process of diabetes management. This includes the tasks and monitoring needed to keep blood glucose levels in a safe range, as well as what happens when they aren't. Courts are required to do an individual assessment of each person by considering how diabetes affects her or him and the impact of medication and any diabetes-related complications. It is important to keep in mind that if you can't show you have a disability, have a record of having a disability, or are regarded as having a disability, then it is legal under federal law for an employer to refuse to hire you, to fire you, or to take other adverse action because you have diabetes.

The employee must also establish that he or she is qualified for the job in question. A qualified applicant possesses the skill, experience, education, and other job requirements of the position he or she would do with or without reasonable accommodation. Employees must also show they were treated unfairly because of their diabetes.

Before these laws were passed, you may have been asked to list any medical conditions on a job application. The employer could then refuse to hire you based on this information. But if you weren't hired, you might not know whether it was because of your qualifications, a bad recommendation, or because of your diabetes.

Current federal law allows an employer to ask an applicant for medical information only after making a job offer and only if all job applicants are asked to provide this information. Then an employer may withdraw a job offer only if the applicant cannot perform the tasks required for the job, even if reasonable accommodations are made by the employer. An employer still has the option of hiring whomever he or she feels is best able to do the job. However, an employer can run into problems if he or she hires someone less qualified while refusing someone with better qualifications who happens to have diabetes or any other disability.

Once you have started working, an employer can only ask medical questions if they are job related and consistent with the needs of the business. For example, if an employee falls asleep on the job, an employer may ask if a medical condition is the cause. However, if an employee doesn't look well, but is performing his or her job adequately, an employer may not ask whether there is a medical problem.

The laws require that employers try to reasonably accommodate people with disabilities. Reasonable accommodation is defined as modification or adjustment of a job or employment practice, to make it possible for a qualified person with a disability to be employed. For people with diabetes, employers may have to allow workers to adjust their work schedule or take breaks to eat or for blood glucose monitoring so that they can manage their diabetes while on the job. People with complications from diabetes might need other accommodations, such as a large-screen computer to deal with retinopathy or the ability to sit on the job to cope with painful neuropathy. The employer must make these accommodations unless they create an undue burden because of cost or other factors.

## Fighting Back against Discrimination

If you believe that you have been discriminated against, either in your job or while seeking employment, the best course of action is first to **educate** and then **negotiate.** If necessary, **litigate,** and last, **legislate.** Sometimes, dealing with a discrimination problem is as simple as teaching people about diabetes. Many employers don't understand the needs or capabilities of people with diabetes. And sometimes they don't understand the laws that protect you from discrimination. By educating employers about your needs, limitations, and strengths and by informing them of your rights and their responsibilities, you can resolve many situations in which you suspect discrimination.

Sometimes education alone may not be enough. You may have to negotiate to secure your rights. Your negotiations may be more effective if you first seek legal advice. Seeking legal advice early will maximize your attorney's ability to help you. Whether you have outside help or not, negotiating involves listening to the concerns of those in the workplace with an open mind and offering solutions to the perceived problems. If your employer is unwilling to take the steps to resolve a problem, you might suggest a trial period in which you can show how your solution may benefit all involved. You might also consider soliciting outside help, such as elected officials or the media.

If this doesn't help, you may have no choice but to litigate. The litigation process begins by filing an administrative complaint with the appropriate agency. If you are discriminated against by a private employer or a local government, you must file a charge with the Equal Employment Opportunity Commission (EEOC) and/or the state agency that handles workplace discrimination issues. The EEOC provides free information booklets. Check the Resources section at the end of this book for more information. If you work for or are seeking a job with the executive branch of the federal government, you must file a complaint with your agency's Equal Employment Opportunity Office. If you have been discriminated against by the legislative branch of the federal government, your claim under the Congressional Accountability Act must be filed with the Office of Compliance.

Be aware that the time limits for filing discrimination claims are very short. Claims with the executive branch of the federal government must be filed within 45 days of the act of discrimination and those with other employers can be due within 180 days of discriminatory treatment. If the agency doesn't resolve the problem to your satisfaction, you can file a lawsuit in federal or state court claiming discrimination on the basis of disability.

If a suit is decided in your favor, the employer may be forced to pay a cash settlement, reverse the discriminatory decision, and pay penalties. To decide on the best course of action, you will want to consult an attorney.

It is up to you to prove that you have been discriminated against because of diabetes. Request a written statement saying why you weren't hired or promoted, or were let go. There may be other reasons for the employer's decision, and you and your attorney should be aware of them.

If an employer is truly discriminating against you on the basis of your diabetes, he or she may not readily admit to it in writing. You may have to do some information gathering to substantiate your claim. Gather materials such as the employer's job application form, policy manuals, and any rules or regulations cited by the employer as the reason you were dismissed or not hired. Save copies of the job advertisement or listing, the job description, and the job performance evaluation criteria.

You should also compile a list of potential witnesses, including work titles and how to contact them. Include some information about their duties at work and how they would know about your situation. Finally, make a diary of events in chronological order.

Sometimes legislative or regulatory changes are necessary. The ADA works to change laws and policies that are unfair to people with diabetes; for example, ADA successfully fought the "blanket ban" that kept people who use insulin from driving a commercial vehicle in interstate commerce.

## Job Hunting

Not everyone discriminates against people with diabetes, so don't let the fear of discrimination in the workplace keep you from seeking or reaching your career goals. But when looking for a new job, keep the following in mind:

- Try not to think of diabetes as a defect. It is a part of your life. Don't be shy about asserting your needs in the workplace.
- Be prepared by knowing your rights. Remember that employers are not allowed to ask about your health before deciding whether to hire you. Once the job has been offered, they can ask about medical conditions only as they relate to the job as part of the pre-employment physical examination.
- If you wait to disclose your diabetes until after the job has been offered, take a positive approach. Be sure to point out how diabetes helps you be a conscientious employee.
- During your physical exam, if required, accurately describe your condition and how you care for your diabetes. Don't try to change your diabetes care plan immediately before any physical examination. Changes in routine can affect your glucose levels. Your company's doctor is probably not

a diabetes specialist, and you may need to educate him or her about how you manage your diabetes. Offer input from your treating diabetes physician to help the examining doctor make an accurate diagnosis.

In time, popular thinking will catch up with what many know already: diabetes doesn't have to keep you from doing what you want to do.

## Diabetes, Commercial Drivers' Licenses, and Blanket Bans

The American Diabetes Association (ADA) has worked for years to overturn the so-called "blanket bans" that sometimes prohibit anyone with diabetes from performing certain jobs or participating in other activities. Thanks to ADA's efforts, the Federal Aviation Administration (FAA) overturned a 36-year-

### To Tell or Not to Tell . . .

Whether you tell your employer or fellow employees about your diabetes is completely up to you. There are reasons to tell—and reasons not to. Much depends on your particular job circumstances and the people involved. Here are some of the pluses and minuses.

#### Reasons to Tell

- If you take insulin or certain oral agents, you may be prone to low blood glucose reactions. This can make you confused and unable to help yourself. If people know you have diabetes, they can help you in the event of such a reaction.

## To Tell or Not to Tell . . . (*Continued*)

- If you need your employer to make accommodations because of your diabetes (for example, providing time for you to check your blood glucose level in a job that doesn't allow breaks at will, your employer needs to know about your diabetes and why you need the accommodation.
- If your employer is not on official notice that you have diabetes and you suspect that some adverse action is the result of your diabetes, it may be very difficult to prove that your employer discriminated against you because of your diabetes.
- Being open helps people to learn more about diabetes. You can help fight prejudice by showing that people with diabetes are just like everyone else. By not telling, you may be sending the message that you have something to be ashamed of.
- When you are open about your diabetes, you may be surprised to learn how many others have diabetes themselves or in their families. You can help each other.
- When you talk about your diabetes, other people can learn about the symptoms and treatment. As a result, people you know get the help they need if they suspect that they may also have diabetes.

### Reasons Not to Tell

- You may want to maintain your privacy. Just as you wouldn't necessarily talk about how much money you make, you might not want to discuss your diabetes, which is just as personal.
- If you don't tell, you are less likely to lose a job promotion or job offer because of your diabetes. However, diabetes can be difficult to hide if you need to take breaks or leave a meeting to monitor blood glucose or take insulin. Although laws protect against discrimination, it is not always easy to prove.

---

### Sources to Contact in Case of Discrimination

- The American Diabetes Association. Call 1-800-DIABETES and ask for the Association's employment discrimination packet. If you have a specific problem, you may also want to fill out a form so that you can talk to the Association's Legal Advocate. A great deal of information is available on the ADA Web site at www.diabetes.org/employmentdiscrimination.
- The Equal Employment Opportunity Commission or your state's anti-discrimination agency. Most states have a commission charged with investigating discrimination.
- Your union representative. If your job is covered by a union contract, your union may be able to help.

---

old blanket ban that prohibited people who use insulin from flying small, private aircraft. For many years, the ADA worked hard to end the blanket ban imposed by the Department of Transportation (DOT) that prevented a person using insulin from driving a commercial vehicle in interstate commerce.

In 2003, the DOT instituted an exemption program to allow some people who use insulin to drive commercial vehicles in interstate commerce. Prior to this change, if you were a truck or bus driver with non–insulin-treated diabetes and later begin using insulin, you would lose your job if it involved driving a commercial vehicle across state lines. As a result of ADA advocacy, this rule was replaced with a system that evaluates each case on an individual basis. However, there are limits on who may apply for a DOT exemption. Currently, only people who have three years of experience driving a commercial vehicle while using insulin are eligible for an exemption. ADA is working to eliminate this "three year rule" legislatively, and it is

## Protecting Your Job with FMLA

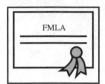

In addition to the Americans with Disabilities Act, the Rehabilitation Act of 1973, and the Congressional Accountability Act, there is another federal law that can help you and your family deal with diabetes in the workplace. The Family and Medical Leave Act (FMLA) was passed in 1993. This law allows workers to take up to 12 weeks of job-protected unpaid leave during any 12-month period to care for their own serious health condition or to care for family members (spouse, child, or parent). FMLA absences may be taken in a single 12-week stretch or in shorter intervals, such as a short period to deal with a diabetes-related illness or emergency or a scheduled doctor's appointment. Employers who normally pay health insurance premiums must continue to do so for an employee on FMLA leave.

FMLA applies to most public employers and to those private companies with 50 or more employees locally (within 75 miles of the workplace). To be eligible, employees must have been with a covered employer for at least 1 year and have worked 1,250 or more hours during the 12 months immediately preceding the date of commencement of FMLA leave. When leave is foreseeable, employees must give 30 days notice. Some high-level company executives—those who are in the top 10 percent salary range—may be ineligible for FMLA leave.

### FMLA offers leave to care for

- yourself
- your spouse
- parents
- step and foster parents
- minor children
- minor step and foster children
- adult children who are incapable of self-care

### FMLA excludes leave to care for:

- unmarried partners
- in-laws
- siblings
- grandchildren
- grandparents

## Fighting Discrimination: A Success Story

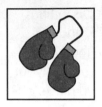 Despite the inherent risks involved with a career in law enforcement, Jeff Kapche knew he wanted to be a police officer. Kapche, fresh out of the police academy, drove to San Antonio and waited in line to receive one of a limited number of applications that were being given out to hopeful candidates. Kapche passed all the tests and the background check required to join the department as a police officer. But then he encountered another hurdle—the doctor the city had assigned to conduct physical examinations of the candidates concluded that Kapche, who has type 1 diabetes, could not do the job because of his diabetes. The doctor disqualified Kapche because driving was an "essential function" of the police job, and San Antonio considered drivers who use insulin to be a safety risk to themselves and others.

Kapche appealed the decision, but after a year he had run out of options for internal appeals. He then turned to the American Diabetes Association for help. ADA put Kapche in touch with Mike Greene, a former chair of the ADA board and the "founding father" of the association's legal advocacy efforts. Greene and John Griffin, an experienced Texas lawyer who had worked on other diabetes discrimination cases, went to work for Kapche. Griffin represented Kapche, and Greene submitted friend of the court (amicus curiae) briefs on behalf of the ADA. The lawyers argued that blanket bans that disqualify all people with diabetes from a given position, such as a law enforcement position, are both unlawful and medically unnecessary.

What seemed like a relatively straightforward case given Kapche's qualifications and excellent diabetes control became a long legal

## Fighting Discrimination: A Success Story (*Continued*)

battle. As the lawsuit continued, Kapche was proving every day that he was qualified for the job—through his work as a deputy at the Fort Bend County Sheriff's Office. Fort Bend recognized that Kapche's diabetes did not prevent him from being a first-rate law enforcement officer and, as the lawsuit against San Antonio worked its way through the courts, Kapche continued to move up the ranks in Fort Bend.

It took more than eight years and two trips to the United States Court of Appeals for the Fifth Circuit, but ultimately Kapche's lawsuit resulted in an important victory for workers with diabetes. The appellate court considered medical evidence and advances in diabetes management and determined that blanket bans against people with diabetes—and specifically Jeff Kapche—were unjustified. Jeff Kapche's struggle helped many people with diabetes who face discrimination on the job.

possible that in the near future more people who use insulin will be able to apply for an exemption.

In addition, the federal government allows individual states to provide waivers to intrastate drivers who use insulin. These waivers allow commercial drivers to travel within a given state, but only if the goods or people being transported are not coming from or going to another state. Contact your state's motor vehicles department to find out if your state has a waiver program for intrastate drivers who use insulin.

The ADA continues to fight for the right for each person with diabetes to be evaluated individually based on how diabetes affects him or her and to not be excluded because of misinformation and stereotypes about diabetes. You can find

more information about employment discrimination at www.
diabetes.org/employmentdiscrimination.

## Diabetes at School

Megan had been diagnosed with diabetes as a toddler.
Adapting to life with diabetes was difficult for her parents.
But Megan seemed to take it all in stride. Under her mother's
watchful eye, Megan eventually learned to check her own blood
glucose and could use her insulin pen to give her own shot once
the dose was set for her. She could even sense when her blood
glucose levels were falling too low. Her parents were finally
beginning to relax until they realized that Megan would be entering school in the fall. They weren't sure how diabetes care would
be provided by Megan's teacher and school staff.

Nick had finally made the transition from elementary school
to middle school. Instead of staying with one teacher all day, he
switched classes every hour. He got to take cool classes that he
really liked, but the best part was gym every afternoon. But then
one day, he passed out during gym class. That's when he was
diagnosed with type 1 diabetes. He and his parents wondered
how he would ever be able to deal with diabetes at school.
Where would he check his blood glucose? Would his teachers
know how to help him if his blood glucose dropped suddenly?
Could he eat the school lunches? What if he had to go to the
bathroom during the middle of class? What would all the other
kids say?

For Nick and Megan, as for all kids with diabetes, adjusting to diabetes in school can be challenging. This is true
whether your child has been living with diabetes and is enter-

ing school for the first time or changing schools, or is already in school and has been recently diagnosed with diabetes. You want to make sure your child is given the same opportunities as other children, but you also want to make sure your child is safe at school and that any special needs are met. And you don't want your child to feel like an outcast.

## Communicate and Educate

The best approach to dealing with diabetes in the schools is to communicate openly with the school's administration and teachers and, if your child agrees, with the kids in your child's class. Make sure your child's school staff understands what it means to have diabetes, how your child manages his or her diabetes, and what needs your child has. Your child's school may already have a policy in effect to deal with the needs of children with chronic illnesses, including diabetes. However, you and your child's health care team will need to develop an individual plan to address your child's specific health care needs. This plan may be called a Diabetes Medical Management Plan (DMMP) but may also be referred to as a health care plan or physician's orders or another name. The information supplied by the health care team is then used to develop a school plan that sets out how your child will be accommodated at school. This plan may be called a Section 504 plan if it is developed under the federal Rehabilitation Act or an Individualized Education Program (IEP) if it is developed under the Individuals with Disabilities Education Act. The plan describes how the DMMP will be implemented in school.

Your child should be able to

■ receive assistance with blood glucose monitoring and insulin or glucagon administration if needed.

- eat whenever and wherever necessary. This includes keeping snacks or glucose tablets close at hand.
- go to the bathroom or water fountain when necessary.
- participate fully in all school activities, including extracurricular activities such as sports or field trips, with diabetes care provided by trained school staff members.
- refrain from exams or physical activity when blood glucose levels are too high or too low.
- eat lunch on schedule, with enough time allotted to finish eating.
- be excused for tardiness in case of a blood glucose problem.
- check blood glucose levels in the classroom or wherever he or she happens to be (if the child is capable of this self-management task).
- be absent, without penalty, for medical appointments and diabetes-related illnesses.

Sitting down with your child's teachers, school nurse, school administrators, and other personnel and discussing your child's needs is important. When schools are reluctant to accommodate a child's diabetes needs, it may be because they do not understand diabetes. While it is the school's job to make sure your child is medically safe and has the same opportunities as other students, you can help by educating your child's school staff about your child's diabetes so that they understand that the needs of a child with diabetes are not unreasonable.

If your child is entering a school for the first time, meet several weeks before school starts with the school principal, school nurse, teachers, and other school personnel who will have direct contact with your child. If your child is already enrolled in school but has been recently diagnosed with diabetes, meet with school personnel before your child returns to school.

Before meeting with school personnel, it is important to meet with your child's health care team and work out a Diabetes Medical Management Plan (DMMP) for your child. This plan spells out the medical care your child should receive at school, including information about blood glucose monitoring, meals and snacks, insulin, and emergency care, which may include the administration of glucagon. Some children are capable of self-care, while other children will need a great deal of help. All children with diabetes will need help in the event of an emergency. ADA has developed a sample DMMP (see p. 521), which is available on the Internet for printing or downloading at www.diabetes.org or by calling 1-800-DIABETES and asking for a school discrimination packet.

In this initial meeting with school personnel, discuss what is in your child's DMMP and how these needs will be met. Provide a brief explanation of diabetes, clarify any misconceptions, and explain the consequences of blood glucose levels that are too high or too low and the appropriate corrective actions. Find out whether there is a nurse on duty to assist with routine care and to handle emergencies and, when a nurse isn't available, which adults will be trained to provide care to your child during the school day and at all school-sponsored extracurricular activities. Determine what time your child will be eating lunch and whether there is a designated snack time for all children. Make sure your child will have immediate access to a snack and a quick-acting form of glucose whenever necessary. Also, it is especially important to talk with school personnel, including your child's physical education teacher, about the impact of food, insulin, and physical activity on blood glucose levels and how to prevent and respond to hypoglycemia.

It is also important to understand how school policies and protocols might affect the diabetes care your child receives while at school and to educate and work with school personnel to make any needed adjustments. Discuss any concerns you might have and be sure to find out what your child is concerned about. Open communication at this stage is critical to establishing a positive working relationship.

Once the DMMP is complete, you will need to develop a Section 504 plan, an IEP, or other written education plan to be sure it is implemented.

## Classroom Blood Glucose Monitoring and Self-Management

Individuals with diabetes must manage their blood glucose levels through the careful balance of food, exercise, and medication. Blood glucose monitoring is an essential component to good health. It is the only way of making sure blood glucose levels are maintained within your child's target range. Because it is extremely important for your child to be able to monitor his or her own blood glucose levels and respond to levels that are too high or too low as quickly as possible, you may want your child to check his or her blood glucose levels and promptly treat wherever he or she is at school or during a school-related activity. Whether this is appropriate depends on your child's age, level of experience and skill, and personal preference. Your child's immediate access to diabetes equipment and self-care is important so that symptoms don't get worse and so that she or he doesn't miss valuable classroom instruction or other school activities.

Unlike many other diseases and chronic medical conditions, good diabetes care depends on self-management. However, because of your child's age, maturity level, or level of experience or skill, he or she may not be able to handle various aspects of diabetes care alone. Because of these factors, or in the event of an emergency, trained school personnel will be needed to check blood glucose levels, to administer insulin or medication, or to recognize and treat hypoglycemia (and administer glucagon) or hyperglycemia.

## Training of School Personnel

Diabetes care training for school nurses and other school personnel should be developed and implemented by diabetes educators, school nurses or other qualified health care providers, and school administrators. School nurses and nonmedical school personnel can be trained to perform and assist with blood glucose and ketone monitoring; insulin, oral medication, and glucagon administration; and recognition and treatment of hypoglycemia or hyperglycemia. There are three levels of training appropriate for school personnel:

1) Training for school personnel who will actually perform diabetes care tasks, such as blood glucose monitoring, insulin administration, glucagon administration, and recognition and treatment of hypoglycemia or hyperglycemia. Training should address the following areas: general overview of diabetes and explanation of type 1 and type 2 diabetes, recognition and treatment of hypoglycemia and hyperglycemia, blood glucose monitoring, insulin and glucagon administration, nutrition and exercise, and explanation of legal rights and responsibilities of parents and schools. Sufficient school personnel should be trained to ensure that a trained person is available during the school day and at all school-sponsored events, field trips, before- and after-school activities, and extracurricular activities.

2) Training for other school staff members who have primary responsibility for a student with diabetes. Such staff members need to understand how to recognize when your child

needs help, what accommodations are needed, and how to locate a diabetes trained person who can provide it.
3) Training for all school personnel, which should include a brief overview of diabetes and how to get help when needed.

Appropriately trained school personnel will help to ensure a safe school environment for your child and will enable her or him to participate in all school-sponsored events and to achieve optimal academic performance.

## Your Child's Rights Are Your School's Responsibilities

Once you have met with school personnel and discussed your child's needs, as set out by his or her Diabetes Medical Management Plan, hopefully the school will accommodate your child. Almost all schools are required by law to provide aids and related services to meet the needs of children with diabetes.

Three federal laws may play an important role at school. Section 504 of the Rehabilitation Act of 1973 protects individuals with disabilities against discrimination in any federally funded program, including public school systems. The Americans with Disabilities Act provides similar protection in all public and private schools, except those schools run by religious institutions. Both laws have been found to protect children with diabetes. The Individuals with Disabilities Education Act (IDEA) guarantees "free appropriate public education including special education and related service programming for all children with disabilities." This law only applies to those children whose diabetes adversely affects their ability to learn. This can occur when your child's blood glucose levels are often very high or low at school, if your child misses a lot of school due to diabetes-related complications, or if your child has

## Your Public School Rights

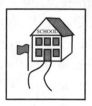 Despite the fact that federal law prohibits discrimination against children with disabilities in public schools, many parents find that their children's needs are still not being met. In working with school officials to meet your child's needs, it helps to know your rights. You have the right to request that your child be evaluated for services, and if eligible

- schedule a meeting with school officials. You have a right to bring an advocate, attorney, or experts to this meeting to better explain your child's diabetes management.
- develop a plan to accommodate the unique needs of your child. This plan should precisely set out the types of special services your child needs to receive.
- withhold signing a plan if it does not meet your child's needs. Be reasonable, but stand firm if your child's needs are not being accommodated.
- be notified and review any proposed changes in your child's plan, be included in any conference or meetings held to review the plan, and review and consider changes before they are implemented.

another disability that affects learning. You can ask your school district to evaluate your child to determine which laws apply.

After you have discussed your child's Diabetes Medical Management Plan with school personnel, the next step is to determine how the school will treat your child. It is important to write down just what steps are going to be taken. That way, everyone from student to parent to school personnel knows their responsibilities. The accommodation may be documented in either a 504 plan or in an IEP. The document should specifically state your child's disability, needs, accommodations, and how these accommodations will be delivered. The plan sets out a blueprint for making sure your child has the same opportunities to participate in all academic and school-sponsored activities as do children without disabilities. Typically, an IEP is more specific than a 504 plan with regard to your child's academic needs.

Make sure to think through what things are important to your child's well-being and include those in the plan. You are more likely to get greater cooperation from the school officials if you show a willingness to understand their concerns, but maintain a firm position on how your child's needs must be met. Try to encourage the attitude that you are all members of the same team.

If you feel that your child's school is not meeting your needs, you have no choice but to take stronger action. You may want to contact an attorney for help in deciding the best course of action. You may consider filing an administrative complaint with the U.S. Department of Education or through the school district or state appeal process. Do not delay in getting legal

## Safe at School Campaign

The American Diabetes Association has long been involved in working to end discrimination against students with diabetes. To further these efforts, ADA launched the Safe at School campaign to ensure that students with diabetes are safe at school and can fully participate in all school activities. You can find more information about the campaign at www.diabetes.org/safeatschool.

help. Administrative appeal and other actions need to be started quickly or you lose the ability to pursue them.

### Further Information from the ADA

The ADA has developed a position statement on the care of children with diabetes in the school and day care setting that provides a basis for a comprehensive school policy that protects both the medical safety and legal rights of students with diabetes. The Association's position statements are reviewed and approved by its Professional Practice Committee and Executive Committee and are peer-reviewed on an ongoing basis. In addition, written materials available from the ADA do an excellent job of explaining diabetes care in a school setting. One example of an ADA pamphlet is *Children with Diabetes: Informa-*

---

### More School Resources

Some resources for school personnel can be easily downloaded from the Internet:

- The National Diabetes Education Program's "Helping the Student with Diabetes Succeed: A Guide for School Personnel," www.ndep.nih.gov/resources/school.htm. This comprehensive guide was developed by the National Institutes of Health, the Centers for Disease Control and Prevention, the U.S. Department of Education, the ADA, and many other diabetes and education organizations.
- ADA's Diabetes Care Tasks School Training Modules, "Diabetes Care Tasks at School: What Key Personnel Need to Know," www.diabetes.org/schooltraining

*tion for Schools and Child Care Providers.* The ADA's packet on school discrimination can be obtained at www.diabetes.org or by calling 1-800-DIABETES. You can also discuss a specific school or day care problem with ADA's legal advocate. A great deal of information is available on the ADA Web site at www. diabetes.org/schooldiscrimination.

# Diabetes on the Go

In today's global marketplace, many jobs require travel. Whether you're circling the globe several times a month or riding the rails every now and then, you're bound to have changes in your daily schedule and routine. That doesn't mean you can't travel if you have diabetes. With a little advance planning, you can go anywhere and do almost anything. But there are a few things you should be aware of that will make your diabetes care that much easier.

## In the Air

*Packing.* Along with everything else, you need to make sure that you have what you need to care for your diabetes. You will want to take enough for your trip plus extras in case you get delayed, you misplace something along the way, or you decide to stay longer. Make sure that all your diabetes supplies are in your carry-on bag. You can't count on your luggage getting to your destination at the same time you do. In addition, the luggage compartments on airplanes are often very cold, and your insulin could freeze. Or your bag could be left in the hot sun and the insulin could get too warm. If you use an insulin pump, take an alternate source of insulin in case your pump stops working while you are away from home. Most pump companies will send another one to your destination by express mail, but you need a way to take insulin in the meantime. You should also be sure to pack snacks to carry with you and have accessible whenever you may feel your blood glucose going low.

*Going through Security.* Although not required, it is a good idea to take a letter from your diabetes care provider saying that you have diabetes. This is particularly helpful if you are traveling overseas. Make sure your insulin, glucagon, and related supplies are clearly identified and labeled. Most people don't have a problem at security, but it is better to be safe than sorry. If you wear an insulin pump, you won't have to take it off to go through security, but security personnel may want to do a visual inspection. For more information or to report unfair treatment by security personnel, contact the Transportation Security Administration at 1-866-289-9673 or www.tsa.gov.

*On the Plane.* Many flights no longer offer food service. Ask at the desk before you board the plane if there will be a meal or snack. You can purchase something at the airport to carry on the plane and eat around your usual mealtime or before you board.

If a meal will be served, you can order a special meal in advance. Most airlines have low-sugar, low-fat, low-salt, and low-cholesterol meals available on request. Most airlines require that you request special meals at least 24 to 48 hours in advance. However, many people prefer to get the regular meals and choose which food to eat.

Mealtimes on the plane can be somewhat unpredictable. So don't inject your premeal insulin until your meal has been served. Bad weather, a bumpy flight, or air traffic can delay service. Take along extra snacks in case your meal is delayed, there is no meal service, or no time to buy food at the airport. You may want to tell your flight attendant that you have diabetes, especially if you are traveling alone. That way, your air-line crew will be prepared should any emergency arise. And if there is a meal delay, he or she may be more willing to see that you get your meal as soon as possible.

Also be aware that air travel can be dehydrating, so you'll feel better at the end if you drink lots of fluids. Avoid alcohol because it can only add to dehydration.

***Time Zones.*** Crossing time zones can sometimes be confusing. Should you be eating according to east coast or west coast time? If you are in the air, when should you inject your next dose of insulin? In general, when you lose hours from your day (traveling from the west coast to the east coast), you may need to reduce or skip a dose of insulin. When adding hours to your day (traveling from the east coast to the west coast), you will probably need an extra dose of insulin. If you are uncertain of how to work your insulin and meals into your travel and business plans, take a copy of your itinerary and work schedule to your diabetes care provider. He or she can suggest some sample routines to try.

Your health care team can help you adjust your intermediate-acting insulins for travel days. Long-, short-, and rapid-acting insulins and insulin pumps are usually easier to manage. If you are crossing several time zones or traveling overseas, it will probably take a day or two to get adjusted to the new schedule.

## On the Ground

If you are traveling by automobile or other types of ground transportation, you often have more flexibility in your schedule, but there are still things to think about. You need to be sure that your insulin is properly stored. Extreme temperatures—

## Eating on the Run

Traveling can throw a monkey wrench in even the most well-thought-out eating plans. Here are some tips for eating while you are traveling:

- Whether driving, flying, or riding the rails, keep snacks on hand in case your blood glucose levels start to drop. Snacks that travel well include cheese, crackers, fruit, and peanut butter.
- Keep glucose tablets, raisins, or other quick sources of sugar close at hand so you can easily treat an insulin reaction.
- If you are traveling by plane, check before you get on to see if food will be served. If it is, wait until you get your meal to take your insulin. If you take your shot and then the meal service is slow, or if it is canceled because of a bumpy flight, your glucose levels can go too low.
- Talk to your health care team about adjusting your insulin and meal schedules when crossing time zones.
- Check your blood glucose levels more often than usual, even if you have type 2 diabetes. Eating different foods and different eating and exercise schedules can affect your blood glucose.
- When dining out, you may get quicker service at off-peak hours. Or reserve a table in advance. Your meal is less likely to be delayed if the restaurant is not crowded.

either hot or cold—may reduce the potency of your insulin. Even backpacks or cycle bags can get too hot in warm weather. You don't have to routinely store open insulin bottles in the refrigerator. But putting insulin in glove compartments and trunks and even in a locked car in a parking lot can cause the insulin to overheat. If there is a danger of overheating, keep insulin in an insulated container. The other caution is very cold weather. Insulin left overnight in a car trunk can freeze. Once insulin freezes it loses all potency and needs to be discarded.

## Exercising on the Road

You've got everything under control. You are exercising regularly and eating well. Then your boss decides to send you out of town at last minute's notice to meet with some prospective clients. Or you go visit your relatives for a long weekend. How will you manage? Fear not. You may not be able to schedule a 2-hour workout session, but here are a few suggestions to keep your exercise program on track:

- Pack a pair of comfortable walking shoes and some athletic socks. It is easier to squeeze a brisk walk into a busy schedule than most other exercises and can be done in almost any locale. If your schedule is jam-packed with long meetings, try getting up a little earlier and squeeze in a walk after breakfast. On long car trips, stop every 2 hours and take a brisk 10-minute walk.
- If you are attending a conference, wear comfortable shoes. You'll be more likely to walk around the exhibit hall, walk outside to a restaurant, or take a stroll in a nearby park if your feet aren't killing you. And you will be less likely to injure your feet.
- Take along your exercise equipment when packing your bags. If space is tight, take a swim suit, walking shoes, or light weights. If you are driving, you might be able to take a racquet and balls, golf clubs, skis, a soccer ball, or even a bicycle.

## Plan in Advance

The key to successful traveling, especially when you have diabetes, is careful planning. Think of all the contingencies that might arise or any particular needs that you might encounter and develop a plan in advance.

- If you travel by plane, you may want to carry a letter from your health care provider, preferably on letterhead stationery, stating that you have diabetes and setting out what diabetes supplies you carry with you. Insulin, glucagon, preloaded syringes, pens, and vials should be clearly identified and labeled. Make sure your lancets are capped and kept with your meter.
- Keep a prescription for insulin on hand. This is especially important if your travel plans are subject to frequent changes.
- Wear a medical ID bracelet or necklace that says you have diabetes.
- If you are traveling abroad, learn how to say "I have diabetes" and "Sugar or orange juice, please," in the language of the country you are visiting.
- If you are overseas and need medical attention—and you have a choice—think about contacting the nearest American consulate, American Express, or a local medical school for a list of English-speaking doctors.
- To be safe, pack twice as much insulin and blood glucose monitoring equipment as you think you will need. Pack your supplies in your carry-on luggage so you'll always have them within reach.
- If you find yourself running low on insulin while abroad, remember that insulin sold outside the United States is often a

*(Continued)*

## Plan in Advance (*Continued*)

buy insulin that is a different strength (U-40 or U-80), you must also buy new syringes to match the new insulin to avoid errors in dosing. If you use U-100 syringes for U-40 or U-80 insulin, you will be taking too little insulin. On the other hand, if you use U-100 insulin in a U-40 or U-80 syringe, you will be taking too much.

- Don't get separated from your supplies. Get used to carrying a tote bag, fanny pack, or backpack with your insulin, syringes, meter, lancets, glucose gel or tablets, glucagon kit and some food.
- You can always look up your local ADA office in the white pages of the phone book if you're traveling in the United States. If you travel frequently to the same cities, keep a list of local ADA offices on hand. This may come in handy if you need to know where to buy supplies or find a doctor in a pinch. If you are going overseas, write to the ADA for a list of International Diabetes Federation groups.

- Suggest that the whole family participate. Play with your children or grandchildren, organize a game of tag or touch football, or go for a walk. Everyone will benefit from the activity, and it's nice to spend time together.
- Before booking your hotel, ask if it has a health club, swimming pool, or exercise room. Some hotels provide access to a nearby fitness center.
- Check with health clubs in the area you are visiting to see if you can buy a few days of use. If you belong to a national health club chain, see if they have clubs in the city you are visiting.

## Carry-On Luggage Checklist

Make sure to bring twice as many supplies and medications as you need, and pack them in your carry-on luggage. That way you won't get stuck without supplies if your luggage gets lost or your trip is unexpectedly delayed or extended.

### Medications

Insulin
Syringes, pens, or pump supplies
Oral diabetes medications
Glucose tablets or other sugar
  source
Snacks, such as dried fruit or
  crackers
Antibiotic ointment
Other prescribed medications
Glucagon kit
Anti-nausea and anti-diarrheal
  medications

### Blood monitoring equipment

Test strips
Lancets
Blood sampling device and
  a spare
Glucose meter
Hand washing gel or
  alcohol wipes
Spare batteries for glucose
  meter
Cotton or tissues

# Working with the Health Care System

15

*You need to be your own advocate, working with your diabetes care team, health insurance company, and hospital, in order to obtain the best possible care.*

Elaine was in a dead-end job with a boss she couldn't stand. But the job had one big bonus: health insurance. She had been living with type 1 diabetes for 25 years and was starting to experience some of the complications. If she switched jobs and health care plans, she was afraid she would lose her insurance and, because of her preexisting condition, have to wait a year to be enrolled. She felt she had no choice but to stay in this miserable job forever.

Chuck had been living with type 2 diabetes for 10 years. He was able to keep his blood glucose levels on target most of the time. But now he was developing some back problems, and he needed suggested surgery. He wondered how the surgery would affect his blood glucose levels and whether his local community hospital could handle someone with diabetes.

He had never really seen anyone besides his primary care doctor for his diabetes and wondered whether he should contact a specialist.

If you have diabetes, you know how high health care costs are. Not only do you have to pay for routine care, but you also have to be prepared for the unexpected. Medical care is expensive for everyone these days, making health insurance an absolute must. Diabetes can make health care even more expensive even if you have insurance. So getting the best insurance coverage possible is critical, not only for your pocketbook, but also for your health.

If you are employed, you may be offered health insurance through your employer. Or maybe you are insured by a health policy obtained through your spouse's employer. Or perhaps you are eligible for Medicare or Medicaid. If you are on your own, you probably already know that finding affordable insurance can be tricky.

Throughout the course of your life, your career, and your diabetes, you need to periodically evaluate your health insurance situation. Ask yourself if your needs are being met. If you are unhappy with your current situation, evaluate the options. But don't be too quick to jump ship. Any change in your health insurance coverage requires careful evaluation. You need to make sure that any new situation provides the health care coverage you need.

There may also be times when you want to make changes in your life. Maybe you want to switch jobs, retire, get married or divorced, or move out of state. Each of these decisions can affect your health insurance coverage. Before you make a change in your life, think about how you will continue to cover your health care expenses.

## Health Insurance

The health insurance landscape for people with diabetes is changing. Although it can be discouraging, it is better than it was just a few years ago. If you change jobs or insurance companies, you will need to talk to your benefits office or the insurer. Read all you can and make a list of questions. You should be prepared to ask for details on the cost of monthly premiums, co-pays, deductibles, and coverage for diabetes-related care and supplies like test strips, diabetes education, durable medical equipment, and so on. Also be sure that your policy covers office visits, laboratory tests, and preventive care. Be prepared and be persistent.

If you allow your insurance to lapse for more than 63 days and then start on a new plan, you may be excluded from coverage for an extended period of time—up to 18 months in a job-based health plan. If you are self-employed or purchase coverage as an individual and are not enrolled in a group plan, you may have to pay more than someone without diabetes. Some insurance companies may even refuse to insure you. Others may offer you insurance but refuse to pay any diabetes-related expenses. So before you leave your old insurance—or the employer who is supplying it—be sure you understand the steps you have to take to protect your coverage. The important thing is not to get caught without insurance, even briefly. Insurance is like having an umbrella in case of rain. The day you forget your umbrella, you can be sure it will rain.

New laws make it easier for people with diabetes to obtain and keep the coverage they need for appropriate treatment.

Some of these laws are federal laws that affect all U.S. residents, but others are state laws that vary from state to state.

## Insurance Options

You can obtain health insurance in many ways. If you are employed or if your spouse is employed, you can usually obtain insurance from your employer. If you leave your job, you can purchase transition coverage such as COBRA or state continuation coverage, or you can purchase coverage through a conversion policy. Other options if you are unemployed or self-employed include individual coverage or high-risk pool coverage.

*Through Employment.* You may have the option of joining a group policy offered by your employer. Group policies are usually open to all employees, regardless of their health. Many policies will also cover your spouse and children for an additional fee. Health care is considered a nontaxable expense, so if you pay a fee for health care coverage, you may have it deducted from your paycheck before taxes are taken out.

*In Transition.* If you are laid off or just striking out on your own for the first time, you may need insurance coverage while you make the transition from school to work, from job to job, or from work to retirement. Fortunately, a federal law called the Consolidated Omnibus Budget Reconciliation Act (COBRA) may help you. Under COBRA, an employer with more than 20 employees must allow you and your dependents to keep your health insurance policy with equal coverage for 18 to 36 months after you leave your job. You will have to pay for the coverage and may be charged up to 2 percent more than the rate the company was charging your employer.

Once you have been laid off, leave a company, or are no longer on your parents' health plan, you have 63 days to accept COBRA benefits. Employers with fewer than 20 employees, the federal government, and churches are exempt from COBRA. But if you are ineligible for COBRA or if your COBRA coverage runs out, you still have some other options.

If you work for an employer with fewer than 20 employees, state continuation coverage may be an option for you when you leave your job. Available in most states, state continuation coverage is similar to COBRA in that it allows you and/or your dependents to continue receiving the health coverage you had as an employee. You will have to pay both your share of the monthly premium as well as what your employer paid toward your health coverage while you were employed, plus an administrative fee of approximately 2%, though it varies from state to state. Not all states offer continuation coverage, and the states that do offer it vary widely in how to sign up for coverage and how long coverage lasts. To find more information on state continuation coverage, contact your state's Department of Insurance.

Many states require employers to offer you a conversion policy regardless of your health or physical condition. In some cases, if you are leaving a job-based health insurance plan, you have the right to purchase a conversion policy as well. When you convert your policy, you remain with the same insurer, but begin paying for your own insurance. Conversion coverage is almost always more expensive than the group plan you may have had while employed, and it usually provides fewer benefits. However, it may be your only choice for coverage and is preferable to going without insurance. Conversion policies are not available in all states, and in some states you must use up any COBRA or state continuation coverage that you are eligible for before purchasing a conversion policy. In other states, you can buy a conversion policy immediately after losing or leaving your job. You will have between 7 and 60 days to accept or reject this type of coverage. If at all possible, be sure to explore all insurance options as far in advance as possible.

The Health Insurance Portability and Accountability Act (HIPAA) of 1996 makes it easier for people with diabetes to get and keep health insurance. According to this act, insurers and employers may not make insurance rules that discriminate against workers because of their health.

HIPAA policies must be offered without preexisting condition exclusions to anyone who 1) has had continuous coverage in a health plan for the previous 18 months, the last day of which must have been under a group health plan; 2) is not currently eligible for coverage under any group plan, Medicare, or Medicaid; and 3) has used up any COBRA or state continuation coverage available to them.

**On Your Own.** If you are self-employed, unemployed, or do not receive health insurance as an employment benefit, you may not be eligible for any form of group insurance. Finding an affordable policy under these circumstances may be difficult. If at all possible, don't forfeit health insurance altogether. Having diabetes makes health insurance an absolute necessity.

Individual policies are contracts between individuals and an insurance company. Companies that enroll in group plans may insure everyone and offer lower rates, because everyone's risks are pooled. That is, if the group is large enough, people with costly health care needs will be balanced out by people with fewer health care needs. If you have a chronic condition such as diabetes, and you are seeking individual coverage, you are a known risk. Insurers will take your medical history into consideration when they decide whether to enroll you. If you are accepted, you may have to pay higher premiums in some states.

If you have been turned down for insurance, you might want to consider high-risk pool health insurance. This kind of insurance is offered in over 30 states to people who have lived in the state for 6 to 12 months and are ineligible for group or individual coverage. Although the coverage is good, the costs can vary widely among the different states that offer it. Some states have waiting lists to buy into the pool.

## Types of Health Care

However you are covered, there are different agreements between insurers and providers as to how services will be provided. Some employers may offer an array of health plans and service options. Other employers may have settled on a single insurance company offering a single type of service. Some agreements limit your choice of providers in exchange for a better-priced plan. This can be a problem, especially if you live far away from work and, often, far from the available hospitals and doctors. The major types of plans are fee-for-service and managed care.

*Fee for Service.* In the past, the vast majority of health insurance companies required you or your employer to pay a set premium each year and allowed you to decide what doctors and hospitals to choose. In these fee-for-service plans, the insurance company pays for some or all of your health care. Usually, you must first pay a small amount for your care as an out-of-pocket deductible. Once you have met your yearly deductible, your insurance company will take over and pay for the remaining expenses during the year, according to the particulars of your contract. Often, insurance companies will also require that you pay a portion of the cost of visits or health care (the co-payment), even after the deductible is met. However, most plans have a maximum out-of-pocket expense, or catastrophic limit. Once you have paid a certain set amount out of your own pocket, they will pay for 100% of all expenses over that amount. When comparing policies, pay special attention to what you may have to pay as a deductible, co-payment, and out-of-pocket limits. Cheaper plans usually have higher deductibles, higher co-payments, and higher catastrophic limits.

The great advantage of the fee-for-service plan is that you are able to choose your own providers among a wide range of health care professionals and hospitals with whom your insurer is affiliated. Check to see whether preventive health care, such as mammograms, Pap smears, or well-child visits, are covered by your plan.

*Managed Care.* Under managed care plans, you or your employer pay a fixed premium and you receive a comprehensive care package, from routine office visits and preventive care to hospitalization. Your cost is generally lowest if you seek care from the network of participating providers and hospitals. Often, you are assigned a primary care practitioner by whom you must first be seen, even for diabetes care. You generally have lower deductibles to satisfy and limited paperwork to process. You also will not be expected to pay large out-of-pocket amounts for services.

The disadvantage to managed care situations is that your choices may be limited. Your primary care provider will usually serve as a gatekeeper in recommending what further care is needed for a particular problem. If you wish to see a health care professional such as an endocrinologist or diabetes educator or have a test that is not approved, you may have to pay much of your own bill.

## Routine Care Coverage

Getting insurance coverage is only the first step. What is covered is just as important for people with diabetes. Today, thanks to the efforts of the American Diabetes Association and its allies, 46 states and the District of Columbia require that state-regulated insurance plans provide comprehensive coverage of diabetes supplies, equipment, and education. But be careful—only about one-half of the private plans in any given state are regulated by the state. The other half are regulated under federal law and are exempt from these laws.

Your insurance policy is a contract between you and the insurance carrier that outlines the services covered. Like any contract, you need to read it carefully to make sure it provides for your needs. It may include coverage for office visits and annual or semi-annual physical exams and laboratory tests. Some insurance companies will only provide partial coverage or will require a co-payment for each visit. Others may not always cover routine physical examinations but will pay for a specific medical problem or medical emergency. Check to see that your carrier considers routine diabetes care part of the treatment for diabetes and provides coverage. Ask if it includes diabetes education and medical nutrition therapy. Many insurers cover blood glucose meters and strips, often under a separate coverage agreement. Read the policy and talk to your human resources department and your insurer to be sure. Purchases of prescription drugs and supplies may require a co-payment. However, if your coverage includes prescription drugs, always ask your provider to write a prescription for insulin. Most insurance plans will reimburse you for insulin with a prescription.

If your health insurance covers durable medical equipment, it should pay for a blood glucose meter, a finger-stick device,

## What You Should Know About Your Health Insurance Plan

When comparison shopping for health care insurance, ask yourself the following:

- Are visits to your diabetes care provider covered? Is there any limit on how many visits are allowed? How much will you have to pay per visit? Will you have to change providers?
- Does the plan reimburse for diabetes education?
- Does the plan cover medical equipment and supplies? This is especially important if you inject insulin or self-monitor your blood glucose.
- Does the plan cover medical nutrition therapy or the services of a dietitian? Managing diet is critical for people with both type 1 and type 2 diabetes.
- What mental health benefits are covered? The services of a social worker or psychologist can help you through the rough spots in coping with diabetes.
- Does the plan cover the services of specialists, such as an endocrinologist, podiatrist, eye doctor, or dentist, whose care is very important to people with diabetes?
- What medications are paid for? Is there a prescription plan to reduce costs? How often can prescriptions be refilled? Is a co-payment required for each prescription?
- What kind of home health care coverage is included? Are there any limitations?

pens, pen needles, syringes, or an insulin injector. Today, more and more plans will pay for an insulin pump if prescribed by your provider as "medically necessary." Check your policy to see that none of these items are specifically excluded. Your provider may have to write a letter explaining why each of these items is necessary. This serves as your "prescription" for these items.

If your insurance covers prescription medications and/or medical supplies, it usually will pay for insulin, lancets, syringes, pens, glucose meter strips, and insulin pump supplies, if you have a prescription for them. It is a good idea to ask the insurance company in advance what is covered. Always keep a record of the name of the person who answers your questions along with the date, in case you need this information to appeal a denied claim.

In addition to visits to your primary care provider, find out if visits to other members of your health care team (see Chapter 13) are covered and under what conditions. Some carriers will provide coverage for routine physicals but will not cover visits to a dietitian, for example. You may recognize that treating your diabetes is a team effort, but not all insurance carriers provide this coverage.

## Medicare and Medicaid

If you are over 65, disabled and unable to work, or have a very low income, you may have other insurance options. The federal insurance program **Medicare** covers a portion of hospital bills, provider fees, and other expenses for people over the age of 65 and for some people with disabilities who cannot work. Even if you get Medicare, you may still have to pay for a portion of your medical bills.

Medicare coverage for people with diabetes has improved dramatically in recent years thanks to the efforts of the American Diabetes Association. You can sign up for Medicare 3 months before the month of your 65th birthday. For more information, contact your local Social Security Administration office, listed under the United States Government listing in your telephone book. Bring your birth certificate when you apply.

Most people over the age of 65 and those with end-stage renal disease are eligible for Medicare. However, some people who have worked at state or local government jobs may not be eligible for Medicare. If you are unsure about coverage, contact your local Social Security Administration office or the Medicare hotline at 1-800-MEDICARE (1-800-633-4227).

If you have a very low income, you might be eligible for **Medicaid,** a joint federal and state health care program. Medicaid regulations vary from state to state, so you will have to contact the Medicaid office in your state to find out whether you qualify. In general, to qualify for Medicaid you must meet certain income limits as well as other criteria. For example, in most states, in addition to having income below a certain level, you must also be a child under age 19, elderly or disabled, a parent, or pregnant. Ask about what health expenses will be covered. If you have questions, a social worker can help you with this.

The health care provisions under Medicaid are constantly changing as more decisions about distributing funds are put in the hands of the individual states. Most provide coverage for important diabetes care, but some states are trying to reduce this coverage. For more information about how these changes may affect you, contact your local Social Security Administration office or call 1-800-772-1213.

## S-CHIP

The State Children's Health Insurance Program (S-CHIP) is available to children, some pregnant women, and some parents whose income may be too high for Medicaid but who cannot access or afford other health insurance options. Each state varies in its eligibility requirements for this program. To find information on S-CHIP in your state, go to www.insurekidsnow.gov or contact 1-877-KIDS-NOW.

## Medicare Benefits

There are two parts to Medicare: Part A and Part B. Part A helps to pay bills for medical care provided in hospitals, skilled nursing facilities, hospices (for people who are terminally ill), and nursing homes. Medicare will not pay for custodial care provided in a nursing home or private home when that is the only kind of care needed. Custodial care includes help in walking, getting in and out of bed, bathing, dressing, eating, taking medicines, and other activities of daily living.

It is critical for people with diabetes to purchase Medicare Part B. Part B helps to pay for health providers' services, ambulance services, diagnostic tests, outpatient hospital services, outpatient physical therapy and speech pathology services, and medical equipment and supplies. Coverage has expanded to include blood glucose meters and strips for people with type 2 diabetes who don't use insulin, as well as insulin pumps and supplies for people who meet certain qualifications. Coverage also includes diabetes education when provided by an ADA-recognized program, and medical nutrition therapy provided by a Medicare-certified dietitian.

Medicare Part B also pays for blood glucose meters, lancets, test strips, and other supplies for the meter, whether you are on insulin or not. Your health care provider must certify in writing that you need all of these items to manage your diabetes. Make copies of your provider's written statement. Give a copy of it to your pharmacist each time you purchase these supplies so that it can be submitted along with your Medicare claim.

Parts A and B will not pay for diabetes pills, insulin if you are not using an insulin pump, or syringes, but Medicare will pay for insulin pumps and the insulin used in the pump for people who meet certain qualifications. Medicare also does not pay for regular eye exams, prescription sunglasses or contact lenses, or routine foot care, such as nail trimming or removal of corns and calluses. Medicare will help pay for therapeutic footwear and shoe inserts, laser surgery for retinopathy, cataract surgery, and kidney dialysis.

Generally, people covered by Medicare get Part A. You can get Part B by paying a monthly fee. Both parts have deductibles and coinsurance amounts that you pay. For more information on Medicare, call the Medicare hotline at 1-800-MEDICARE (1-800-633-4227). For a more detailed explanation of Medicare, ask for a free copy of *Medicare and You* and the *Medicare Personal Plan Finder* at www.medicare.gov.

## Medigap and Medicare Part C *(Medicare Advantage)*

Even in its present state, Medicare does not cover everything you will need for your diabetes care. To fill gaps in your coverage, you can choose from the many so-called Medigap plans available from private insurance companies. These plans pick up some of the charges that Medicare won't cover. You cannot be denied Medigap coverage if you apply within 6 months of first applying for Medicare Part B. To be designated as a Medicare supplement policy, insurance policies must meet certain federal standards. If you are considering one of these plans, be sure to read the policy carefully and comparison shop before purchasing anything.

The booklet *Guide to Health Insurance for People with Medicare*, written by the National Association of Insurance Commissioners and the Centers for Medicare and Medicaid Services (CMS) of the Department of Health and Human Services, is updated every year and is available at www. medicare.gov or through any insurance company. Ask for it, or call Social Security to have it sent to you. It will be especially helpful in face of the changes that regularly occur in Medicare. It contains the federal standards for Medigap policies and general information about Medicare.

If you choose to purchase a Medicare Advantage plan (formerly called Medicare + Choice), you will not need to purchase a Medigap policy. Medicare Advantage plans require you to purchase Medicare parts A and B, but they cover many of the same services and benefits as a Medigap policy would. Medicare Advantage plans are not available everywhere, and you may have to pay a monthly premium for these policies. While Medicare Advantage plans may provide additional health care benefits, you usually have to see a provider who has been assigned to you or who is in your plan network instead of choosing your own physician.

Please be aware that beginning January 1, 2006, Medigap plans will no longer exist in their current form due to major changes in the Medicare program. See Medicare Part D, below, for more information.

## Medicare Part D

In December 2003, the Medicare Modernization Act (MMA) was enacted. The MMA offers several new programs and benefit options available to all Medicare beneficiaries. Here are some of the key changes:

*Medicare-Approved Drug Discount Cards.* People who currently have Medicare can now enroll to receive a Medicare-Approved Drug Discount Card. These cards may help you save money on your prescription drugs until the new Part D prescription drug benefit begins in January 2006. Call 1-800-MEDICARE for more information about these drug discount cards.

*Preventive Care Coverage.* In 2005, Medicare began offering diabetes screening tests. Certain Medicare beneficiaries who are at risk for diabetes are eligible for these tests. Some people with Medicare coverage may also get diabetes self-management training and cardiovascular screening blood tests. Talk with your diabetes care provider to see if you qualify for these tests, or call 1-800-MEDICARE for more information.

*Part D Prescription Drug Benefit.* Starting January 1, 2006, Medicare will work with private companies to offer optional prescription drug coverage. If you would like to obtain prescription drug coverage through this program, you must choose the plan that best suits your needs and enroll. Enrollment begins November 15, 2005. Medicare may charge you a higher premium if you do not enroll within six months of the date you become eligible for Part D coverage. People who are currently on Medicare should enroll during the initial enrollment period (November 15, 2005–May 15, 2006) to avoid a penalty.

The benefits offered by the new Part D plan require that beneficiaries

- pay the first $250 in drug costs per year;
- pay 25% of total drug costs between $250 and $2,250 per year;
- pay 100% of the total drug costs between $2,250 and $5,100 per year (which equals $3,600 in out-of-pocket costs for each beneficiary);
- pay $2 for generics, $5 for brand name drugs, or 5% of the cost of each prescription after reaching the $3,600 out-of-pocket limit per year.

The "total drug cost" is the total amount of money your prescription drugs cost, regardless of who is paying for them.

In other words, it is the amount you would spend on your prescription drugs if you had no drug coverage at all. As the above details indicate, there is a gap in coverage where Medicare will not pay for your medications. This occurs when your total drug costs reach between $2,250 and $5,100. Once you exceed $2,250 in total drug costs, you will be responsible for paying for all your prescriptions out-of-pocket until your total drug costs reach $5,100. After you reach $5,100 in total drug costs ($3,600 out-of-pocket), Medicare Part D will pick up 95% of the cost of any additional prescription drugs for the year.

Your drug costs under Medicare Part D may differ from these amounts. Depending on your income, you may be eligible for one of the prescription drug subsidies available to some beneficiaries under Medicare Part D. Individuals who are eligible for both Medicare and Medicaid will be sent information in the mail about choosing a Medicare Part D plan. If you do not choose a Part D plan, Medicare will choose for you, without consideration of your particular health care needs. Be sure to find the best plan available to you.

For information on whether you qualify for a subsidy, please contact Medicare directly. For individuals with Medicare Part B coverage, diabetes supplies and services such as blood glucose meters, blood glucose testing strips, lancets, diabetes education, and medical nutrition therapy will remain Medicare Part B benefits even after Medicare Part D drug coverage begins in 2006. Contact Medicare at 1-800-MEDICARE for more information.

## When Your Claim Is Denied

It's bound to happen at one time or another. You have done all your homework and think you know just what is and what is not covered by your health insurance. So you may be surprised to someday receive a claim marked DENIED. To resolve the situation most fairly and efficiently, it will help if you have all the paperwork on hand to support your claim.

When your claim is denied, you will receive an explanation of benefits from your insurance company, which should include a reason for the denial of your claim. If you do not understand the reason for the denial, you may want to call a company representative for a thorough explanation. Make sure to ask and record the name of the person to whom you are speaking. Understanding what the problem is may help you to better organize the papers and documents you need to support your claim. Contact your human resources department if your policy is through your employer. They can often explain why it wasn't covered or help you work through the system more quickly.

Make sure the claim form has been completed correctly. If this checks out, get the rest of your paperwork in order. If the denial is for your diabetes medications or supplies, make sure you have a prescription for every piece of equipment you need, even if it does not require a prescription at the pharmacy. Sometimes, just submitting the prescription and receipt will be enough. Some companies may also want a letter of explanation from your provider. Never send any original documents to your insurance company. Make copies of everything you plan to submit. Send in the copies and keep the originals. Send all pertinent paperwork by registered mail so that you have a record that they have been received.

Once you have received the statement telling you that your claim has been denied, you will have a certain period of time in which to appeal this decision. State laws vary on the amount of time allowed to appeal, so make sure to check the law in your state. Your next step will be to write to the claims manager of your insurance company, explaining what is wrong. It helps to address the claims manager by name. Point out the items that have been denied payment and ask for a written response to your request. Give your address and phone number and that of your provider. Also, send your provider a copy of your appeal request for his or her records. State that you will call the insurance company on a certain date if you have not received a response by that time. On that date, call the claims manager and discuss your case. Two or 3 weeks is a reasonable period of time to wait.

Sometimes claims are denied for simple reasons. Maybe a clerk was unfamiliar with the newest equipment for diabetes care. Requesting an appeal moves the decision out of the clerk's hands and into those of people who should have greater familiarity with blood meters, test strips, and other equipment. Even if you are denied again, don't give up! Request an insurance hearing.

If you work for a company that is self-insured, appeal directly to your personnel manager or to the head of the company first. Often they can easily remedy the situation. If the claim is still denied, write to the state labor department.

Your state insurance commissioner acts as a consumer complaint department. Do not hesitate to contact this office. They can also provide you with an opportunity for a hearing. This is where your paperwork is most important. When writing to the state commission, be sure to list the following:

- the name of your insurance company
- the coverage provided in your policy as you understand it, along with a copy of your policy
- a description of what happened (this should include copies of all letters or details of phone conversations between you and the insurance company)
- a specific request for a hearing to determine the insurance company's responsibility for payment

An insurance hearing is like a court hearing in many respects. Both you and the insurance company will be allowed to state your case. You must also submit copies of all the documents you sent to the commission. Some people represent themselves, while others have lawyers. A decision may be made right away or within the ensuing few weeks. If you are dissatisfied with the decision, you still have the option of taking your case to small-claims court.

Check with your local small-claims court, because each system has a different way of handling cases. You can find a listing in the city or county government section of the telephone book. The judges there understand that most people represent themselves. The judge will want to hear your side of the story and see copies of your documents.

You can also seek the help of two organizations who will advise you of your situation: The National Insurance Consumer Helpline, operated by insurance industry associations, and the National Insurance Consumer Organization, a nonprofit, non-partisan consumer organization.

## Hospital Stays

No one likes to think about it. After all, a hospital stay means there is a problem. This can include anything from routine elective surgery to a life-threatening emergency. Once you are admitted to a hospital, you may feel that you are no longer in charge. All of a sudden, your daily routine is disrupted, and you may have to face a recovery period that lasts from days to weeks or even months.

As unpleasant as it seems now, taking time to plan for how to handle hospital visits will pay off in the long run. You can take steps that will help get you the best possible care, whether you face an emergency situation or one for which you can plan

## Getting Admitted

Here are some tips to keep in mind when you are checking into the hospital:

- Make sure all doctors and nurses and other caregivers are aware that you have diabetes.
- Tell them what medications you are taking for diabetes and any other medications you are taking, including any over-the-counter drugs. It helps to keep a list of these ahead of time, including how often you take them and in what doses.
- Explain any allergies or other conditions you may have that could affect the actions of medications.
- Speak up about any other medical conditions you may have, including complications of diabetes. High blood pressure may require special treatment before and during surgery. Heart disease medications may require adjustment.
- Tell them about any recent or frequent low blood glucose reactions. Bring your self-monitoring records with you.
- Tell them about your meal plan. Ask to see the hospital's dietitian and explain what type of meal plan you're using, including any special modifications such as less salt, less cholesterol, or less fat.

ahead. Because, the truth is, the people who get the best care are the ones who take a proactive role in their health care, are well informed, and know what questions to ask.

***Plan Ahead.*** The first place to start is to learn something about your local hospitals. Which ones are accepted by your health insurance? Does your primary care provider have privileges at a particular hospital? If he or she has privileges at several local hospitals, which is preferred? Are there advantages or disadvantages to a particular hospital depending on the situation?

There are three types of hospitals: city or county hospitals, private community hospitals, and hospitals that serve as teaching centers, usually affiliated with a medical school. But these types of hospitals are not mutually exclusive. A county or private hospital can also be a affiliated with a medical school.

To learn about a hospital's general reputation, as well as its reputation for treating people with diabetes, talk to your diabetes care provider. Discuss the steps you should take in the event of an emergency and agree on which hospital to use. Ask your provider where he or she would go or would send a family member. Or ask any friends, neighbors, or relatives who have recent hospitalizations. You can also check with your local ADA office, diabetes educator, or support group for further input.

When evaluating the reputation of a hospital, try to find out the following:

- Are there endocrinologists on the staff?
- Does the hospital have diabetes education and dietitians with expertise in diabetes on the staff? Are they available to both inpatients and outpatients?
- Is there a diabetes education program within the hospital or affiliated with the hospital?
- What other types of support services are available to people with diabetes?
- What is the protocol for managing blood glucose levels in the hospital? Will you be able to do any of your own care, such as blood glucose monitoring?

Ask your health insurance company which hospital services they cover and for how much. Also, many insurance companies require you to notify them in advance for any service, except emergencies, so they can pre-approve your treatment.

## Diabetes Management in the Hospital

Whether you are admitted for illnesses or surgeries related to your diabetes or for other health issues, there is growing evidence that intensive diabetes management makes a difference in how quickly you recover, how long you are hospitalized, and whether you experience complications during your hospitalization.

When you are critically ill, it is recommended that your blood glucose be kept as close to 110 mg/dl as possible and go no higher than 180 mg/dl. As you recover, ADA-recommended targets for premeal blood glucose levels are 90–130 mg/dl and less than 180 mg/dl after meals. Your blood glucose will be checked frequently during this time. It is a good idea to talk to your provider before any scheduled hospitalization about the plan for achieving these targets during your stay.

Insulin is the most effective and efficient way to keep blood glucose levels in this range. Even if you are not on insulin at home, you may need insulin during your hospitalization. You can often go back to oral medications after you get better. If you are acutely ill, need to be in an intensive care unit, or are recovering from surgery, you should receive insulin intravenously. That way, the nursing staff can react very quickly to blood glucose levels that are too high or low and make adjustments in your dose. Once you are beginning to recover or your illness becomes less acute, you can often take insulin injections and achieve the same results. You will receive routine doses of both basal and bolus insulins and corrective doses if your blood glucose level goes out of range.

Other aspects of your care may change as well. Your meal plan will be adjusted to give you adequate nutrition for healing. The type of illness or surgery you have will also influence what you are able to eat. If you are unable to eat solid foods, you will be given adequate nutrition through your IV.

If you are used to managing your diabetes at home, you may prefer to give your own injections and do your own blood glucose checks. Ask your provider if that is possible in your hospital and to write an order so that the rest of the staff will know.

## Handling Surgery

If you are facing surgery, it's perfectly normal to feel apprehensive. And when you have diabetes, there is even more to think about. The good news is that people with diabetes can recover about as quickly as anyone. But blood glucose levels can get out of hand around the time of an operation, and high levels can complicate your recovery and prolong your hospital stay. Regardless of the cause of your hospital stay, it's essential that your diabetes be closely managed the entire time you are there. By taking an active role and by doing everything you can, you can help yourself recover on schedule.

The first question you will probably ask yourself is whether the surgery is necessary. This may not be possible in an emergency situation, but if surgery is recommended, ask the following questions:

### Seeking a Second Opinion

You may want a second opinion when a provider recommends surgery, long-term medication, or other treatments that will affect your life. Or, if you have a specific problem or needs that are not being addressed, a second opinion may also be in order—if your

## Seeking a Second Opinion (*Continued*)

provider says there is no known therapy or calls the condition incurable, for example. Sometimes insurance companies require a second opinion. Ask your insurer what costs for the recommended procedure are covered and whether they will cover the cost of a second opinion. Also ask if they pay only if you see one of the consultants they recommend.

When seeking a second opinion, ask someone you trust. Look for a doctor who is board certified in the field in which you are seeking information, such as cardiology or surgery. Make sure to tell the physician you have diabetes. One option is to call the appropriate department of a major medical center or teaching hospital and ask for the name of a specialist in the field.

Prepare a list of questions for your visit. Here are some things you may want to ask:

- What is the diagnosis and how was it determined?
- What treatments are available and which are most often used?
- Why do you suggest this particular treatment?
- What is the success rate of the treatment?
- What are the potential side effects and complications of treatment and how likely are they? Are they reversible?
- Is the problem or treatment likely to affect my blood glucose levels or any complications of diabetes?
- How long will I have to be in the hospital or undergo treatment? Will I need follow-up care?
- Are there other costs associated with this treatment, such as repeated blood tests, physical therapy, or postoperative nursing care?
- Is there research in this area in which I can participate?

■ Are there alternatives? What are the consequences of not having the surgery? If you are still in doubt, get a second opinion.

■ What is the risk involved? Feel free to ask questions. Even the most minor surgeries have some degree of risk. You have the right to have that spelled out in advance. If you want an explanation of tests or other procedures to expect, ask. Unanswered questions can produce anxiety.

■ Who will manage your diabetes before, during, and after surgery? Will you be under the care of your diabetes care provider, endocrinologist, or a hospital physician who specializes in diabetes?

■ What is the protocol for managing glucose levels before, during, and after surgery?

If your surgery is elective, try to bring your A1C levels as close to normal as possible before you are hospitalized. This will help you withstand the stress of the surgery and may help reduce the chances of infection and speed healing after the operation. You will receive an intravenous insulin drip prior to and during surgery to keep your blood glucose on target. Ask your diabetes provider to work with your surgeon as much as possible.

Certain medications need to be stopped before surgery, some as much as a week ahead of time. Make sure you discuss all the medications you are taking with your surgeon.

If you are scheduled for surgery, here's what you are likely to experience. The surgeon will meet with you at least once before your operation to explain the surgery and what to expect afterward. It's a good idea to have a list of questions ready. The anesthesiologist, who administers the anesthesia to keep you pain free and manages your insulin drip during surgery, will also visit you to tell you what to expect and, sometimes, to offer alternatives. The nurses caring for you will also be able to answer questions or address concerns you may have.

After the operation, don't hesitate to ask for medication for pain or nausea. Short-term use of these medications does not affect blood glucose levels.

## Home Health Care and Nursing Homes

With an emphasis on shorter hospital stays, many people today are turning to home health care for a variety of reasons. Home health care services include nursing care and physical, respiratory, occupational, or speech therapy; chemotherapy; nutritional guidance; personal care such as bathing or dressing; and homemaker care. Home health care can include health professionals who help you when you are bedridden with a long illness or housebound for a short period. They may provide blood testing or send a nurse into your home to administer medicines and other treatments. Home health care workers include professionals, trained aides who help professionals, and volunteers.

Check with your health insurance plan or your company's benefits officer to see if home health care benefits are covered. Don't hesitate to ask the agency you are considering hiring how much they charge for each service, and ask your insurance carrier what services will be covered. If you are covered by Medicare, some limited coverage may apply to you. These benefits apply only to those 65 or older or those under 65 who need kidney dialysis and/or transplants. Usually, Medicare home health care benefits are restricted to the homebound and bedridden. Veterans Affairs, the military, and worker's compensation can be other sources of help for home health care.

If full-time care is needed, an extended-care or nursing home is often the best option. If you are researching nursing homes, here are some good sources of help:

- private or public case management social workers
- your local office on aging
- the county or state department of health
- your primary care provider
- your religious leader or pastoral counselor
- local organizations or law firms for the retired or elderly

It is important that you visit prospective sites. It is also a good idea to talk to friends, family, neighbors, or coworkers who have family members in nursing homes.

Nursing homes can be very expensive. There are four possible sources of payment: private insurance, Medicare, Medicaid, and self-pay or private pay. Different facilities ask for different types of payments. It is important that you understand what you get for the required fees. The admissions coordinator should provide details of regular monthly charges and exactly what they do—and do not—include. Ask if there is something specific you should know about that is not covered. Ask about how they routinely care for diabetes and how they handle acute situations related to high or low glucose values.

As an alternative to nursing homes, many people are turning to assisted-living communities or foster care homes. Many of these facilities are suitable for people who do not require full-time nursing care but who might enjoy the benefit of nursing staff and neighbors close at hand. Check to see what nursing or other services are provided before you choose an assisted-living community. There is a wide array of living situations, from communities that function much like individual apartments, to individual units that provide nursing services, to full-time nursing centers. Check to see whether any of these facilities might meet your needs.

# Glossary

**A1C (glycated hemoglobin):** Describes the attachment of glucose to the hemoglobin in red blood cells. When blood glucose levels are high, the percentage of glucose attached to red blood cells increases. A1C levels can be measured in a laboratory, with a fingerstick, or with a mail-in kit.

**Autoimmunity:** A condition in which the body's own immune system attacks cells of the body. Type 1 diabetes is an autoimmune disease in which the immune system attacks the beta cells of the pancreas, and insulin is no longer produced.

**Basal insulin:** Sometimes called background insulin. An intermediate- or long-acting insulin that is absorbed slowly and gives the body a steady, low level of insulin to manage blood glucose levels between meals. This mimics the body's natural low-level steady background release of insulin. Also used to describe the low-level steady background release of insulin by an insulin pump.

**Beta cells:** Cells that make and release insulin. These cells are found in the islets of Langerhans in the pancreas.

*Blood glucose meter:* A handheld instrument that tests the level of glucose in the blood. A drop of blood (obtained by pricking a finger or other site) is placed on a small strip that is read by the meter. The meter calculates and displays the blood glucose level.

*Bolus insulin:* Rapid- or fast-acting insulin injected before meals that gives the body a quick rise in insulin levels. This mimics the body's natural after-meal release of insulin that controls the rise in blood glucose from eating. Also used to describe the before-meal insulin dose given with an insulin pump.

*Calories:* Units that represent the amount of energy provided by food. Carbohydrate, protein, and fat are the primary sources of calories in the diet, but alcohol also contains calories. If all calories consumed aren't used as energy, they may be stored as fat.

*Carbohydrate:* One of the three major sources of calories in the diet (4 calories per gram). Carbohydrate comes primarily from sugar and starch. Carbohydrate is broken down into glucose during digestion and is the main nutrient that raises blood glucose levels.

*Cholesterol:* A waxy, fat-like substance used by the body to build cell walls and make certain vitamins and hormones. The liver produces enough cholesterol for the body, but cholesterol also comes from animal products. Eating too much cholesterol, trans-fatty acids, and saturated fats can cause the blood cholesterol to rise and accumulate along the inside walls of blood vessels. This is a risk factor for heart attack and stroke.

*DCCT:* The Diabetes Control and Complications Trial. This was a 10-year study sponsored by the National Institutes of Health. More than 1,400 people with type 1 diabetes were divided into two groups: those who intensively managed blood glucose levels and those who used standard care. The study showed that keeping the blood glucose level closer to normal reduces the risk of diabetes complications (eye, kidney, and nerve disease).

*Diabetes:* A disease in which the body cannot produce insulin or cannot use insulin properly. It is characterized by high blood glucose levels.

*DPP:* The Diabetes Prevention Program. This was a 3-year study sponsored by the National Institutes of Health and the American Diabetes Association, involving 3,234 people with impaired glucose tolerance (IGT). People with IGT are at high risk for type 2 diabetes. The results showed that a 5 to 7 percent weight loss and 30 minutes of exercise 5 days a week reduced the incidence of diabetes by 58 percent. Treatment with metformin reduced the incidence of diabetes by 31 percent.

*Endocrinology:* The study of hormones produced by the body. Hormones are substances produced in one part of the body that can travel to remote sites and affect other parts of the body. Because insulin is a hormone, diabetes is a disease of the endocrine system. Many "diabetes doctors" are endocrinologists.

*Exchanges:* The food groups used in the American Diabetes Association and the American Dietetic Association Exchange Lists for Meal Planning. There are six basic food groups: Starch/Bread, Meat and Meat Substitutes, Vegetables, Fruits, Milk, and Fat. Any food in a given group can be exchanged for any other food in that group in the appropriate amount.

*Fats:* The most concentrated source of calories in the diet (9 calories per gram). All fats contain different percentages of saturated, polyunsaturated, and monounsaturated fat. Saturated fats are found primarily in animal products. Unsaturated fats mainly come from plants and can be monounsaturated (olive or canola oil) or polyunsaturated (safflower, sunflower, corn, or other oils). Polyunsaturated and monounsaturated fats can be processed to make trans-fatty acids. Both trans-fatty acids and saturated fats are damaging to cardiovascular health.

*Fiber:* Consists of both soluble and insoluble fiber. Insoluble fiber is found in the parts of plants that the body can't digest, such as wheat bran and fruit and vegetable skins. It aids in the normal functioning of the digestive system. Soluble fiber is found in foods such as oats, barley, fruits, and vegetables. It can help improve serum lipid levels. Twenty-five to 30 grams of fiber per day are generally recommended.

*Gestational diabetes:* Diabetes that develops during pregnancy. The mother's blood glucose rises in response to hormones secreted during pregnancy, and the mother cannot produce enough insulin to handle the higher blood glucose levels. Although gestational diabetes usually goes away after pregnancy, about 60 percent of women who have had gestational diabetes eventually develop type 2 diabetes.

*Glucagon:* A hormone produced by the pancreas that raises blood glucose levels. An injectable preparation is available by prescription for use in treating severe insulin reactions.

*Glucose:* A simple form of sugar that serves as fuel for the body. It is produced when carbohydrate is broken down in the digestive system. It can also be made from protein or fat in the liver and kidney. Glucose is carried by the blood to cells. The amount of glucose in the blood is known as the blood glucose level.

*Health care team:* The group of health care professionals who helps patients manage diabetes. This team may include a physician, registered dietitian, and certified diabetes educator. (A certified diabetes educator can be a registered nurse, pharmacist, registered dietitian, or physician.) Ophthalmologists, podiatrists, exercise physiologists, psychologists, and other specialists can also be part of the team and may also be certified diabetes educators.

*Heart disease:* A condition in which the heart cannot efficiently pump blood. Coronary artery disease is one type of heart disease. It occurs when the arteries that nourish the heart muscle narrow or become blocked. This can lead to a heart attack. People with diabetes have a higher risk than the general population for developing heart disease.

*Hyperglycemia:* A condition in which blood glucose levels are too high (generally, fasting levels above 130 mg/dl and above 180 mg/dl 2 hours after a meal). Symptoms include frequent urination, increased thirst, and weight loss.

*Hypoglycemia:* Also called an insulin reaction; a condition in which blood glucose levels drop too low (generally, below 70 mg/dl). Symptoms include moodiness, numbness in the arms and hands, confusion, and shakiness or dizziness. When left untreated, this condition can become severe and lead to unconsciousness.

*Immunosuppression:* Suppression of the immune system. The immune system protects the body from foreign invaders. People who receive islet cell, kidney, and pancreas transplants take immunosuppressive drugs to prevent the immune system from attacking the new organ.

*Impaired glucose tolerance:* Also called pre-diabetes; a condition diagnosed when blood tests show that a person's blood glucose level falls between normal and diabetes levels. It isn't considered a form of diabetes, but people with this condition are at an increased risk for developing diabetes.

*Insulin:* A hormone produced by the pancreas that helps the body use glucose. It is the "key" that unlocks the "doors" to cells and allows glucose to enter. The glucose then fuels the cells.

*Insulin resistance:* A condition in which the body cannot use insulin to lower blood glucose levels to normal ranges. This is the most common cause of type 2 diabetes.

*Intensive diabetes management:* A way of managing diabetes to achieve near-normal blood glucose levels. The approach may involve multiple daily injections of insulin, frequent blood glucose monitoring, exercise, and diet.

*Ketoacidosis or diabetic coma:* A severe condition caused by a lack of insulin or an elevation in stress hormones. It is marked by high blood glucose levels, ketones in the urine, low blood pressure, and breath with a sweet, fruity odor. It occurs almost exclusively in those with type 1 diabetes.

*Ketones:* Chemicals produced when the body breaks down fat for fuel. This occurs when there is not enough insulin to permit glucose to enter the cells to be used for energy or when there are too many stress hormones.

*Metabolism:* Term used to describe the body's capture and use of energy and nutrients to sustain life. Diabetes is a metabolic disease because it affects the body's ability to capture glucose from food for use by the cells.

*mg/dl:* Milligrams per deciliter. This is the unit of measure used in the U.S. when referring to blood glucose levels.

*Nephropathy:* Kidney damage. This condition can be life-threatening. When kidneys fail to function and waste materials build up in the bloodstream, dialysis (filtering blood through a machine) or kidney transplantation becomes necessary.

*Neuropathy:* Damage to the nerves. Peripheral neuropathy, which affects the nerves outside the brain and spinal cord, is the most common form of neuropathy. Peripheral neuropathy can damage motor nerves (which affect voluntary movement, such as walking), sensory nerves (which affect touch and feeling), and autonomic nerves (which affect bodily functions such as digestion).

*Obesity:* An abnormal and excessive amount of body fat. Most obese people are significantly overweight. However, obesity also occurs in people who are not overweight, but have more body fat than muscle. Obesity is considered a chronic illness. It is on the rise and is a risk factor for type 2 diabetes. Body mass index, skin fold measurements, and bioelectrical impedance are common ways to assess obesity.

*Oral diabetes medications or oral hyperglycemic medications:* Medications taken orally that are designed to manage blood glucose levels. They are used by some people with type 2 diabetes and are not to be confused with insulin.

*Pancreas:* A comma-shaped gland located just behind the stomach. It produces enzymes for digesting food and hormones that regulate the use of fuel in the body, including insulin and glucagon. In a fully functioning pancreas, insulin is produced and released through special cells (beta cells) located in clusters called islets of Langerhans.

*Protein:* One of three major sources of calories in the diet. Protein provides the body with material for building blood cells, body tissue, hormones, muscle, and other important substances. It is found in meats, eggs, milk, beans, legumes, vegetables, starches, and nuts.

*Receptors:* Molecules that often sit on cell surfaces as attachment sites. Insulin binds to its receptors on the cell surface to allow glucose to enter the cell.

*Retinopathy:* Damage to small blood vessels in the eye that can lead to vision problems. In background retinopathy, the blood vessels bulge and leak fluids into the retina and may cause blurred vision. Proliferative retinopathy is more serious and can cause vision loss. In this condition, new blood vessels form in the retina and branch out to other areas of the eye. This can cause blood to leak into the clear fluid inside the eye and can also cause the retina to detach.

*Stress hormones or counter-regulatory hormones:* Hormones released during stressful situations, such as an illness or infection. These hormones include glucagon, epinephrine (adrenaline), norepinephrine, cortisol, and growth hormone. They cause the liver to release glucose and the cells to release fatty acids for extra energy. If there's not enough insulin present in the body, these extra fuels can build up and lead to hyperglycemia and ketoacidosis.

*Sugar:* A carbohydrate that provides calories (4 calories per gram) and is converted to glucose. There are a variety of sugars, such as white, brown, confectioner's, and raw. Glucose is one type of sugar. Fructose, lactose, sucrose, maltose, dextrose, glucose, honey, corn syrup, molasses, and sorghum are also sugars.

*Sugar substitutes:* Sweeteners used in place of sugar. Note that some sugar substitutes have calories and will affect blood glucose levels, such as fructose (a sugar, but often used in "sugar-free" products) and sugar alcohols, such as sorbitol and mannitol. Others have very few calories and will not affect blood glucose levels, such as saccharin, acesulfame-K, aspartame (NutraSweet), and sucralose (Splenda).

*Triglycerides:* Simple fatty acids found in both plants and animals. Vegetable oils contain triglycerides with unsaturated fatty acids and tend to be liquid at room temperature. Animal sources of triglycerides contain mostly saturated fatty acids and tend to be solid at room temperature.

*Type 1 diabetes:* Also called immune-mediated diabetes. A form of diabetes that tends to develop before age 30 but may occur at any age. It's usually caused when the immune system attacks the beta cells of the pancreas and the pancreas can no longer produce insulin. People who have type 1 diabetes must take insulin to survive.

*Type 2 diabetes:* Also called insulin-resistant diabetes. This form of diabetes usually occurs in people over the age of 40, but may develop in younger people, especially among certain ethnic groups. Almost all people who develop type 2 diabetes are insulin resistant, and most have a problem with insulin secretion. Some simply cannot produce enough insulin to meet their bodies' needs, and others have a combination of these problems. Many people with type 2 diabetes initially manage the disease through diet and exercise but, as the ability of the pancreas to secrete insulin decreases, progress to oral medications and/or insulin.

*UKPDS:* The United Kingdom Prospective Diabetes Study. This was a 20-year study of over 5,000 people with type 2 diabetes. The study showed that people with type 2 who used intensive diabetes management experienced fewer diabetes-related complications.

*Urine tests:* Tests that measure substances in the urine. Urine tests for blood glucose levels do not provide the timely information that is important in blood glucose management. Monitoring urine for ketones is important in preventing ketoacidosis.

# Appendix

## Self-Monitoring Technique

Follow your meter manufacturer's instructions for calibrating, setting date and time, and using control solutions. Check to make sure your strips are not outdated, and store them within the proper temperature limits. Strips can be ruined if they are kept outside the range of acceptable temperatures. If you have problems, there is a toll-free number on the back of the meter that you can call for help. Read the instructions for possible test sites.

### Equipment

- lancet (blood-letting device)
- test strip
- cotton ball or tissue
- blood glucose meter
- logbook

1. Make sure your hands and skin are clean and dry. Soap or lotion on your skin can cause incorrect test results.

2. Puncture the skin where testing is to be done with the lancing device. If there is a problem with potential hypoglycemia, use your finger for testing.

3. Squeeze or milk out the amount of blood needed by the individual meter. With alternative sites, follow manufacturer's instructions.

4. Follow instructions to see if blood needs to be dropped on the test strip or if the finger or other site should be held so the strip can absorb the blood.

5. Apply firm pressure with a cotton ball or tissue to the lanced site until bleeding stops.

6. Dispose of the lancet and test strip according to local waste disposal laws.

7. Record your test results in your logbook. Make sure your name and telephone numbers are in your logbook in case you lose it.

## Ketone Testing (Type 1)

Perform this test to check for ketones in the urine or blood if a blood glucose test is 300 mg/dl or higher, particularly if you have symptoms of illness.

### Equipment

- ketone test strip
- cup or clean container for sample, if desired
- a watch or other timing device

1. Dip a ketone test strip in a urine sample or pass it through the stream of urine.

2. Time test according to the directions on the package.

3. The strip will change colors if ketones are present. Compare test strip to package color chart.
4. Record the results.
5. Contact your provider as recommended based on your results.

## Preparing Insulin Injections

### Equipment

- syringe, insulin pen, and needle
- insulin bottle

1. Wash hands
2. Choose injection site. Do not inject insulin into a callused or hard, lumpy site. Rotate site as instructed by your health care professional.
3. Check the bottle of insulin to make sure you are using the right kind. For an insulin pen, screw on the needle. Use a new needle every time with an insulin pen.
4. For cloudy insulin, gently roll the bottle of insulin between your palms or rotate the pen slowly from end to end to mix. Make sure it is mixed thoroughly. Shaking the bottle can cause air bubbles. Do not use if it has clumps or particles in it.
5. For an insulin syringe, hold the syringe with the needle pointing up and draw air into it by pulling down on the plunger to the amount that matches the dose to be given. For an insulin pen, perform an "air shot" by pushing 1–2 drops of insulin through the needle. Set the insulin dose according to manufacturer's directions. Proceed to instructions on injecting insulin.

6. Remove the cap from the needle. Hold the insulin bottle steady on a tabletop and push the needle straight down into the rubber top on the bottle. Push down on the plunger to inject the air into the insulin bottle.

7. Keep the needle in and turn the bottle and syringe upside down so that the insulin is on top. Pull the correct amount of insulin into the syringe by pulling back on the plunger.

8. Check for air bubbles on the inside of the syringe. If you see air bubbles, keep the bottle upside down and push the plunger up so the insulin goes back into the bottle.

9. Pull down on the plunger to refill the syringe. If necessary, empty and refill until all air bubbles in the syringe are gone.

10. Remove the needle from the bottle after checking again that you have the correct dose.

11. If you need to set the syringe down before giving your injection, recap and lay it on its side. Make sure the needle doesn't touch anything.

## Mixing Insulins

Glargine (Lantus) insulin has a lower pH level and cannot be mixed in the same syringe with any other insulin.

### Equipment

- syringe, the correct size for the total units of insulin
- bottles of insulin

1. Be clear on the amounts of each insulin and the total units you want. To find the total units, add the units of rapid- or short-acting insulin to the units of intermediate- or long-acting insulin.

2. Wash your hands.
3. For cloudy insulin, gently roll the bottle of insulin slowly between your palms to mix. Make sure it is mixed thoroughly. Do not use if it has clumps or particles in it. Shaking the bottle can cause air bubbles.
4. Draw air into the syringe equal to the intermediate- or long-acting dose.
5. Hold the bottle steady on the table and put the needle through the rubber stopper. Inject the air into that bottle. Take out the needle without drawing up any insulin.
6. Draw air into the syringe equal to the dose of rapid- or short-acting insulin and inject the air into the bottle of rapid- or short-acting insulin.
7. With the needle still in the rapid- or short-acting insulin bottle, turn it upside down so that insulin covers the tip of the needle.
8. Pull the correct amount of insulin into the syringe by pulling back on the plunger. Check for air bubbles in the syringe. If you see air bubbles, keep the bottle upside down and push the plunger up so the insulin goes back into the bottle. If necessary, empty and refill until all air bubbles in the syringe are gone. Remove the syringe.
9. Insert the syringe into the bottle of intermediate- or long-acting insulin. (You have already injected the right amount of air into this bottle.)
10. Slowly pull the plunger down to draw in the right dosage of intermediate- or long-acting insulin. This will be the total units of the short- and intermediate- or long-acting insulins.
11. Do not return any extra insulin back to this bottle. It's now a mixture. Double check for the correct total amount of insulin. If incorrect, discard the insulin in the syringe and start over.

12. Take the needle out of the bottle, recap, and lay the syringe carefully on a table without it touching anything.

## Storing Insulin Mixtures

1. Follow manufacturer's instructions for storing insulin pens.
2. Only mix insulins made by the same company. For instance, don't mix regular made by Lilly with NPH made by Novo Nordisk.
3. If you prefill the syringe, the mixture will remain stable for 21–30 days when refrigerated.
4. Keep the prefilled syringes capped and horizontal or vertical. Positioning with the syringe pointing downward can cause the needle to plug.
5. Before injecting, roll the syringe gently between your palms to remix the insulin.
6. Premixed insulins are stable and can be stored according to the manufacturer's directions.
7. Mixture of regular and lente insulins is not recommended unless your diabetes is already adequately managed on such a mixture. The lente insulin delays the onset of action of the regular insulin in an unpredictable way. If regular-lente mixtures are to be used, the time between mixing and administration should be standardized.

## Injecting Insulin

### Equipment

- prepared syringe or insulin pen
- cotton ball, gauze square, or Kleenex, if desired, to cover the injection site for a few seconds after the injection

1. Choose an injection site with fatty tissue, such as the abdomen except for a 2-inch circle around the belly button, the back of the arm, the top and outside of the thigh, or the buttocks. Make sure the site and your hands are clean and dry.
2. Gently pinch a fold of skin between your thumb and forefinger and inject straight in if you have a normal amount of fatty tissue. For a thin adult or a small child, you may need to inject on a 45-degree angle.
3. Push the needle through the skin as quickly as you can.
4. Relax the pinch and push the plunger in to inject the insulin.
5. Pull the needle straight out.
6. Cover the injection site with your finger or a cotton ball or gauze and apply slight pressure for 5 to 8 seconds—but do not rub. Rubbing may spread the insulin too quickly or irritate your skin.
7. Write down how much insulin you injected and the time of day.

## Reusing Syringes

Always use a new needle with an insulin pen.

1. Carefully recap the syringe when you are finished using it.
2. Don't let the needle touch anything but clean skin and your insulin bottle stopper. If it touches anything else, don't reuse it.
3. Store the used syringe at room temperature.
4. There will always be a tiny, even invisible, amount of insulin left in the syringe. If you use glargine insulin, be careful not to use the glargine syringe for other insulins.

5. Do not reuse a needle that is bent or dull, as this can make the injection more painful. However, just because an injection is painful doesn't mean the needle is dull. You may have hit a nerve ending.

6. Do not clean the needle with alcohol. This removes some of the coating that makes the needle go more smoothly into your skin.

7. When you're finished with a syringe, dispose of it properly according to the laws in your area. Contact the city or county sanitation department for information.

## Injecting Glucagon

Glucagon is a prescription that needs to be available to others if you have severe hypoglycemia and are not able to treat yourself. Because you will not be able to give glucagon to yourself, others need to be trained to give the injection. The doses for children and adults might be different. Ask your provider in advance of an emergency how much to use.

1. A glucagon kit has a syringe filled with diluting fluid and a bottle of powdered glucagon. You must mix the diluting fluid with the powder immediately before it is to be injected. The instructions for mixing and injecting glucagon are included in the kit.

2. Inject glucagon into the buttock, arm, or thigh.

3. Turn the person on his or her side so if there is vomiting he or she will not choke.

4. Feed the person with appropriate carbohydrate immediately when he or she wakes up and is able to swallow. Start with nondiet soda, juice, glucose tablets or gels, and then additional carbohydrate.

5. Check blood glucose. If the person does not wake up within 15 minutes, call for an ambulance. The dose may be repeated.

6. Always call your provider and emergency personnel when a severe reaction occurs in order for help to arrive and appropriate care to be administered. Ask for instructions on emergency procedures when you get the prescription. Read the instructions that come with the glucagon and share them with friends, family, and coworkers.

# Resources

## For the Visually Challenged

### American Council of the Blind
1155 15th Street, NW, Suite 1004
Washington, DC 20005
202-467-5081
800-424-8666
e-mail: info@acb.org
Web site: www.acb.org

National information clearing-house and legislative advocate that publishes a monthly magazine in Braille, large-print, cassette, and computer disk versions.

### American Foundation for the Blind
11 Penn Plaza, Suite 300
New York, NY 10001
212-502-7600
800-232-5463
e-mail: afbinfo@afb.net
Web site: www.afb.org

Works to establish, develop, and provide services and programs that assist visually challenged people in achieving independence.

### American Printing House for the Blind
1839 Frankfort Avenue
P.O. Box 6085
Louisville, KY 40206-0085
502-895-2405
502-899-2274 (*fax*)
800-223-1839
e-mail: info@aph.org
Web site: www.aph.org

Concerned with the publication of literature in all media (*Braille, large type, recorded*) and manufacture of educational aids. Newsletter provides information on new products.

**National Association for Visually Handicapped (NAVH)**
22 W. 21st Street
New York, NY 10010
212-889-3141
e-mail: staff@navh.org
Web site: www.navh.org

or

**NAVH San Francisco regional office**
(*for states west of the Mississippi River*)
3201 Balboa Street
San Francisco, CA 94121
415-221-3201
e-mail: staff@navh.org

A list of low-vision facilities is available by state. Visual aid counseling and visual aids, peer support groups, and more intensive counseling are offered at both offices. Some counseling is done by mail or phone. Maintains a large-print loan library.

**National Federation of the Blind**
1800 Johnson Street
Baltimore, MD 21230
410-659-9314 (*for general information*)
800-414-5748 (*for job opportunities for the blind*)

e-mail: nfb@nfb.org
Web site: www.nfb.org

Membership organization providing information, networking, and resources through 52 affiliates in all states, the District of Columbia, and Puerto Rico. Some aids and appliances available through national headquarters. The Diabetics Division publishes a free quarterly newsletter, Voice of the Diabetic, in print or on cassette.

**National Library Service (NLS) for the Blind and Physically Handicapped**
Library of Congress
1291 Taylor Street, NW
Washington, DC 20542
202-707-5100
202-707-0744 (TDD)
800-424-8567 (*to speak with a reference person*)
800-424-9100 (*to leave a message*)
e-mail: nls@loc.gov
Web site: www.loc.gov/nls

Encore, a monthly magazine on flexible disk (*record*), includes articles from *Diabetes Forecast*. It is available on request through the NLS program to individuals registered with the talking book program.

Recording for the Blind &
Dyslexic (RFBD)
20 Roszel Road
Princeton, NJ 08540
609-452-0606
609-987-8116 (*fax*)
800-221-4792 (weekdays 8:30
   a.m. to 4:45 p.m. EST)
Web site: www.rfbd.org

Library for people with print disabilities. Provides educational
materials in recorded and computerized form; 80,000 titles on cassette. Registration fee of $50.00
includes loan of cassettes for up to
a year.

The Seeing Eye, Inc.
P.O. Box 375
Morristown, NJ 07963-0375
973-539-4425
973-539-0922 (*fax*)
e-mail: info@seeingeye.org
Web site: www.seeingeye.org

Offers guide-dog training and
instruction on working with a
guide dog.

## For Amputees

American Amputee Foundation
P.O. Box 250218
Little Rock, AR 72225
501-666-2523
501-666-8367 (*fax*)

Offers peer counseling for new
amputees and their families.
Provides information and referral
to vendors. Sponsors Give-a-Limb
program. Has local chapters.
Maintains a list of support groups
throughout the United States.
Publishes newsletter.

National Amputation Foundation
40 Church Street
Malverne, NY 11565
516-887-3600
516-887-3667 (*fax*)
e-mail: amps76@aol.com
Web site:
   www.nationalamputation.org

Sponsor of Amp-to-Amp program,
in which new amputee is visited by
amputee who has resumed normal
life. A list of support groups
throughout the country is available.

## For Finding Long-Term or Home Care

**National Association for Home Care (NAHC)**
228 7th Street, SE
Washington, DC 20003
202-547-7424
202-547-3540 (*fax*)
Web site: www.nahc.org

Free information for consumers about how to choose a home care agency. Call and leave address or send a self-addressed, stamped envelope.

## For Finding Quality Health Care

**American Association for Marriage and Family Therapy**
112 S. Alfred Street
Alexandria, VA 22314
703-838-9808
e-mail: memberservice@aamft.org
Web site: www.aamft.org

Information on marriage and family therapists in your area.

**American Association of Diabetes Educators**
100 W. Monroe Street, Suite 400
Chicago, IL 60603
312-424-2426
312-424-2427 (*fax*)
800-832-6874 (*referral line*)
Web site: www.aadenet.org

Referral to a local diabetes educator.

**American Association of Sex Educators, Counselors, and Therapists**
P.O. Box 238
Mount Vernon, IA 52314-0238
e-mail: aasect@aasect.org
Web site: www.aasect.org

For a list of certified sex therapists and counselors in your state, send a self-addressed, stamped, business-size envelope (*you may request lists from more than one state*).

**American Board of Medical Specialties**
1007 Church Street, Suite 404
Evanston, IL 60201-5913
866-275-2267 (866-ASKABMS)
Web site: www.abms.org

Record of physicians certified by
24 medical specialty boards. Only
certification status of physicians is
available to callers. Directories of
certified physicians organized by
city of medical practice and alpha-
betically by physician names are
available in many libraries.

**American Board of Podiatric
Surgery**
445 Fillmore Street
San Francisco, CA 94117-3404
415-553-7800
415-553-7801 (*fax*)
e-mail: info@abps.org
Web site: www.abps.org

Referral to a local board-certified
podiatrist.

**American Dietetic Association**
120 South Riverside Plaza,
    Suite 2000
Chicago, IL 60606-6995
800-877-1600
800-366-1655 (*Consumer
    Nutrition Hotline; 9 a.m. to
    4 p.m. CST, M–F only*)
Web site: www.eatright.org

Information, guidance, and referral
to a local dietitian.

**American Medical Association**
515 N. State Street
Chicago, IL 60610
312-464-4818
800-621-8335
Web site: www.ama–assn.org

Referral to your county or state
medical society, which may be able
to refer you to a local physician.

**American Optometric Association**
243 N. Lindbergh Boulevard
St. Louis, MO 63141
314-991-4100
314-991-4101 (*fax*)
Web site: www.aoanet.org

Referral to your state optometric
association for referral to a local
optometrist.

**American Psychiatric Association**
1000 Wilson Boulevard,
    Suite 1825
Arlington, VA 22209
703-907-7300
888-357-7924
e-mail: apa@psych.org
Web site: www.psych.org

Referral to your state psychiatric
association for referral to a local
psychiatrist.

**American Psychological Association**
750 First Street, NE
Washington, DC 20002-4242
202-336-5500 (*main number*)
202-336-5700 (*public affairs*)
202-436-5800 (*professional practice*)
800-374-2721
Web site: www.apa.org

Referral to your state psychological association for referral to a local psychologist.

**National Association of Social Workers (NASW)**
750 First Street, NE, Suite 700
Washington, DC 20002-4241
202-408-8600
800-638-8799
Web site: www.naswdc.org

Referral to your state chapter of NASW for referral to a local social worker.

**Pedorthic Footwear Association**
7150 Columbia Gateway Drive, Suite G
Columbia, MD 21046
410-381-7278
410-381-1167 (*fax*)
800-673-8447

Web site: www.pedorthics.org

Referral to a local certified pedorthist (a person trained in fitting prescription footwear).

## For Miscellaneous Health Information

**American Academy of Ophthalmology**
Customer Service Department
P.O. Box 7424
San Francisco, CA 94120-7424
415-561-8500
415-561-8533 (*fax*)
Web site: www.aao.org

For brochures on eye care and eye diseases, send a self-addressed, stamped envelope.

**American Heart Association**
7272 Greenville Avenue
Dallas, TX 75231
800-242-8721
Web site: www.americanheart.org

For referral to local affiliate's Heartline, which provides information on cardiovascular health and disease prevention.

**Medic Alert Foundation**
2323 Colorado Avenue
Turlock, CA 95382
209-668-3331
209-669-2450 (*fax*)
888-633-4298
Web site: www.medicalert.org

To order a medical ID bracelet.

**National AIDS Hotline**
Centers for Disease Control and
    Prevention
800-342-2437 (24 hours)
800-344-7432 (Spanish)
800-243-7889 (TTY)
Web site: www.ashastd.org/nah

Information on HIV and AIDS,
including pamphlets and
brochures, counseling, and referral
to local test sites, case managers,
and medical services.

**National Chronic Pain Outreach
Association**
P.O. Box 274
Millboro, VA 24460
540-862-9437
540-862-9485 (*fax*)
e-mail: ncpoa@cfw.com
Web site: www.chronicpain.org

To learn more about chronic pain
and how to deal with it.

**National Kidney Foundation**
30 E. 33rd Street
New York, NY 10016
212-889-2210
212-689-9261 (*fax*)
800-622-9010
e-mail: info@kidney.org
Web site: www.kidney.org

For donor cards and information
about kidney disease and transplants.

**The Neuropathy Association**
60 E. 42nd Street, Suite 942
New York, NY 10165
212-692-0662
212-692-0668 (*fax*)
e-mail: info@neuropathy.org
Web site: www.neuropathy.org

For information about disorders
that affect the peripheral nerves.

**United Network for Organ Sharing**
P.O. Box 2484
Richmond, VA 23218
804-782-4800
800-355-SHARE or
    800-24-DONOR
    (*for information on becoming
    a donor*)
Web site: www.unos.org

For information about organ transplants and a list of organ transplant centers in the U.S.

## For Travelers

### Centers for Disease Control and Prevention
Travelers' Health Hotline
877-FYI-TRIP
888-232-3299 (fax)
Web site: www.cdc.gov/travel

Provides health information for international travelers.

### International Association for Medical Assistance to Travelers
1623 Military Road, #279
Niagara Falls, NY 14304
716-754-4883
e-mail: info@iamat.org
Web site: www.iamat.org

For a list of doctors in foreign countries who speak English and who received postgraduate training in North America or Great Britain.

### International Diabetes Federation
Avenue Emile De Mot 19
B-1000 Brussels, Belgium
e-mail: info@idf.org
Web site: www.idf.org

For a list of International Diabetes Federation groups that can offer assistance when you're traveling.

## For Exercisers

### American College of Sports Medicine
P.O. Box 1440
Indianapolis, IN 46206-1440
317-637-9200
317-634-7817 (fax)
Web site: www.acsm.org

For information about health and fitness.

### Diabetes Exercise and Sports Association
8001 Montcastle Drive
Nashville, TN 37221
800-898-4322
615-673-2077 (fax)
e-mail: desa@diabetes-exercise.org
Web site: www.diabetes-exercise.org

For people with diabetes and for health care professionals interested in exercise and fitness at all levels. Newsletter.

President's Council on Physical
Fitness and Sports
Department W
200 Independence Avenue, SW
Room 738-H
Washington, DC 20201-0004
202-690-9000
202-690-5211 (*fax*)
e-mail: pcpfs@osophs.dhhs.gov
Web site: www.fitness.gov

For information about physical
activity, exercise, and fitness.

## For Schools and Students

Disability Rights Education and
Defense Fund
2212 Sixth Street
Berkeley, CA 94710
510-644-2555
Web site: www.dredf.org

Law and policy center dedicated to
protecting and advancing the civil
rights of people with disabilities.

National Dissemination Center for
Children with Disabilities
P.O. Box 1492
Washington, DC 20013-1492
800-695-0285
202-884-8441 (*fax*)
Web site: www.nichcy.org

Provides information on disabilities in children, laws relating to
children with disabilities, and effective educational practices.

National Diabetes Education
Program (NDEP)
1 Diabetes Way
Bethesda, MD 20892-3600
800-438-5383
Web site: www.ndep.nih.gov

The NDEP school guide can be
found at http://www.ndep.nih.
gov/resources/school.htm.

United States Department of
Education
400 Maryland Avenue
Washington, DC 20202

Office of Civil Rights
800-421-3481
Web site: www.ed.gov/ocr

Office of Special Education and
Rehabilitative Services
202-205-5507
Web site: www.ed.gov/osers

## For People Over 50

**AARP (American Association of Retired Persons)**
601 E Street, NW
Washington, DC 20049
888-687-2277
Web site: www.aarp.org

Over-the-counter and prescription drugs delivered to your door in 7 to 10 days. Competitive prices that are the same for members and non-members. May pay by credit card or be billed.

**National Council on the Aging**
300 D Street, SW, Suite 801
Washington, DC 20024
202-479-1200
202-479-0735 (*fax*)
800-424-9046
e-mail: info@ncoa.org
Web site: www.ncoa.org

Advocacy group concerned with developing and implementing high standards of care for the elderly. Referral to local agencies concerned with the elderly.

## For Equal Employment Information

**American Bar Association Commission on Mental and Physical Disability Law**
740 15th Street, NW
Washington, DC 20005-1009
202-662-1570
202-662-1032 (*fax*)
202-662-1012 (TTY)
e-mail: cmpdl@abanet.org
Web site:
www.abanet.org/disability

Provides information and technical assistance on all aspects of disability law.

**Disability Rights Education and Defense Fund, Inc.**
2212 6th Street
Berkeley, CA 94710
510-644-2555 (voice/TDD)
510-841-8645 (*fax*)
800-466-4232 (voice/TDD)
e-mail: dredf@dredf.org
Web site: www.dredf.org

Provides technical assistance and information to employers and individuals with disabilities on disability rights legislation and policies. Assists with legal representation.

**Equal Employment Opportunity Commission (EEOC)**
1801 L Street, NW
Washington, DC 20507
For technical assistance and filing a
   charge:
202-663-4900
202-663-4912 (fax)
202-663-4494 (TTY)
800-669-4000 (connects to nearest
   local EEOC office)
800-669-3362 (for publications)
800-669-6820 (TDD)
Web site: www.eeoc.gov

**National Dissemination Center for Children and Youth with Disabilities**
P.O. Box 1492
Washington, DC 20013-1492
202-884-8200 (voice and TTY)
202-884-8441 (fax)
800-695-0285 (voice and TTY)
e-mail: nichcy@aed.org
Web site: www.nichcy.org

Provides technical assistance and information on disabilities and disability-related issues.

**For Health Insurance Information**

**American Association of Retired Persons (AARP)**
Health Insurance
601 E Street, NW
Washington, DC 20049
800-523-5800
800-232-7773 (TTY)
Web site:
   www.aarp.healthcare.com

The AARP administers 10 health insurance plans. For some plans, individuals with diabetes or other chronic illnesses are eligible within 6 months after enrolling in Medicare Part B. For other plans, a 3-month waiting period is required for those with conditions preexistent in the 6 months preceding the effective date of the insurance, if not replacing previous coverage.

**Medicare Hotline**
U.S. Department of Health and
   Human Services
Centers for Medicare and
   Medicaid Services
7500 Security Boulevard
Baltimore, MD 21244-1850
1-800-MEDICARE
Web site: www.medicare.gov

For information and various publications about Medicare.

## Social Security Administration
1-800-772-1213
Web site: www.ssa.gov

For information and various publications about Medicare.

## Helpful Web Sites

### ADA
www.diabetes.org

### National Diabetes Information Clearinghouse
diabetes.niddk.nih.gov

### Children with Diabetes
Resources for kids, families, and adults with diabetes. Created by a father; offers chat rooms and answers to more than 3,000 questions online.
www.childrenwithdiabetes.com

### Diabetes Monitor
Supplies information on new medications and research; features a mentor section.
www.diabetesmonitor.com

### David Mendosa's Diabetes Directory
Provides a list of online diabetes resources.
www.mendosa.com/diabetes.htm

You can also subscribe to the following list servers (groups of people who share information about a topic)

### listserv@lehigh.edu
To subscribe, send an e-mail to the list serve. In the message box, write the words "subscribe diabetic [your name]" (write your name here).

### majordomo@world.std.com
To subscribe, send an e-mail to the list serve. In the message box, write the words "subscribe diabetes."

## ADA National Office

### American Diabetes Association
1701 North Beauregard Street
Alexandria, VA 22311
800-DIABETES (800-342-2383)

## ADA Division Offices

### Midwest Division

2323 North Mayfair Road, Suite 502
Wauwatosa, WI 53226
414-778-5500

Iowa, Illinois, Indiana, Michigan, Minnesota, Nebraska, North Dakota, Ohio, South Dakota, West Virginia, Wisconsin

### Mountain/Pacific Division

2480 West 26th Avenue, Suite 120B
Denver, CO 80211
720-855-1102

Alaska, Arizona, Colorado, Idaho, Montana, New Mexico, Oregon, Utah, Washington, Wyoming

### Northeastern Division

149 Madison Avenue, 8th Floor
New York, NY 10016
212-725-4925

Connecticut, Delaware, District of Columbia, Maine, Maryland, Massachusetts, New Hampshire, New Jersey, New York, Northern Virginia, Pennsylvania, Rhode Island, Vermont

### South Central Division

4425 West Airport Freeway, Suite 130
Irving, TX 75062
972-255-6900

Arkansas, Kansas, Louisiana, Missouri, Oklahoma, Texas

### Southeast Division

2 Hanover Square
434 Fayetteville Street Mall, Suite 165
Raleigh, NC 27601
919-743-5400

Alabama, Florida, Georgia, Kentucky, Mississippi, North Carolina, South Carolina, Tennessee, Virginia (except Northern Virginia)

### Western Division

2720 Gateway Oaks Drive, Suite 110
Sacramento, CA 95833
916-924-3232

California, Hawaii, Nevada

# Diabetes Medical Management Plan

Date of Plan: _____

*This plan should be completed by the student's personal health care team and parents/guardian. It should be reviewed with relevant school staff, and copies should be kept in a place that is easily accessed by the school nurse, trained diabetes personnel, and other authorized personnel.*

Effective Dates: _____

Student's Name: _____

Date of Birth: _____

Date of Diabetes Diagnosis: _____

Grade: _____ Homeroom Teacher: _____

Physical Condition: ☐ Diabetes type 1 ☐ Diabetes type 2

## Contact Information

Mother/Guardian:_____

Address: _____

_____

Telephone: Home _____ Work _____

Cell _____

Father/Guardian:_____

Address: _____

_____

Telephone: Home _____ Work _____

Cell _____

### Student's Doctor/Health Care Provider:

Name:_____

Address: _____

_____

Telephone: _____

Emergency Number: _____

### Other Emergency Contacts:

Name:_____

Relationship: _____

Telephone: Home _____ Work _____

Cell _____

Notify parents/guardian or emergency contact in the following situations: _____

_____

## Blood Glucose Monitoring

Target range for blood glucose is    ☐ 70–150    ☐ 70–180

Other _____

Usual times to check blood glucose _____

Times to do extra blood glucose checks (*check all that apply*)

☐ before exercise
☐ after exercise
☐ when student exhibits symptoms of hyperglycemia
☐ when student exhibits symptoms of hypoglycemia
☐ other (explain):_____

_____

Can student perform own blood glucose checks?    ☐ Yes   ☐ No

Exceptions:_____

_____

Type of blood glucose meter student uses:_____

_____

## Insulin

### Usual Lunchtime Dose

Base dose of Humalog/Novolog/Regular insulin at lunch (*circle type of rapid-/short-acting insulin used*) is _____ units or does flexible dosing using _____ units/ _____ grams carbohydrate.

Use of other insulin at lunch: (*circle type of insulin used*): interme-diate/NPH/lente _____ units or basal/Lantus/Ultralente _____ units.

### Insulin Correction Doses

Parental authorization should be obtained before administering a correction dose for high blood glucose levels.   ☐ Yes   ☐ No

_____ units if blood glucose is _____ to _____ mg/dl

_____ units if blood glucose is _____ to _____ mg/dl

_____ units if blood glucose is _____ to _____ mg/dl

_____ units if blood glucose is _____ to _____ mg/dl

_____ units if blood glucose is _____ to _____ mg/dl

Can student give own injections?   Yes   No

Can student determine correct amount of insulin?   ☐ Yes ☐ No

Can student draw correct dose of insulin?   ☐ Yes ☐ No

_____ Parents are authorized to adjust the insulin dosage under the following circumstances: _____

_____

_____

### For Students with Insulin Pumps

Type of pump: _____

Basal rates:_____ 12 am to _____

_____ _____ to _____

_____ _____ to _____

Type of insulin in pump: _____

Type of infusion set: _____

Insulin/carbohydrate ratio: _____

Correction factor: _____

### *Student Pump Abilities/Skills:*                    *Needs Assistance*

| | | |
|---|---|---|
| Count carbohydrates | ☐ Yes | ☐ No |
| Bolus correct amount for carbohydrates consumed | ☐ Yes | ☐ No |
| Calculate and administer corrective bolus | ☐ Yes | ☐ No |
| Calculate and set basal profiles | ☐ Yes | ☐ No |
| Calculate and set temporary basal rate | ☐ Yes | ☐ No |
| Disconnect pump | ☐ Yes | ☐ No |
| Reconnect pump at infusion set | ☐ Yes | ☐ No |
| Prepare reservoir and tubing | ☐ Yes | ☐ No |
| Insert infusion set | ☐ Yes | ☐ No |
| Troubleshoot alarms and malfunctions | ☐ Yes | ☐ No |

## For Students Taking Oral Diabetes Medications

Type of medication: _____

                    Timing: _____

Other medications: _____

                    Timing: _____

## Meals and Snacks Eaten at School

Is student independent in carbohydrate calculations and management?   ☐ Yes ☐ No

| Meal/Snack | Time | Food content/amount |
|---|---|---|
| Breakfast | _____ | _____ |
| Mid-morning snack | _____ | _____ |
| Lunch | _____ | _____ |
| Mid-afternoon snack | _____ | _____ |
| Dinner | _____ | _____ |

Snack before exercise?    ☐ Yes   ☐ No

Snack after exercise?    ☐ Yes   ☐ No

Other times to give snacks and content/amount: _____

_____

Preferred snack foods: _____

_____

Foods to avoid, if any: _____

_____

Instructions for when food is provided to the class (e.g., as part of a class party or food sampling event):

_____

_____


## Exercise and Sports

A fast-acting carbohydrate such as _____
should be available at the site of exercise or sports.

Restrictions on activity, if any: _____
student should not exercise if blood glucose level is below

_____ mg/dl or above _____ mg/dl
or if moderate to large urine ketones are present.

## Hypoglycemia (Low Blood Sugar)

Usual symptoms of hypoglycemia: _____

_____

Treatment of hypoglycemia: _____

_____

Glucagon should be given if the student is unconscious, having a
seizure (convulsion), or unable to swallow.

Route _____, dosage _____, site for glucagon injection:
_____arm, _____thigh, _____other.

If glucagon is required, administer it promptly.  Then, call 911 (or
other emergency assistance) and the parents/guardian.

## Hyperglycemia (High Blood Sugar)

Usual symptoms of hyperglycemia: _____

_____

Treatment of hyperglycemia: _____

_____

Urine should be checked for ketones when blood glucose levels
are above _____ mg/dl.

Treatment for ketones: _____

_____

## Supplies to Be Kept at School

_____Blood glucose meter, blood glucose test strips, batteries for meter

_____Lancet device, lancets, gloves, etc.

_____Urine ketone strips

_____Insulin pump and supplies

_____Insulin pen, pen needles, insulin cartridges

_____Fast-acting source of glucose

_____Carbohydrate containing snack

_____Glucagon emergency kit

## Signatures

**This Diabetes Medical Management Plan has been approved by:**

_____    _____

Student's Physician/Health Care Provider        Date

I give permission to the school nurse, trained diabetes personnel, and other designated staff members of _____
School to perform and carry out the diabetes care tasks as outlined by
_____'s Diabetes Medical Management Plan. I also consent to the release of the information contained in this Diabetes Medical Management Plan to all staff members and other adults who have custodial care of my child and who may need to know this information to maintain my child's health and safety.

**Acknowledged and received by:**

_____    _____

Student's Parent/Guardian                        Date

_____    _____

Student's Parent/Guardian                        Date

# Index

## About the American Diabetes Association

The American Diabetes Association is the nation's leading voluntary health organization supporting diabetes research, information, and advocacy. Its mission is to prevent and cure diabetes and to improve the lives of all people affected by diabetes. The American Diabetes Association is the leading publisher of comprehensive diabetes information. Its huge library of practical and authoritative books for people with diabetes covers every aspect of self-care—cooking and nutrition, fitness, weight control, medications, complications, emotional issues, and general self-care.

**To order American Diabetes Association books:** Call 1-800-232-6733 or log on to http://store.diabetes.org

**To join the American Diabetes Association:**
Call 1-800-806-7801 or log on to www.diabetes.org/membership

**For more information about diabetes or ADA programs and services:**
Call 1-800-342-2383. E-mail: AskADA@diabetes.org or log on to www.diabetes.org

**To locate an ADA/NCQA Recognized Provider of quality diabetes care in your area:** www.ncqa.org/dprp

**To find an ADA Recognized Education Program in your area:**
Call 1-800-342-2383. www.diabetes.org/for-health-professionals-and-scientists/recognition/edrecognition.jsp

**To join the fight to increase funding for diabetes research, end discrimination, and improve insurance coverage:** Call 1-800-342-2383. www.diabetes.org/advocacy-and-legalresources/advocacy.jsp

**To find out how you can get involved with the programs in your community:**
Call 1-800-342-2383. See below for program Web addresses.
*American Diabetes Month:* educational activities aimed at those diagnosed with diabetes—month of November. www.diabetes.org/communityprograms-and-localevents/americandiabetesmonth.jsp

*American Diabetes Alert:* annual public awareness campaign to find the undiagnosed—held the fourth Tuesday in March. www.diabetes.org/communityprograms-and-localevents/americandiabetesalert.jsp

*The Diabetes Assistance & Resources Program (DAR):* diabetes awareness program targeted to the Latino community. www.diabetes.org/communityprograms-and-localevents/latinos.jsp

*African American Program:* diabetes awareness program targeted to the African American community. www.diabetes.org/communityprograms-and-localevents/africanamericans.jsp

*Awakening the Spirit: Pathways to Diabetes Prevention & Control:* diabetes awareness program targeted to the Native American community. www.diabetes.org/community programs-and-localevents/nativeamericans.jsp

**To find out about an important research project regarding type 2 diabetes:**
www.diabetes.org/diabetes-research/research-home.jsp

**To obtain information on making a planned gift or charitable bequest:**
Call 1-888-700-7029. www.wpg.cc/stl/CDA/homepage/1,1006,509,00.html

**To make a donation or memorial contribution:** Call 1-800-342-2383.
www.diabetes.org/support-the-cause/make-a-donation.jsp